Management of Gastroesophageal Reflux Disease

Santiago Horgan • Karl-Hermann Fuchs

Editors

Management of Gastroesophageal Reflux Disease

Surgical and Therapeutic Innovations

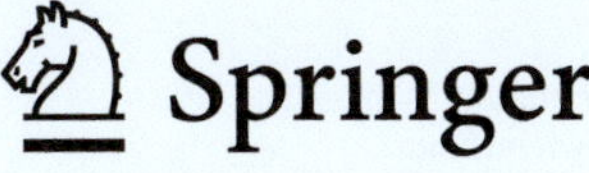

Editors
Santiago Horgan
University of California, San Diego
Center for the Future of Surgery
La Jolla, CA
USA

Karl-Hermann Fuchs
University of California, San Diego
Center for the Future of Surgery
La Jolla, CA
USA

ISBN 978-3-030-48011-0   ISBN 978-3-030-48009-7   (eBook)
https://doi.org/10.1007/978-3-030-48009-7

This Springer imprint is published by the registered company Springer Nature Switzerland AG
The registered company address is: Gewerbestrasse 11, 6330 Cham, Switzerland

Foreword

The diagnosis and management of Gastroesophageal Reflux Disease (GERD) has changed substantially over the course of the past decades. GERD is a highly prevalent disease in western industrial countries and accounts for a large part of healthcare budgets in these countries. As a consequence, many doctors, technicians, nursing staff, and other caretakers are involved in diagnosis and therapy of GERD. New developments and insights have shown a multifactorial pathophysiologic background, emerging new diagnostic technologies, and a variety of therapeutic options. Each of these requires significant expertise to adequately diagnose and respond to a patient's needs. This book provides an overview on the new aspects of GERD for all involved specialties and disciplines.

The close association with related diseases such as functional dyspepsia, gastrointestinal motility disorders, and somatoform tendencies creates a diagnostic challenge. Detailed knowledge is therefore required to manage GERD, especially as the diagnostic modalities combined with innovations in endoscopic and surgical treatment are developing/emerging quickly. This work provides a comprehensive state-of-the art overview in the field of GERD, as well as a current insight into new algorithms for diagnosis and treatments (endoscopic and surgical). The book is a valuable as resource of knowledge for clinicians, surgeons, nurses, technicians, students, and researchers with an interest in esophageal and upper gastrointestinal disease.

We want to thank all authors and co-authors for their excellent work and dedication to make this project possible. We also want to express our gratitude to all involved at Springer publishing company for their assistance and professionalism through the publishing process.

Finally, we would like to express our gratitude for the outstanding, supportive environment at UC San Diego that made this possible. We are extremely excited and grateful for this project.

La Jolla, CA, USA
Santiago Horgan
Karl-Hermann Fuchs

Contents

Contributors

Wolfram Breithaupt Agaplesion Markus Krankenhaus, Department of General and GI-Surgery, Frankfurt am Main, Germany

Ryan C. Broderick Division of Minimally Invasive Surgery, Department of Surgery, University of California San Diego, La Jolla, CA, USA

Department of Surgery, Center for the Future of Surgery, University of California San Diego, La Jolla, CA, USA

Karel Caca Department of Gastroenterology, Hospital Ludwigsburg, Ludwigsburg, Germany

Joslin N. Cheverie Division of Minimally Invasive Surgery, Department of Surgery, University of California San Diego Medical Center, La Jolla, CA, USA

Robert F. Cubas Division of Minimally Invasive Surgery, Department of Surgery, University of California San Diego Medical Center, La Jolla, CA, USA

Steven R. DeMeester Thoracic and Foregut Surgery, The Oregon Clinic, Portland, OR, USA

Karima Farrag Department of Gastroenterology, Krankenhaus Sachsenhausen, Frankfurt am Main, Germany

Sean M. Flynn Division of Minimally Invasive Surgery, Department of Surgery, University of California San Diego, La Jolla, CA, USA

Karl-Hermann Fuchs University of California San Diego, Center for the Future of Surgery, La Jolla, CA, USA

Hans Friedrich Fuchs Department of General, GI- and Tumor Surgery, University of Cologne, Cologne, Germany

Santiago Horgan Division of Minimally Invasive Surgery, Department of Surgery, University of California San Diego, La Jolla, CA, USA

David C. Kunkel University of California San Diego, Department of Medicine Gastroenterology, La Jolla, CA, USA

Arielle Lee University of California San Diego, Center for the Future of Surgery, La Jolla, CA, USA

Kai Neki University of California San Diego, Center for the Future of Surgery, La Jolla, CA, USA

José Bezerra Câmara Neto University of California San Diego, Center for the Future of Surgery, La Jolla, CA, USA

Edy Soffer Department of Medicine, Keck School of Medicine, University of Southern California, Los Angeles, CA, USA

Jürgen Stein Department of Gastroenterology, Krankenhaus Sachsenhausen, Frankfurt am Main, Germany

Gabor Varga Agaplesion Markus Krankenhaus, Department of General and GI-Surgery, Frankfurt am Main, Germany

Andreas Wannhoff Department of Gastroenterology, Hospital Ludwigsburg, Ludwigsburg, Germany

Definition and Pathophysiology of Gastroesophageal Reflux Disease

Karl-Hermann Fuchs

Introduction and Definition

Gastroesophageal reflux disease (GERD) is a multifactorial determined disease with a high prevalence in Western industrial populations [1–4]. Several attempts have been made in the past to define this disease and at the same time create a definition, which can clinically be used for decision-making [5, 6]. The problem with a definition is the complex pathophysiologic process on one side and the necessity to have a feasible solution for clinical practice. The Montréal classification and definition for GERD is accepted worldwide; however, a definition using symptoms has its limitations and has led to some criticism in several guidelines [1–4].

Symptoms are quite unreliable and, therefore, a definition based on symptoms could be not precise enough for some applications [7, 8]. Symptoms of GERD have a large overlap with other functional disorders of the upper GI tract and, therefore, there is lack of precision. On the other hand, a definition of a disease should be helpful for diagnostic and therapeutic decision-making, which in the case of GERD may lead to controversies.

As a consequence, GERD should be best defined with clinical parameters, visible endoscopic damage, and functional quantitative assessment in order to be used for therapeutic decisions [4, 5]. The latter sort of definition would respond to the multifactorial character of the disease. Critics of such controversial thinking claim that this would lead to a complex definition, which could hardly be applied in daily practice. The European Association of Endoscopic Surgery has demonstrated in its guidelines that the Montréal definition can be a basis for defining the disease but must be expanded by objective criteria [3].

Gastroesophageal reflux disease is present when a given person suffers from troublesome symptoms by reflux of gastric contents into the esophagus, and this process can be objectified by diagnostic investigations such as endoscopic visible

K.-H. Fuchs (✉)
University of California San Diego, Center for the Future of Surgery, La Jolla, CA, USA

© Springer Nature Switzerland AG 2020
S. Horgan, K.-H. Fuchs (eds.), *Management of Gastroesophageal Reflux Disease*,
https://doi.org/10.1007/978-3-030-48009-7_1

damage in the esophagus and by quantitative functional assessments. With this definition, it must be noted that in rare cases, asymptomatic pathophysiologic pathologic reflux can occur without visible damage, which can only be detected by impedance-pH monitoring.

The clinical presentation of the disease can occur with so-called typical symptoms such as heartburn and regurgitation. These symptoms have been demonstrated as quite specific in the past [9]. More recent evidence shows that these symptoms are not reliable as final proof of the presence of the disease because of tremendous overlap with other functional esophageal disorders [8, 10].

The disease can be described by the endoscopic visible damage in the esophageal mucosa differentiating between nonerosive reflux disease (NERD), erosive reflux disease (ERD), and Barrett's esophagus [1–4]. However, only less than half of patients with GERD show endoscopic visible damage at the time of investigation [11]. As a consequence, the definition should be more complex, representing the complexity of the disease.

The Anatomy of the Esophagus and Stomach

The esophagus is a muscular tube which connects the pharynx with the stomach through the mediastinum [12]. The essential function of the esophagus is transport of fluid and nutrition to ensure sufficient alimentation of the body. On its oral and distal end, the esophagus has special closure mechanisms, which are important to fulfill the complex function of this organ [13]. The most proximal part of the esophagus carries the upper esophageal sphincter, which is integrated into the complex swallowing system of the pharyngo-laryngeal and pharyngoesophageal junction. The oral third of the esophagus consists of skeletal muscle, while the lower two-thirds of the esophagus and the lower esophageal sphincter consist of smooth muscle. Between these two segments of different muscular origin, there is a junctional zone, which is characterized by a somewhat minor muscular strength during peristalsis. The lower esophageal sphincter (LES) represents, together with the muscles and ligamentous structures of the diaphragm at the esophageal hiatus, the antireflux barrier between esophagus and stomach.

The functional coordination of these different anatomical structures by their hormonal and neurologic regulatory mechanisms controls the complex physiologic processes of swallowing, belching, and vomiting next to breathing and coughing. In addition, the limitation of gastroesophageal reflux is secured within its physiologic borders. These complex functions of the two esophageal sphincters and the muscular body is regulated and influenced by neural innervations, the intraluminal pressure coordination, hormonal and chemical influences, and external as well as possible psychologic factors [4, 5, 12, 13].

The high-pressure zone at the lower end of the esophagus should be seen as a functional unit between the lower esophageal sphincter (LES) and the elements of the diaphragm [4, 12, 13]. The exact dimension of the LES can hardly be recognized as a visible anatomical structure under direct intra-abdominal vision because there is not much difference between sphincter area and esophageal body, when inspected from the outside. The LES can be estimated in its position during intraluminal, endoscopic inspection, since a narrowing of the lumen can be noticed inside the esophagus at the cardia. During longer, endoscopic inspection of the cardia, one can notice a changing tension of the LES with spontaneous openings under air insufflation allowing for short sights through the sphincter into the gastric lumen. This narrowing of the distal esophagus can also be noticed during radiographic studies and under fluoroscopy.

The LES is best assessed quantitatively by esophageal manometry [14]. The physiologic role of the high-pressure zone (LES and diaphragm) is the closure of the gastric lumen and reservoir toward its oral end, thus preventing reflux of gastric contents and fluids in large amounts back into the esophagus. The latter is of extreme importance for preservation of esophageal integrity, since gastric juice, especially the mixture of gastric acid and duodenal juice, is extremely toxic and damaging for the esophageal mucosa [4].

The structure of the LES has been studied intensively by anatomical evaluations [12]. These studies show very clearly that the lower esophageal muscular wall has an inner, circular and an outer, longitudinal muscle layer. This can be currently demonstrated extremely well during transesophageal myotomy in the POEM technique in achalasia patients [15, 16]. Furthermore, Liebermann-Meffert has shown that special-shaped muscle fibers or clasps and oblique muscle bundles are responsible for the structure of the LES as shown in Fig. 1.1 [12]. At the smaller curvature,

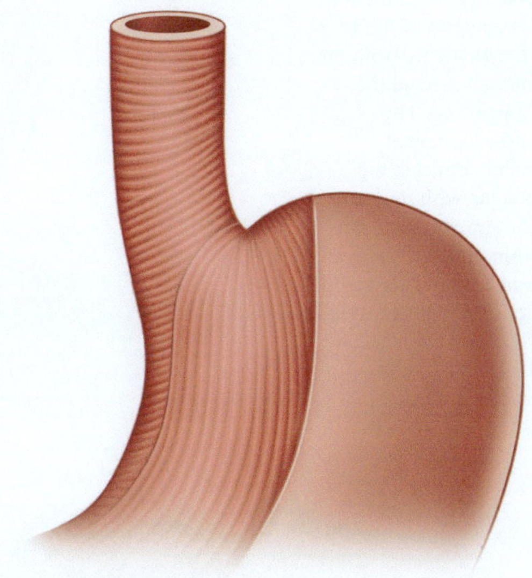

Fig. 1.1 Anatomical structure of the esophagogastric junction according to Liebermann-Meffert [2]. The semicircular muscle bundles from the greater curvature (oblique fibers) reach over to the semicircular muscle claps from the smaller curvature and create together the lower esophageal sphincter (LES)

the inner, circular muscle layers of the distal esophagus transform at the transition zone at the cardia and proximal stomach into half-circular muscle clasps (Fig. 1.1). On the greater curvature, the muscle fibers below the angle of His transform into bundles of oblique fibers. Both types of muscle bundles from each side create U-shaped, half-circular muscle structures that together form the LES. As a result, the LES consists of two structural entities and is therefore not symmetric. Branches of the vagal nerve regulate the neurologic function of the LES.

A second important structure at the gastroesophageal junction are the elements of the diaphragm around the esophagus [12, 13]. The hiatus consists of the right and left crus, the hiatal arch as the ventral border of the hiatus, and the muscular and ligamentous structures of the diaphragm around the hiatus with the phreno-esophageal ligament. The phreno-esophageal ligament secures the position of the LES within the hiatus. With this fixation of the distal esophagus, the esophageal body is kept under a certain tension within the thorax and the mediastinum, since its longitudinal muscle tends to contract and thus tends to shorten its position. In the physiologic situation, a 2–3 cm long intra-abdominal segment of the LES is secured by the phreno-esophageal ligament (Fig. 1.2).

Inspiration will cause a negative pressure in the thoracic pressure environment and at the same time an elevated pressure in the abdominal pressure system [4]. Any physical body activity can elevate intra-abdominal pressure in humans. The latter circumstance causes, based on the pressure distribution between mediastinum and abdominal cavity, an increased pressure and tension on the phreno-esophageal

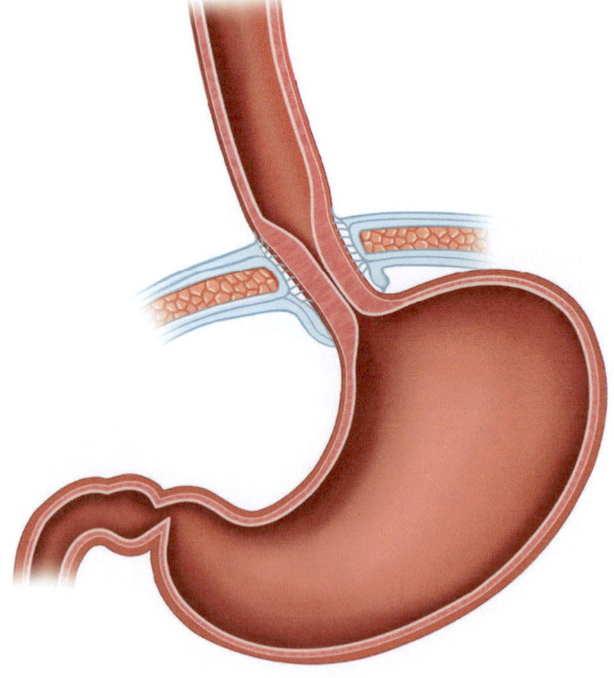

Fig. 1.2 The esophagogastric junction (EGJ) consists of the LES and the elements from the diaphragm around the hiatal opening. The phreno-esophageal ligament connects the esophagus with the diaphragm and fixes its position, thus securing an intra-abdominal segment of the LES. The pressure at the EGJ is established by the LES, the diaphragm, and the intra-abdominal pressure environment

ligament and the esophagus from the abdominal cavity. As a result, there is a permanent stress on the gastroesophageal junction and its anatomical elements because the positive intra-abdominal pressure and respiratory-based temporary negative intrathoracic pressure will tend to push the gastroesophageal junction further into the mediastinum. The latter will eventually lead to wearing out of these tissues over the years.

This phreno-esophageal ligament is in the physiologic situation not a circular structure, since the hiatal opening in the diaphragm is not a circular opening. Depending on the size of an individual, the hiatus can be different in size [4, 12, 13]. The crura are not circular but are established from cranial and ventral to caudal and posterior and surround the esophagus. Anteriorly, the crura come together at the hiatal arch, and posteriorly, the crura unite at the arcuate ligament on the aorta. All these structures and the esophagus are connected with each other by the phreno-esophageal ligament or membrane. As clinical evidence shows, there are a large number of individual, anatomical norm variations in this area. These tissue connections between the crura and the ligaments can be quite different from person to person. The phreno-esophageal ligament has a less solid base, if these connecting structures have less stability. A reduced stability or durability of these structures may cause a failure and insufficiency of the ability of phreno-esophageal ligament to keep the esophagus in a stable position.

In addition, individual factors may even worsen this physiologic situation; for example, a large amount of intra-abdominal fat can weaken the insertions of the phreno-esophageal ligament. Another example could be an individual who had to perform hard physical labor during many decades, which would also encumber the muscular and ligamentous structures at the hiatus, creating a risk for insufficiency.

Normal anatomical variations may create conditions in which the optimal stabilization of the esophageal position within the hiatus may suffer over time and the posterior located aorta may function as a perfect sliding area for the esophagus. Clinical evidence has shown that in some young individuals, the left crus may be created by nature shorter and weaker than the right one. This means that the anchoring point of the phreno-esophageal ligament is weaker at that point and may deteriorate earlier in life with subsequent less stabilization of the esophagus and possible higher risk of GERD in the future of this individual. Similarly, an individual with a preaortic lipoma could be predisposed for earlier GERD development, since the lipoma on the aorta will have the potential to function as a perfect sliding cushion for the esophagus and, thus, facilitate the development of an early hiatal hernia.

The closure mechanism of the LES is not a one-way valve. On the one hand, nutrition must pass the sphincter into the stomach and stay there, and on the other hand, LES must prevent massive reflux of gastric contents into the esophagus. In addition, the system must be flexible enough in special situations, for example, in excessive bloating of the stomach, to allow for passage of air from the gastric lumen into the esophagus and further up outside. Also in a situation of a gastrointestinal infection, the system must allow for vomiting of contaminated food to preserve the person's health. The LES is regulated in the physiologic configuration by several mechanisms influenced by neurologic and hormonal and possibly psychologic factors. The coordinated concert of these different regulatory mechanisms creates enough room to allow for physiologic reflux [4].

In the physiologic situation, the LES moves during the act of swallowing about 1–2 cm up and down, which also puts strain on the holding structures of the LES [4]. The structures securing the position of the LES, especially the phreno-esophageal ligament and the crura, must keep the esophagus in its intra-abdominal position during swallowing, during physical activity, and during a meal with increase of intra-abdominal pressure and shortening of the LES due to fundic accommodation (Fig. 1.2).

The nutritional habits of many people in Western industrialized countries with daily overeating put much strain on the fundus, which is the storage area of the stomach [4, 17]. Figure 1.3 demonstrates the effacement of the fundus during mealtime and its influence on the LES. Since the gastric fundus has to enlarge without pressure increase (fundic accommodation), this will cause a stepwise shortening of the LES due to the pull of the fundic wall on the LES [4, 17–19]. In addition, there will be an increase in intra-abdominal pressure, leading to more strain on the phreno-esophageal ligament and pushing the cardia into the mediastinum. It is not surprising that after many years of strain on these structures of the LES and the diaphragm, mechanical insufficiency will develop and functional regulatory mechanism may wear out too, resulting in the development of hiatal hernia and gastro-esophageal reflux disease.

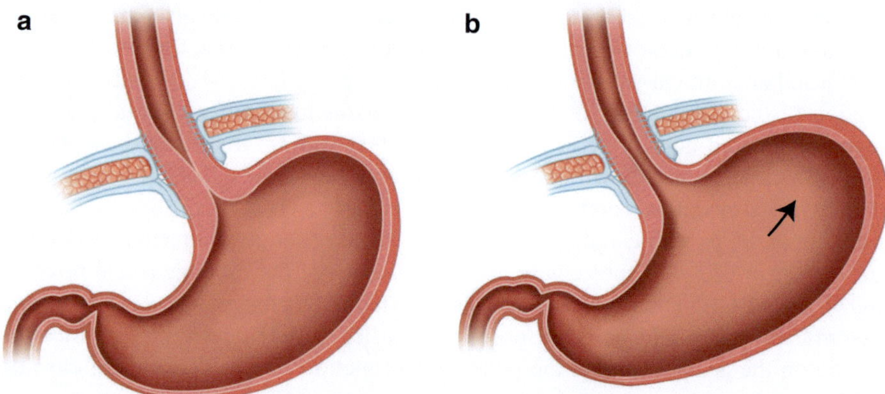

Fig. 1.3 The strain on the esophagogastric junction (a = normal) can be caused by repetitive, excessive overeating and overfilling of the gastric fundus, which leads to effacement of LES and weakening of all structures (b = effacement). Eventually, this process will end in shortening of the LES, with subsequent incompetence of the sphincter as well as strain and enlargement of the phreno-esophageal ligament with subsequent migration of the cardia into the mediastinum and the development of a hiatal hernia

Pathophysiology of GERD

The central, pathologic problem in GERD is an increased passage of refluxate of gastric contents into the esophagus above the physiologic level. This leads to a pathologic exposure of the esophageal mucosa to gastric acid and possibly duodenal contents, which can cause symptoms and/or damage of the esophagus [4, 5].

Scientific work around the gastroesophageal junction and its function over the past four decades has produced two major concepts of thinking to describe this process. A first concept was developed mainly by the "DeMeester school" and which is characterized by a more "surgical and mechanical thinking" and interpretation of the involved processes based on manometric parameters [4, 5, 13, 14, 20]. A second concept is mainly developed by gastroenterologists Dent and Dodds, who created a more dynamic concept of LES function in measuring and describing the "spontaneous transient relaxations" of the LES (TLESRs) [21–23].

It must be emphasized that the manometric systems of the past century were limited and did basically allow only for an intraluminal measurement of pressure changes in the LES, mostly missing out the pressure influences of the diaphragm, which limited the complete mechanical assessment of the gastroesophageal junction as composed by more than one anatomical structure. As a consequence, both concepts did focus more on the intraluminal pressure changes in the esophagus, and the assessments were limited to the LES. In contrast, today with high-resolution manometry, there is the possibility to also monitor on a routine basis functional and mechanical influences of the diaphragm together with the LES [24, 25].

The Incompetence of the LES

Following the "DeMeester school," a more mechanical interpretation of the LES function and anatomy is described by three manometric criteria: the overall length, the sphincter pressure, and the sphincter position expressed as the remaining intra-abdominal length of the sphincter in the hiatal position [4, 5]. This concept was developed using traditional perfusion manometry [5, 14]. In the physiologic situation, the high-pressure zone has a length of 3–5 cm and an average pressure of around 14 mmHg [5, 14]. As described above, the LES must create a sufficient and effective pressure environment over a certain length within the distal esophagus to maintain enough resistance against gastric pressure and prevent excessive acid reflux over 24 hours a day. In this concept, it is evident that the shorter the sphincter is, the higher the pressure must be within the high-pressure zone to maintain a sufficient closure to prevent reflux [4, 5]. The LES is supported by the external mechanical pressure of the diaphragm and the intra-abdominal pressure, of which the intra-abdominal segment of the distal esophagus is exposed causing also compression (Fig. 1.2). The longer the intra-abdominal esophageal segment is, the larger the compression area is and the more the intra-abdominal pressure can support the LES in keeping reflux in a physiologic level.

It must be emphasized that the incompetence of the LES is defined by its short length, by its weak pressure, and by its altered position expressed as short intra-abdominal length [4, 5, 14]. It is not just a weak pressure alone, which characterizes LES incompetence, even though this is often used by mistake.

Since this mechanism was described by functional assessments with perfusion manometry, one could argue that this technique was probably too limited with only five points of measurement at the openings of the perfusion catheter [4, 5, 14, 25, 26]. However, the bulk of knowledge generated by this system and its interpretations together with a vast amount of clinical evidence has shown that these findings had a serious clinical relevance [4, 5, 14, 20]. A major finding has been in GERD that the more advanced this disease is associated with complications such as esophagitis, ulcerations, and Barrett's esophagus, the more frequent an incompetent LES is present in these patients [27–29]. Today, there is enough evidence to state that these three criteria are important in the characterization of severe and progressive GERD and, in addition, that these criteria can be used for therapeutic decision-making in the clinical setting [4, 27–29]. It has been shown that these criteria have a prognostic value in that patients with a documented LES incompetence have a higher probability that their GERD will persist for the next 6–10 years [30].

There is a higher prevalence of GERD in Western industrialized societies compared to other populations [1, 4, 6]. One explanation has been the association between the rising prevalence of GERD and the nutritional habits of people in Western countries [1, 4, 6]. The process of repetitive overeating in our daily life will cause mechanical and functional alterations in the upper GI tract [4]. When a person is eating a large meal, the ability of the stomach and especially the fundus allows for an enlargement of the gastric lumen to ingest the complete meal by fundic accommodation. Figure 1.3 demonstrates both, the enlargement by fundic accommodation and at the same time the mechanical strain on the LES, since the strong pull of the gastric wall on the LES at the angle of His will shorten eventually the sphincter area and its lower segment while at the same time the physiologic sphincter function needs to keep the high-pressure zone closed to prevent excessive postprandial reflux.

If this process is repeated on a daily basis over several decades and an individual is wearing out the structures at the esophagogastric junction, it is not surprising that the strain on the tissue weakens these structures such as the sphincter (repetitively forced into mechanical shortening) and the phreno-esophageal ligament (repetitively exposed to increased intra-abdominal pressure by large meals and increased amount of intra-abdominal fat).

In addition, there is evidence that during and shortly after a meal, the acid secretion is massively stimulated by several mechanisms, and newly secreted acid collects in the subcardial region, creating an "acid pocket" [18, 31, 32]. This acid pocket is directly located below the LES, being under strain by shortening through fundic accommodation. Thus, reflux can occur easily after large meals. The progression from physiologic amounts of reflux to excessive and pathologic gastro-esophageal acid reflux is well understood [4]. Again, if this process is maintained over several decades, the competence of the esophagogastric junction is fading and the progression toward functional, histologic, and anatomical changes is possible up to fully established mechanical and functional defects.

The Transient Lower Esophageal Sphincter Relaxations (TLESRs)

The second concept of the esophagogastric junction, created and propagated by Dent and Dodds, describes a spontaneous opening of the LES as the most important mechanism for the development of gastroesophageal reflux [21–23]. This occurs in healthy persons and also in patients with GERD and was considered a physiologic mechanism to evacuate ingested air from the gastric lumen [21–23]. However, if the LES is open during such relaxations, acid reflux can occur. Transient lower esophageal sphincter relaxations (TLESRs) develop without previous swallowing and may be increased in pathologic reflux [33]. In contrast, LES relaxations are triggered in the process of swallowing. In TLESRs, a vagal reflex is caused by stimulation at the cardia and by fundic distension [21–23, 34–36].This signal reaches, via afferent vagal lines, the central nervous system and further causes an inhibition of the LES and diaphragm, leading to a TLESR [21–23, 34–36]. The relaxation develops with a pressure drop of >1 mmHg/sec and continues for approximately 10 sec [21–23, 34–36]. TLESRs were detected and recorded by a special manometric device, a sleeve catheter that is inserted in the high-pressure zone and assesses the complete length of the sphincter [21]. The sleeve catheter is able to characterize the intraluminal and integral pressure changes over the complete length of the high-pressure zone. It must be emphasized that these TLESRs occur without previous swallowing, and the opening of the sphincter will allow for reflux of gastric contents into the esophagus.

There has been, over the years, a controversial discussion between gastroenterologists and surgeons about the interpretation of this phenomenon. A main criticism of this concept has been based on the fact that studies have shown that TLESRs are not necessarily increased in its frequency between individuals without reflux problems and those with reflux problems, which raises the question whether there is a connection [4]. TLESRs are especially increased in patients with GERD in the postprandial phase [23, 34–36]. In contrast, in patients with progressive and advanced GERD, TLESRs may not necessarily be increased, which raises again the question whether this parameter can really describe the severity of the functional defect in GERD and whether this phenomenon is really the basis of pathologic gastroesophageal reflux [35, 36].

Manometric studies have shown that in the postprandial phase, an effacement of the LES and the cardia occurs, and at the same time, a shortening of the LES can be detected due to the fundic accommodation as described above (Fig. 1.3) [4, 17]. Since physiologic LES function depends on its intra-abdominal segment, both in pressure and intra-abdominal length, a spontaneous shortening of the sphincter in the postprandial phase will create a temporary incompetency, leading to a temporary spontaneous opening of the sphincter. The latter could fully explain the manometric observations of a TLESR in the postprandial phase [4, 34].

These considerations have led, among critics of the TLESR concept, to the interpretation that possibly TLESRs could be rather not active relaxations of the muscle but could be more transient LES shortenings due to postprandial shortening by strain on the LES due to enlargement of the stomach. This would explain why TLESRs are increased in the postprandial phase. Nevertheless, it remains controversial that patients with advanced GERD may not have any increase in TLESRs compared to other patients, which weakens this parameter's ability to be used as discriminator between health and disease.

With the introduction of high-resolution manometry, a better and more precise evaluation may be possible to accurately describe the esophagogastric junction with its functional and mechanical features due to the large amount of assessment points [37, 38]. This technology allows for an integral measurement of all pressure changes in the esophageal corpus, at the LES, and its surrounding anatomical structures also displaying the pressure influences of the diaphragm (Fig. 1.4). Experience of the past years has shown that different interpretations of the pressure components are possible and may provide more explanation about the precise mechanisms of anatomical and functional changes of the antireflux barrier [37–39].

Histopathologic Considerations

An important element of the pathophysiology of GERD can be followed on the histopathologic level. This concept is currently also discussed quite controversially. It is known since many years that histologic changes in the squamous epithelium of

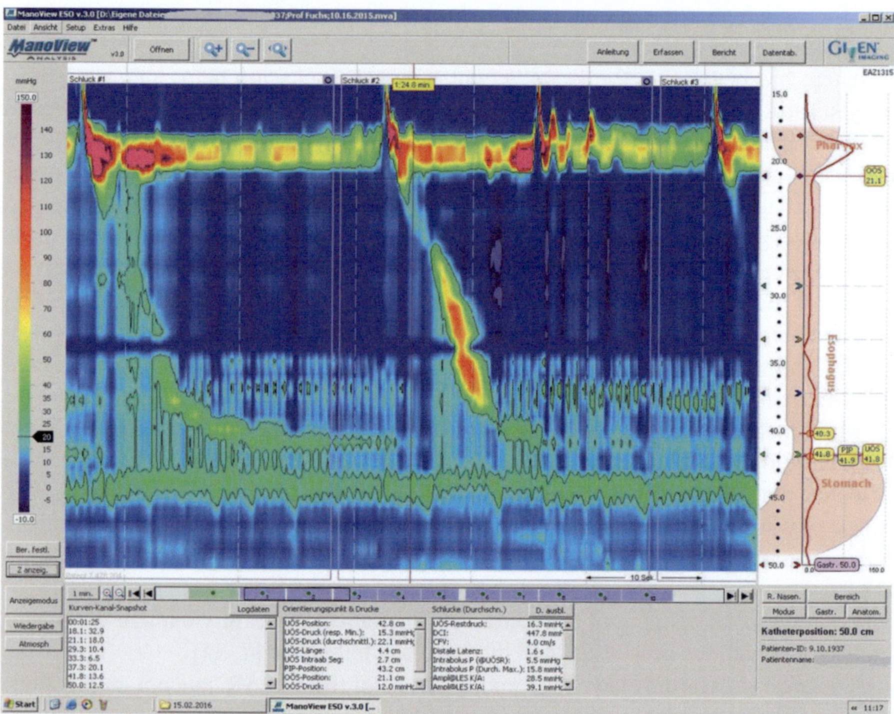

Fig. 1.4 High-resolution manometry of a patient with GERD and hiatal hernia demonstrating the patient's altered esophageal anatomy and function. The separation between remaining weakened pressure of the LES and remaining pressure of the diaphragm at the hiatal opening is shown

the distal esophagus can occur by acid reflux [1, 4, 40]. There is some evidence that even more severe damage can occur by the mixture of acid and duodenal contents in the esophageal mucosa, which can lead to intestinal metaplasia and Barrett's esophagus [41, 42]. In the past, the gastroesophageal junction was described on the histologic level by different types of columnar-lined epithelium such as fundic cells, cardia cells, and intestinal metaplasia [43, 44].

Chandrasoma et al. have investigated the histopathologic changes in the cardia from the normal physiologic setting to more specific changes in patients with incompetent LES and GERD [45–49]. In the physiologic situation, squamous epithelium is directly connected at the transition zone to the gastric epithelium (gastric oxyntic mucosa). In the process of strain on the LES and esophagogastric junction, increased acid exposure of the distal esophagus will damage the squamous epithelium, which may no longer withstand the acid aggression and develops changes. Figure 1.5a, b demonstrate these changes over time. These changes have an anatomical component and a histopathologic component. The anatomical component is represented by the shortening of the LES due to strain by gastric enlargement and fundic accommodation after overeating [4].

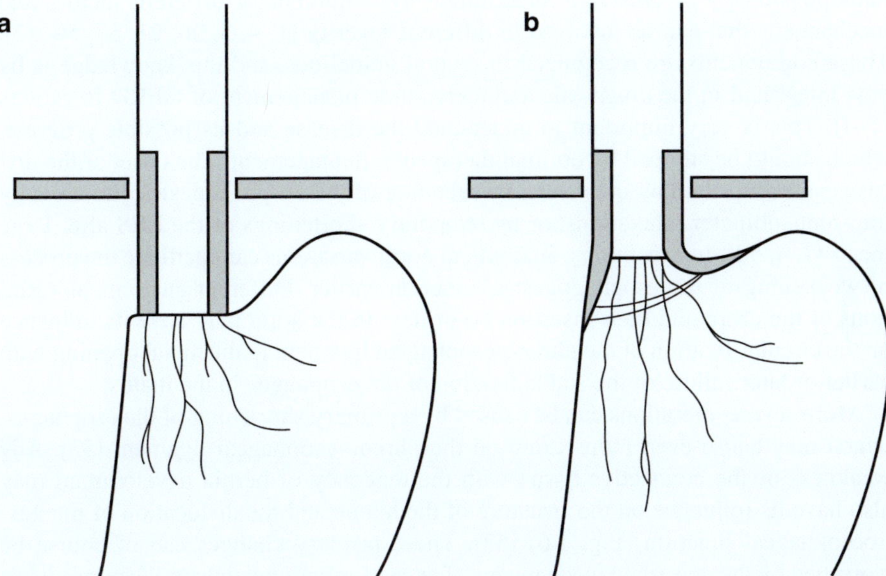

Fig. 1.5 (**a**) Physiologic situation: Esophageal squamous epithelium reaches to the transit zone toward the stomach. (**b**) The damage of acid exposure after shortening of the LES: Below the squamous epithelium, a short zone develops with intestinal metaplasia, and further below, a zone of carditis has developed as the initial step of damage. The changes are not obvious for superficial endoscopic inspection, since the EGJ may look like a "normal" transition zone; however, the distal part of the LES has been widened and has become part of the gastric lumen. This most distal part of the LES used to be a regular tubular part of the LES, participating in the EGJ-pressure profile to establish antireflux barrier function. This function of this segment is now lost

The histopathologic component is a change from squamous epithelium (Fig. 1.5a) in the distal esophagus to a columnar-lined epithelium also called "carditis" [4, 45, 46]. During this process, the very distal part of the esophagus and LES is dilated, and the former squamous cell epithelium is taken over by cardiac mucosa, which can be detected histologically as carditis (Fig. 1.5b).

Macroscopically, for a "superficial" endoscopist, it will be very difficult to recognize these changes, if not focused on and if not assessed histologically, because the longitudinal folds of the stomach will expand eventually upward in the very distal part of the widened LES [37]. The latter will widen and develop mucosal folds and carry endoscopic aspects of the most proximal part of a stomach. At least inexperienced endoscopists may not recognize any difference, unless proof will be taken by biopsy. This process will be recognized by endoscopy latest, when the altered segment of the very distal part of the LES is taken over by columnar-lined epithelium, the visible aspect can be diagnosed as Barrett's esophagus, and proof is gained by histologic documentation of intestinal metaplasia [4, 44–49].

Pathophysiologic Overview and Summary

Pathophysiology of GERD is determined by a number of different factors and mechanisms that can be involved in different severity [1, 4, 5, 20, 21, 37, 50–52]. These components are recognized in several guidelines, and this knowledge is by now integrated in the diagnostic and therapeutic management of GERD in centers [1–4]. This is very important to understand the disease and its possible progress, which should be stopped by optimal therapeutic management. The onset of the disease can occur often by mechanical weakening of the esophagogastric junction, by transient sphincter relaxations, or by temporary shortenings of the LES after large meals [1, 4, 50]. In exceptions, anatomical norm variations can facilitate the process of weakening of the esophagogastric junction earlier. Different anatomical variations of the crura and their insertion on or next to the aorta may have its influence on the circular fixation of the phreno-esophageal ligament in the hiatal opening with earlier or later failure of the stable fixation of the esophagus in the hiatus.

More severe alterations can be caused by a primary shortening of the esophagus, which may cause even more strain on the phreno-esophageal ligament [53]. Any weakness of the connective tissue with the tendency of hernia development may also have its influence on the structure of the hiatus and the dislocation of the gastroesophageal junction (Fig. 1.6) [53]. These primary changes can of course be worsened by the described mechanisms of excessive eating habits in Western societies. Mechanical strain by overeating, development of obesity, and increased intra-abdominal fat will cause intra-abdominal pressure increase, which both will weaken the stable position of the esophagus in the hiatus. Thus, it is not surprising that GERD has a high prevalence in Western societies with their specific eating habits.

The natural course of the disease is determined by the chronic character and the progressive development in some of the involved patients [4, 50–52]. Studies with thousands of patients have shown that most patients stay within a certain level of

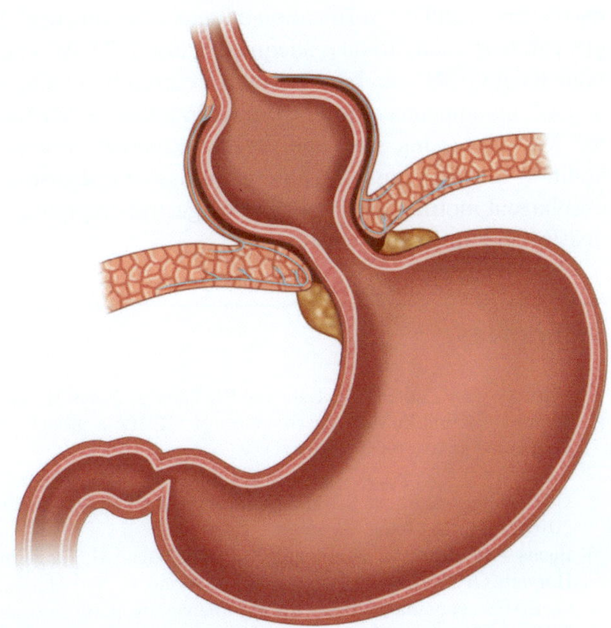

Fig. 1.6 The initial firm and taut phreno-esophageal ligament has developed into a soft, fatty hernia sac. The latter allows for a sliding hernia and further migration of the esophagogastric junction into the mediastinum. The process can be quite progressive, if all pathophysiologic factors can continue their effect on the EGJ. The result will be a permanent dislocation of the stomach into the chest

Table 1.1 Presence of significant role of pathophysiologic components and rates of progression in GERD [14, 40]

Endoscopic visible damage	Normal mucosa	NERD	ERD LA A + B	ERD LA C + D	Barrett's mucosa
Hiatal hernia				0.001	
LES incompetence				0.02	0.001
Pathologic acid exposure		0.05		0.03	0.03
Pathologic duodeno-gastroesophageal reflux					0.03
Rate of progression		5.9	12.1	19.7	

severity of the disease over decades (malfert). This characterizes the benign nature of this functional disorder [11, 54]. However, evidence has shown from these studies that there is a smaller group of patients with a potential of progression to more severe forms of GERD [54]. The latter can not only ruin the quality of life of these patients but also can progress to complicated forms of the disease and, in a minority, even to cancer [4, 55]. Table 1.1 demonstrates these findings that were published from the ProGERD study [4, 11, 29, 54, 55]. Table 1.1 correlates the rates of progression toward more severe disease with the endoscopic findings and objective functional defects. This enlightens the importance of early detection of these patients with more progressive disease in order to provide them with an improved attention and earlier management of diagnosis and therapy [56]. Early detection and interpretation of findings signaling the presence of progressive disease, for example, patients with years of reduced quality of life, the presence of a hiatal hernia, an incompetent LES, a massive increased acid exposure, or even exposure to duodenal gastric juice, and the verification of detectable mucosal damage in the distal esophagus can help today to take adequate action [57]. All known pathophysiologic components of GERD can be investigated currently by diagnostic assessment, detecting an LES incompetence or an increase in transient relaxations, detecting a hiatal hernia with increasing size, and detecting increasing exposure to gastric contents in addition to other possible functional associated disorders such as an insufficient esophageal motility and/or a delayed gastric emptying, which all can aggravate the disease and the patient's status.

References

1. Vakil N, van Zanten SV, Kahrilas PJ, Dent J, Jones R, the global consensus Group. The Montreal definition and classification of GERD: a global evidence-based consensus. Am J Gastro. 2006;101:1900–20.
2. Stefanidis D, Hope WW, Kohn GP, Reardon PR, Richardson WS, Fanelli RD, SAGES Guideline committee. SAGES guidelines for surgical treatment of GERD. Surg Endosc. 2010;24(11):2647–69.
3. Fuchs KH, Babic B, Breithaupt W, Dallemagne B, Fingerhut A, Furnee E, Granderath F, Horvath OP, Kardos P, Pointner R, Savarino E, Van Herwarden-Lindeboom M, Zaninotto G. EAES recommendations for the management of gastroesophageal reflux disease. Surg Endosc. 2014;28:1753–73.
4. DeMeester TR. Etiology and natural history of gastroesophageal reflux disease and predictors of progressive disease. In: Yeo CJ, DeMeester SR, McFadden DW, editors. Shackelford's surgery of the alimentary tract. 8th ed. Philadelphia: Elsevier; 2019. p. 204–20.
5. DeMeester TR. Definition, detection and pathophysiology of gastroesophageal reflux disease. In: DeMeester TR, Matthews HR, editors. International trends in general thoracic surgery, Benign esophageal disease, vol. vol. 3. St. Louis: Mosby; 1987. p. 99–127.
6. Dent J, El-Serag HB, Wallander MA. Epidemiology of gastroesophageal reflux disease: a systematic review. Gut. 2005;54:710.
7. Costantini M, Crookes PF, Bremner RM, Hoeft SF, Ehsan A, Peters JH, Bremner CG, DeMeester TR. Value of physiologic assessment of foregut symptoms in a surgical practice. Surgery. 1993;114(4):780–6.
8. Fuchs KH, Musial F, Ulbricht F, Breithaupt W, Reinisch A, Schulz T, Babic B, Fuchs HF, Varga G. Foregut symptoms, somatoform tendencies, and the selection of patients for antireflux surgery. Dis Esophagus. 2017;30:1–10.
9. Klauser AG, Schindlbeck NE, Müller-Lissner SA. Symptoms in gastro-esophageal reflux disease. Lancet. 1990;335:205–8.
10. Broderick R, Fuchs KH, Breithaupt W, Varga G, Schulz T, Babic B, Lee A, Musial F, Horgan S. Clinical presentation of GERD: a prospective study on Symptom Diversity and Modification of Questionnaire Application. Dig Dis. 2019. https://doi.org/10.1159/000502796.
11. Malfertheiner P, Nocon M, Vieth M, Stolte M, Jaspersen D, Koelz HR, Labenz J, Leodolter A, Lind T, Richter K, Willich SN. Evolution of gastro-oesophageal reflux disease over 5 years under routine medical care – the ProGERD study. Aliment Pharmacol Ther. 2012;35(1):154–64.
12. Liebermann-Meffert D, Duranceau A. Anatomy and embryology of the esophagus. In: Orringer MB, Zuidema GD, editors. Shackelford's surgery of the alimentary tract, vol 1, the esophagus. 4th ed. Philadelphia/London/Toronto/Montreal/Sydney/Tokyo: Saunders; 1996. p. 3–38.
13. Fuchs KH, Babic B, Fuchs HF. Esophageal Sphincters in Health and Disease. In: Yeo CJ, DeMeester SR, McFadden DW, editors. Shackelford's surgery of the alimentary tract. 8th ed. Philadelphia: Elsevier; 2019. p. 2–10.

14. Zaninotto G, DeMeester TR, Schwizer W, Johansson KE, Cheng SC. The lower esophageal sphincter in health and disease. Am J Surg. 1988;155:104–11.
15. Inoue H, Minami H, Kobayashi Y, et al. Peroral endoscopic myotomy (POEM) for esophageal achalasia. Endoscopy. 2010;42:265–71.
16. von Renteln D, Fuchs KH, Fockens P, Bauerfeind P, Vassiliou M, Breithaupt W, Heinrich H, Bredenoord A, Verlaan T, Trevisonno M, Rösch T. PerOral endoscopic myotomy for the treatment of achalasia: prospective international multi center study. Gastroenterology. 2013;145:309–11.
17. Ayazi S, Tamhankar A, DeMeester SR, Zehetner J, Wu C, Lipham JC, Hagen JA, DeMeester TR. The impact of gastric distension on the lower esophageal sphincter and its exposure to acid gastric juice. Ann Surg. 2010;252:57–62.
18. Wilson RL, Stevenson CE. Anatomy and physiology of the stomach. In: Yeo CJ, DeMeester SR, McFadden DW, editors. Shackelford's surgery of the alimentary tract. 8th ed. Philadelphia: Elsevier; 2019. p. 634–46.
19. Bredenoord AJ, Chial HJ, Camilleri M, Mullan BP, Murray JA. Gastric accommodation and emptying in evaluation of patients with upper gastrointestinal symptoms. Clin Gastroenterol Hepatol. 2003;1:264–72.
20. Fuchs KH, Freys SM, Heimbucher J, Fein M, Thiede A. Pathophysiologic spectrum in patients with gastroesophageal reflux disease in a surgical GI function laboratory. Dis Esophagus. 1995;8:211–7.
21. Dent J, Holloway RH, Toouli J, Dodds WJ. Mechanisms of lower oesophageal sphincter incompetence in patients with symptomatic gastro-oesophageal reflux. Gut. 1988;29:1020–8.
22. Mittal RK, Holloway RH, Penagini R, Blackshaw A, Dent J. Transient lower esophageal sphincter relaxations. Gastroenterology. 1995;109:601–10.
23. Mittal RK, Holloway R, Dent J. Effect of atropine on the frequency of reflux and transient lower esophageal sphincter relaxation in normal subjects. Gastroenterology. 1995;109:1547.
24. Kahrilas Peter J. Sifrim Daniel: high-resolution manometry and impedance-pH/manometry: valuable tools in clinical and investigational esophagology. Gastroenterology. 2008;135(3):756–69.
25. Kahrilas PJ. Esophageal motor disorders in terms of high-resolution esophageal pressure topography: what has changed? Am J Gastroenterol. 2010;105:981–7.
26. Ayazi S, Hagen JA, Zehetner J, Ross O, Wu C, Oezcelik A, Abate E, Sohn HJ, Banki F, Lipham JC, DeMeester SR, DeMeester TR. The value of high-resolution manometry in the assessment of the resting characteristics of the lower esophageal sphincter. J Gastrointest Surg. 2009;13:2113–20.
27. Stein HJ, Barlow AP, DeMeester TR, Hinder RA. Complications of gastroesophageal reflux disease. Role of the lower esophageal sphincter, esophageal acid and acid/alkaline exposure, and duodenogastric reflux. Ann Surg. 1992;216(1):35–43.
28. Fein M, Ritter M, DeMeester TR, Oberg S, Peters JH, Hagen JA, Bremner CG. Role of lower esophageal sphincter and hiatal hernia in the pathogenesis of GERD. J Gastrointest Surg. 1999;3(4):405–10.
29. Lord RVN, DeMeester SR, Peters JH, Hagen JA, Elyssnia D, Sheth CT, DeMeester TR. Hiatal hernia, lower esophageal sphincter incompetence, and effectiveness of Nissen fundoplication in the spectrum of gastroesophageal reflux disease. J Gastrointest Surg. 2009;13:602–10.
30. Kuster E, Ros E, Toledo-Pimentel V, Pujol A, Bordas JM, Grande IC. Predictive factors of the long term outcome in gastro-oesophageal reflux disease: six year follow up of 107 patients. Gut. 1994;35(1):8–14.
31. Clarke AT, Wirz AA, Seenan JP, Manning JJ, Gillen D, McColl KE. Paradox of gastric cardia: it becomes more acidic following meals while the rest of stomach becomes less acidic. Gut. 2009;58:904–9.
32. Beaument H, Benninck RJ, de Jong J, Boeckxstaens GE. The position of the acid pocket as a major risk factor for acidic reflux in healthy subjects and patients with GORD. Gut. 2010;59:441–51.

33. Holloway RH, Kocyan P, Dent J. Provocation of transient lower esophageal sphincter relaxations by meals in patients with symptomatic gastroesophageal reflux. Dig Dis Sci. 1991;36:1034–9.
34. Schoeman MN, Tippett MD, Akkermans LM, Dent J, Holloway RH. Mechanisms of gastroesophageal reflux in ambulant healthy human subjects. Gastroenterology. 1995;108(1):83–91.
35. Van Herwaarden MA, Samson M, Smout AJP. Excess gastroesophageal reflux in patients with hiatal hernia is caused by mechanisms other than transient LES relaxations. Gastroenterology. 2000;119:1439.
36. Trudgill NJ, Riley SA. Transient lower esophageal sphincter relaxations are no more frequent in patients with gastroesophageal reflux disease than in asymptomatic volunteers. Am J Gastroenterol. 2001;96(9):2569–74.
37. Kahrilas PJ, Kim HC, Pandolfino JE. Approaches to the diagnosis and grading of hiatal hernia. Best Pract Res Clin Gastroenterol. 2008;22(4):601–16. https://doi.org/10.1016/j.bpg.2007.12.007.
38. Kahrilas PJ, Bredenoord AJ, Fox M, Gyawali CP, Roman S, Smout AJPM, Pandolfino JE, The Chicago Classification of esophageal motility disorders, v3.0. International HRM Working Group. Neurogastroenterol Motil. 2015;27:160–74.
39. He S, Jell A, Hüser N, Kohn N, Feussner H. 24-hour monitoring of transient lower esophageal sphincter relaxation events by long-term high-resolution impedance manometry in normal volunteers: the "mirror phenomenon". Neurogastroenterol Motil. 2019;31(3):e13530. https://doi.org/10.1111/nmo.13530.
40. Oberg S, Peters JH, DeMeester TR, Lord RV, Johannsson J, Crookes P, Bremner CG. Endoscopic grading of the gastroesophageal valve in patients with symptoms of GERD. Surg Endosc. 1999;13:1184–8.
41. Fein M, Ireland AP, Ritter MP, Peters JH, Hagen JA, Bremner CG, DeMeester TR. Duodenogastric reflux potentiates the injurious effects of gastroesophageal reflux. J Gastrointest Surg. 1997;1(1):27–32.. discussion 33
42. Oberg S, Ritter MP, Crookes PF, Fein M, Mason RJ, Gadensytätter M, Brenner CG, Peters JH, DeMeester TR. Gastroesophageal reflux disease and mucosal injury with emphasis on short-segment Barrett's esophagus and duodenogastroesophageal reflux. J Gastrointest Surg. 1998;2(6):547–53.. discussion 553–4
43. Barrett NR. Chronic peptic ulcer of the oesophagus and oesophagitis. Br J Surg. 1950;38:175–82.
44. Paull A, Trier JS, Dalton MD. The histologic spectrum of Barrett's esophagus. N Engl J Med. 1976;295:476–80.
45. Chandrasoma P, Lokuhetty DM, DeMeester TR, Bremner CG, Peters JH, Oberg S, Groshen S. Definition of histopathologic changes in GERD. Am J Surg Pathol. 2000;24:344–51.
46. Chandarsoma P, Wijetunge S, DeMeester SR, Hagen J, DeMeester TR. The Chicago Classification of esophageal motility disorders, v3.0. Am J Surg Pathol. 34:15741581.
47. Oberg S, Peters JH, DeMeester TR, Chandrasoma P, Hagen JA, Ireland AP, Ritter MP, Mason RJ, Crookes P, Bremner CG. Inflammation and specialized intestinal metaplasia of cardiac mucosa is a manifestation of gastroesophageal reflux disease. Ann Surg. 1997;226:522–30.
48. Oberg S, Peters JH, DeMeester TR, Lord RV, Johansson J, DeMeester SR, Hagen JA. Determinants of intestinal metaplasia within the columnar-lined esophagus. Arch Surg. 2000;135:651–5.
49. Theisen J, Oberg S, Peters JH, Gastal O, Bremner CG, Mason R, DeMeester TR. Gastroesophageal reflux disease confined to the sphincter. Dis Esophagus. 2001;14:235–8.
50. Boeckxstaens GEE. Review: the pathophysiology of gastro-esophageal reflux disease. Aliment Pharmacol Ther. 2007;26:149–60.
51. Herbella FA, Patti MG. Gastroesophageal reflux disease: from pathophysiology to treatment. World J Gastroenterol. 2010;16(30):3745–9.
52. Herregods TVK, Bredenoord AJ, Smout AJPM. Pathophysiology of GERD: new understanding in a new era. Neurogastroenterol Motil. 2015;27:1202–12.
53. Mattioli S, Lugaresi ML, Costantini M, Del Genio A, Di Martino N, Fei L, Fumagalli U, Maffettone V, Monaco L, Morino M, Rebecchi F, Rosati R, Rossi M, Sant S, Trapani V,

Zaninotto G. The short esophagus: intraoperative assessment of esophageal length. J Thorac Cardiovasc Surg. 2008;136:1610.

54. Leodolter A, Nocon M, Vieth M, Lind T, Jaspersen D, Richter K, Willich S, Stolte M, Malfertheiner P, Labenz J. Progression of specialized intestinal metaplasia at the cardia to macroscopically evident Barrett's esophagus: an entity of concern in the ProGERD study. Scand J Gastroenterol. 2012;47(12):1429–35. https://doi.org/10.3109/00365521.2012.733952.

55. Labenz J, Chandrasoma PT, Knapp LJ, DeMeester TR. Proposed approach to the challenging management of progressive gastroesophageal reflux disease. World J Gastrointest Endosc. 2018;10(9):175–83. https://doi.org/10.4253/wjge.v10.i9.175.

56. Maret-Ouda J, Wahlin K, Artama M, Brusselaers N, Färkkilä M, Lynge E, Mattsson F, Pukkala E, Romundstad P, Tryggvadóttir L, von Euler-Chelpin M, Lagergren J. Risk of esophageal adenocarcinoma after antireflux surgery in patients with gastroesophageal reflux disease in the nordic countries. JAMA Oncol. 2018;4(11):1576–82. https://doi.org/10.1001/jamaoncol.2018.3054.

57. Fuchs KH, Lee AM, Breithaupt W, Varga G, Babic B, Horgan S. Pathophysiology of GERD – which factors are important? Transl Gastroenterol Hepatol. 2020. inprint.

Symptom Spectrum in Gastroesophageal Reflux Disease

2

Ryan C. Broderick and Karl-Hermann Fuchs

Introduction

The Montreal classification has described the presentation of symptoms in patients with gastroesophageal reflux disease (GERD) extensively [1]. The authors of the Montreal classification define the disease with symptoms: "GERD is a condition which develops when the reflux of stomach contents causes troublesome symptoms and/or complications" [1]. These symptoms can reduce patient's well-being [2–4]. Klauser et al. have stated that heartburn and regurgitation are the most typical symptoms characterizing GERD [5]. In clinical practice, a variety of esophageal and extraesophageal symptoms can be documented in patients referred for the diagnostic confirmation or exclusion of GERD. GERD may present with a large variety of symptoms such as heartburn, regurgitation, thoracic pain, epigastric pain, respiratory symptoms, globus, and others. There can be an overlap with symptoms from other esophageal and gastric disorders such as dyspepsia, esophageal motility disorders, functional heartburn, hypersensitive esophagus, irritable stomach and bowel, and somatoform disorders [1, 6–10]. While the symptom spectrum is complex, the use of objective studies can help further diagnose GERD.

R. C. Broderick
Division of Minimally Invasive Surgery, Department of Surgery, University of California San Diego, La Jolla, CA, USA

University of California San Diego, Department of Surgery, Center for the Future of Surgery, La Jolla, CA, USA

K.-H. Fuchs (✉)
University of California San Diego, Center for the Future of Surgery, La Jolla, CA, USA

© Springer Nature Switzerland AG 2020
S. Horgan, K.-H. Fuchs (eds.), *Management of Gastroesophageal Reflux Disease*,
https://doi.org/10.1007/978-3-030-48009-7_2

Diagnostic Workup for Patients with Symptoms Indicative of GERD

In a dedicated center for gastrointestinal functional disorders, patients with a suspicion for GERD should undergo a number of functional investigations to verify or exclude the disease and to possibly determine another diagnosis [2, 11]. All patients should undergo an upper GI endoscopy, a high-resolution manometry, a 24-h impedance-pH monitoring, and selectively other investigations such as gastric emptying studies and/or dynamic radiographic studies. The presence of pathologic reflux should be documented by impedance-pH monitoring with symptom correlation. The objective workup from the tests listed above may show functional defects or visible esophageal damage. Objectively, the studies can be used to characterize the severity of GERD [1, 2, 11].

The Variety of Symptoms in Patients with GERD

Klauser showed that heartburn and regurgitation are the most typical symptoms characterizing GERD [5]. Figure 2.1 demonstrates these findings. While it is interesting that heartburn and regurgitation are the most frequent and specific symptoms in GERD, it was also shown that heartburn and regurgitation are often present in other disorders [6]. In literature, heartburn is reported to be present in patients with pathologic esophageal acid exposure in up to 99% [1, 2, 6, 12–16]. However, heartburn is also seen in 6–20% of dyspepsia patients [1–16]. Regurgitation has a prevalence of 33–86% [1, 2, 6, 10, 12–16]. Epigastric pain may be present in patients with foregut symptoms in 70% and in those with documented GERD in 12–67% [1, 10, 12–16].

In our recently published study, we showed that heartburn and regurgitation are very often the chief complaints in patients with GERD; however, other symptoms associated with "gas" problems such as belching, bloating, and flatulence are also commonly present [10]. Figure 2.2 demonstrates the chief complaints in GERD patients, with chief complaint being the symptom marked with maximum intensity [10]. Figure 2.3 shows the overall presence of any symptoms noted by patients in

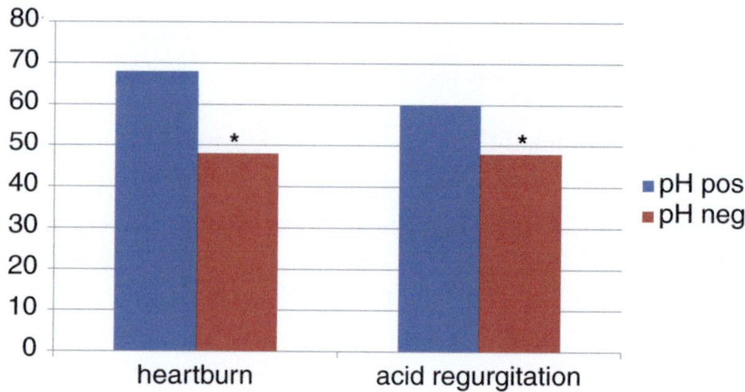

Fig. 2.1 Clinical presentation of heartburn and regurgitation in a group of patients with foregut symptoms, divided up in those with and those without pathologic esophageal acid exposure (Klauser et al. [5])

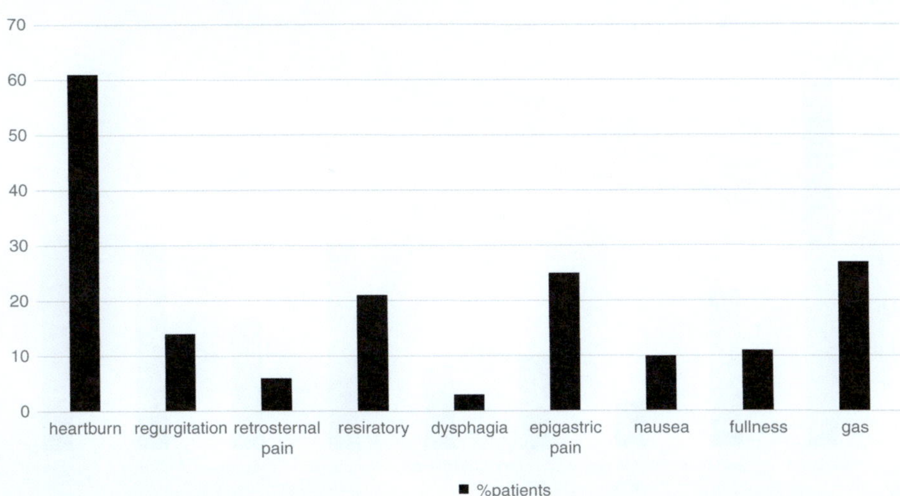

Fig. 2.2 Overview on the prevalence of chief complaints (most severe symptom with maximal intensity). The most important chief complaint is heartburn in GERD, followed by respiratory symptoms and gas-related symptoms (Broderick et al. [10])

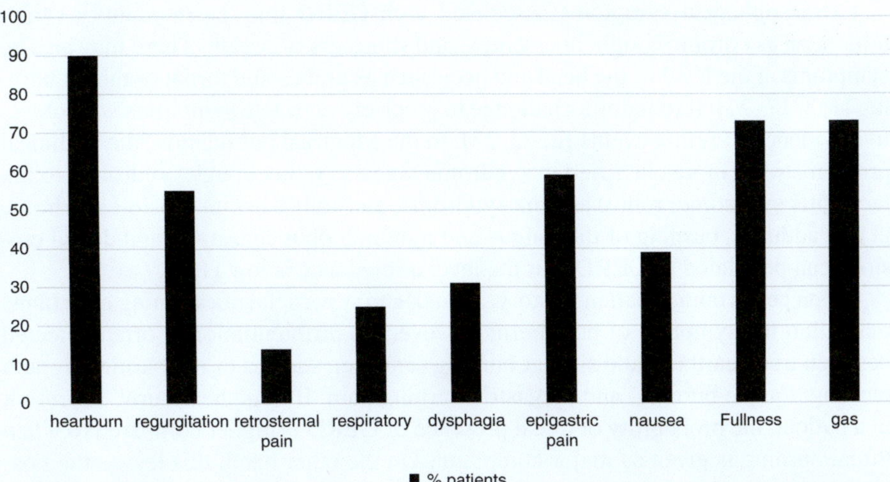

Fig. 2.3 Overview on the prevalence of all presenting symptoms. Heartburn is the most frequent presenting symptom, followed by gas-related symptoms, fullness, and epigastric pain (Broderick et al. [10])

our study [10]. A wide diversity of symptoms are present, such as respiratory symptoms and gas-related symptoms [10]. Despite the diversity of symptoms, many are reported in incidence as often as heartburn; however, the level of symptom intensity is not as high (Fig. 2.4).

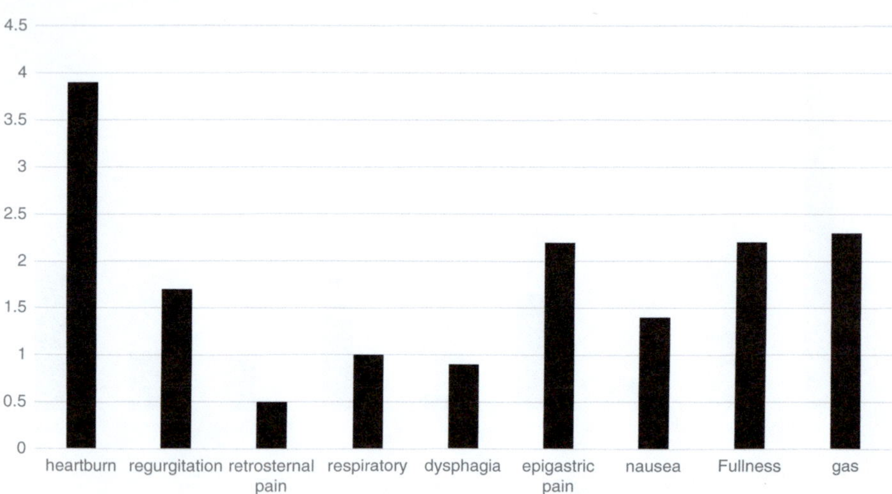

Fig. 2.4 Demonstration of the mean intensity of the documented GERD symptoms. Most intense and disturbing symptoms are heartburn, regurgitation, epigastric pain, fullness, and gas-related symptoms (Broderick et al. [10])

Extraesophageal symptoms associated with GERD may be respiratory symptoms such as chronic cough, hoarseness, and shortness of breath. There may also be symptoms at the level of the head and neck such as globus and throat or mouth burning [1, 2, 17–21]. It remains a challenge to precisely correlate symptoms with objective evidence of reflux events [2, 22, 23]. In the Montreal publication, these clinical problems were more classified in syndromes such as reflux cough syndrome, reflux laryngitis syndrome, reflux asthma syndrome, and reflux dental erosion syndrome [1]. In addition, burning of the tongue and mouth, globus sensation, and dental erosions can be related to GERD, but the level of evidence is low [1, 2].

When performing a patient history, a quick and superficial questioning of patients may elicit the symptom of heartburn; however, no differentiation is often detected between true heartburn and similar burning sensation such as throat burning, mouth burning, tongue burning, and epigastric burning/pain. If "true heartburn" is present in a patient, the probability of a real presence of GERD is higher compared to when throat burning is given as major complaint. On the other hand, this leaves the possible overlap with other disorders such as hypersensitive esophagus or somatoform disorders unaddressed [6–9]. It is important to perform a detailed history of patients with special attention and accuracy to the symptom evaluation while also letting the patients document their symptoms independently in order to elicit a complete symptom profile [10].

When the intensity of symptoms is evaluated in GERD, the most intense and disturbing symptoms are usually heartburn, regurgitation, and epigastric pain [2, 10]. GERD remains a disease with a wide variety of symptoms experienced by the patient. Heartburn and regurgitation are continual mainstays of symptom profile while other symptoms show a high diversity. The variety of symptoms experienced also shows the importance of a full objective workup including upper GI endoscopy, high-resolution manometry, and impedance-pH monitoring to assist with accurate diagnosis and identification of patients who may need surgical therapy for their reflux disease.

Symptom Profile of Esophageal Motility Disorders

Several years ago, a very detailed investigation was performed to evaluate the symptom profile of esophageal motility disorders especially assessing those symptoms that are usually also present in patients with GERD [24]. Figure 2.5 demonstrates the distribution of symptoms in these conditions such as achalasia, esophageal spasm, nutcracker esophagus, and other nonspecific motility disorders. The results show an opposite pattern of symptoms compared to reflux. Motility disorders have high prevalence of dysphagia, while heartburn was infrequent compared to GERD symptom profiles (Fig. 2.5). These results also demonstrate the variety of reflux-like symptoms in other disorders of the upper gastrointestinal tract, indicating the importance of objective studies for diagnosis [24].

GERD Symptoms and Somatoform Disorders

Somatoform disorders can also present similar to GERD [9]. In this study, patients with foregut symptoms and GERD, documented by positive esophageal acid exposure, were tested with a psychodiagnostic instrument SOMS (screening test

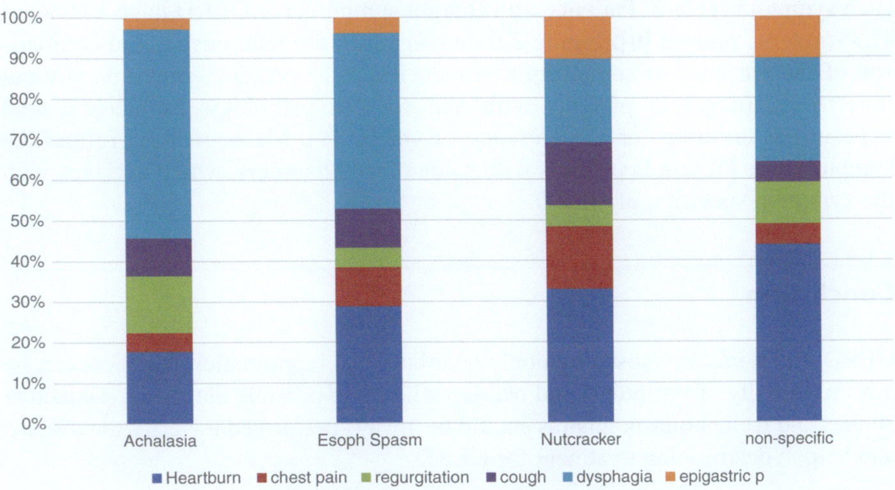

Fig. 2.5 Distribution of symptoms, often presenting in GERD, in patients with esophageal motility disorders such as achalasia, esophageal spasm, nutcracker, and nonspecific esophageal motility disorders (Tsuboi et al. [24])

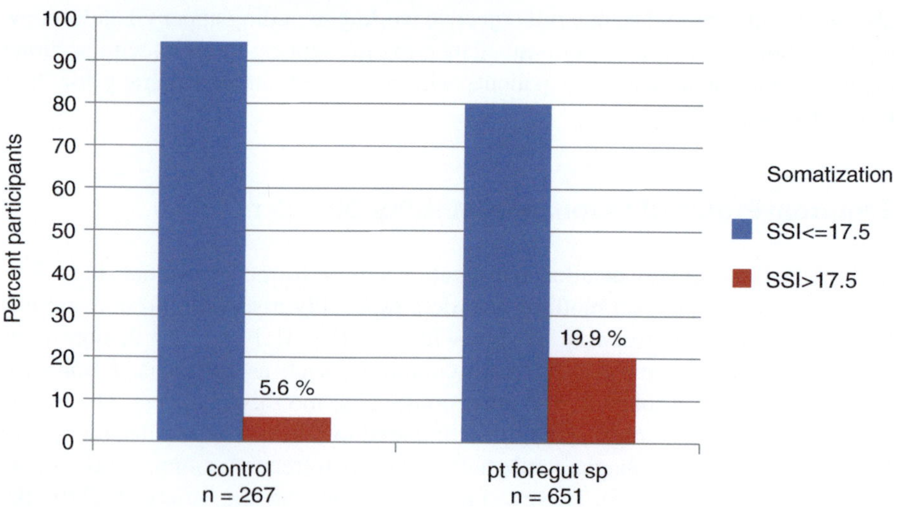

Fig. 2.6 Comparison of the presence of somatoform tendencies (Somatoform Symptom Index [SSI] > 17) in patients without (20,6%) and with pathologic esophageal acid exposure as criterion for GERD (19,5%) (Fuchs KH et al. [9])

for somatoform symptoms). This helped determine the probability of somatoform tendencies [9]. The study confirmed that in patients with foregut symptoms and GERD, the presence of a somatoform disorder was significantly higher than in normal individuals [9]. Somatization is characterized by the scenario of a given patient complaining about symptoms which cannot be explained by pathophysiologic or objective findings [25, 26]. In normal individuals, the mean number of such symptoms is 5–6. Patients with foregut symptoms or GERD have a mean of 12 symptoms present [9]. Figure 2.6 demonstrates the relationship and comparison of the presence of somatoform tendencies (> 17 present symptoms without objective findings) in patients with and without pathologic esophageal acid exposure as criterion for the presence of GERD [9]. Many of these reflux-like symptoms are present in patients with somatoform disorders, which overlaps with the symptom spectrum of GERD.

Conclusion

GERD symptoms are most commonly heartburn and regurgitation, but there can be a wide diversity of symptoms and overlap with other possible diagnoses. Objective studies and patient questionnaires should be always performed to verify the disease and help in determining treatment for GERD.

References

1. Vakil N, van Zanten SV, Kahrilas PJ, Dent J, Jones R, the global consensus Group. The Montreal definition and classification of GERD: a global evidence-based consensus. Am J Gastro. 2006;101:1900–20.
2. Fuchs KH, Babic B, Breithaupt W, Dallemagne B, Fingerhut A, Furnee E, Granderath F, Horvath OP, Kardos P, Pointner R, Savarino E, Van Herwarden-Lindeboom M, Zaninotto G. EAES recommendations for the management of gastroesophageal reflux disease. Surg Endosc. 2014;28:1753–73.
3. Kamolz T, Granderath F, Pointner R. Laparoscopic antirefluxsurgery: disease-related quality of life assessment before and after surgery in GERD patients with and without Barrett's esophagus. Surg Endosc. 2003;17:880–5.
4. Dallemagne B, Weertz J, Markiewicz S, Dewandre JM, Wahlen C, Monami B, Jehaes C. Clinical results of laparoscopic fundoplication ten years after surgery. Surg Endosc. 2006;20:159–65.
5. Klauser AG, Schindlbeck NE, Müller-Lissner SA. Symptoms in gastro-esophageal reflux disease. Lancet. 1990;335:205–8.
6. Costantini M, Crookes PF, Bremner RM, Hoeft SF, Ehsan A, Peters JH, Bremner CG, DeMeester TR. Value of physiologic assessment of foregut symptoms in a surgical practice. Surgery. 1993;114(4):780–6.
7. Tack J, Caenepeel P, Arts J, Lee KJ, Sifrim D, Janssens J. Prevalence of acid reflux functional dyspepsia and its association with symptom profile. Gut. 2005;54(10):1370–6.
8. Savarino E, Pohl D, Zentilin P, Dulbecco P, Sammito G, Sconfienza L, Vigneri S, Camerini G, Tutuian R, Savarino V. Functional heartburn has more in common with functional dyspepsia than with non-erosive reflux disease. Gut. 2009;58(9):1185–91.
9. Fuchs KH, Musial F, Ulbricht F, Breithaupt W, Reinisch A, Schulz T, Babic B, Fuchs HF, Varga G. Foregut symptoms, somatoform tendencies, and the selection of patients for antireflux surgery. Dis Esophagus. 2017;30:1–10.
10. Broderick R, Fuchs KH, Breithaupt W, Varga G, Schulz T, Babic B, Lee A, Musial F, Horgan S. Clinical presentation of GERD: a prospective study on symptom diversity and modification of questionnaire application. Dig Dis. 2019. https://doi.org/10.1159/000502796.
11. Jobe BA, Richter JE, Hoppo T, Peters JH, Bell R, Dengler WC, DeVault K, Fass R, Gyawali CP, Kahrilas PJ, Lacy BE, Pandolfino JE, Patti MG, Swanstrom LL, Kurian AA, Vela MF, Vaezi M, DeMeester TR. Preoperative diagnostic workup before antireflux surgery: an evidence and experience-based consensus of the Esophageal Diagnostic Advisory Panel. J Am Coll Surg. 2013;217(4):586–97. https://doi.org/10.1016/j.jamcollsurg.2013.05.023.
12. Bradley LA, Richter JE, Pulliam TJ, et al. The relationship between stress and symptoms of gastroesophageal reflux: the influence of psychological factors. Am J Gastroenterol. 1993;88(1):11–9.
13. Johnston BT, Lewis SA, Love AH. Stress, personality and social support in gastro-oesophageal reflux disease. J Psychosom Res. 1995;39(2):221–6.
14. Oustamanolakis P, Tack J. Dyspepsia – organ versus functional. J Clin Gastroenterol. 2012;46:175–90.
15. Kahrilas PJ, Jonsson A, Denison H, Wernerson B, Hughes N, Howden CW. Concomitant symptoms itemized in the reflux disease questionnaire are associated with attenuated heartburn response to acid suppression. Am J Gastroenterol. 2012;107(9):1354–60.
16. Kahrilas PJ, Jonsson A, Denison H, Wernersson B, Hughes N, Howden CW. Regurgitation is less responsive to acid suppression than heartburn in patients with gastroesophageal reflux disease. Clin Gastroenterol Hepatol. 2012;10(6):612–9.
17. Kiljander TO, Salomaa ERM, Hietanen EK, et al. Chronic cough and gastro-esophageal reflux: a double-blind placebo-controlled study with omeprazole. Eur Respir J. 2000;16:633–8.
18. Allen CJ, Anvari M. Gastro-esophageal reflux related cough and its response to laparoscopic fundoplication. Thorax. 1998;53:963–8.

19. Smith JA, Decalmer S, Kelsall A, et al. Acoustic cough-reflux associations in chronic cough: potential triggers and mechanisms. Gastroenterology. 2010;139:754–62.
20. Pacheco-Galvan A, Hart SP, Morice AH. Relationship between gastro-oesophageal reflux and airway diseases: the airway reflux paradigm. Arch Broncopneumol. 2011;47:195–203.
21. Kahrilas PJ, Altman KW, Chang AB, et al. Chronic cough due to gastroesophageal reflux in adults: chest guideline and expert panel report. Chest. 2016;150:1341–60.
22. Ayazi S, Lipham JC, Hagen JA, et al. A new technique for measurement of pharyngeal pH: normal values and discriminating pH threshold. J Gastrointest Surg. 2009;13:1422–9.
23. Fuchs HF, Muller DT, Berlth F, et al. Simultaneous laryngopharyngeal pH monitoring (Restech) and conventional esophageal pH monitoring-correlation using a large patient cohort of more than 100 patients with suspected gastroesophageal reflux disease. Dis Esophagus. 2018; https://doi.org/10.1093/dote/doy018.
24. Tsuboi K, Hoshino M, Srinivasan A, Yano F, Hinder RA, Demeester TR, Filipi CJ, Mittal SK. Insights gained from symptom evaluation of esophageal motility disorders: a review of 4,215 patients. Digestion. 2012;85(3):236–42. https://doi.org/10.1159/000336072.
25. Rief W, Heuser J, Mayrhuber E, Stelzer I, Hiller W, Fichter MM. The classification of multiple somatoform symptoms. J Nerv Ment Dis. 1996;184(11):680–7.
26. Hiller W, Cuntz U, Rief W, Fichter MM. Searching for a gastrointestinal subgroup within the somatoform disorders. Psychosomatics. 2001;42(1):14–20.

Diagnostic Investigations in GERD

3

David C. Kunkel

Introduction

Functional disorders in the upper gastrointestinal tract present with a large diversity of different symptoms [1–7]. Among these, gastroesophageal reflux disease (GERD) is no exception. Despite typical symptoms such as heartburn and regurgitation, GERD may cause also a variety of different symptoms such as chest pain, chronic cough, hoarseness, epigastric pain, and/or nausea [5–7]. The Montréal classification of GERD has described the presence of symptoms in GERD and also demonstrated the variety of symptoms in several groups [8]. Furthermore, other functional and somatoform disorders may also present with "reflux-like" symptoms, creating an overlap with the clinical presentation of GERD [6, 8]. Therefore, symptoms may be in some cases misleading regarding a sufficient diagnosis for therapeutic decision-making [5–9].

Diagnostic Investigations

As a consequence, diagnostic investigations in GERD are very important [8, 10]. Current technology allows for a very comprehensive assessment and understanding of the morphologic, anatomical, and functional alterations that emerge with the development of GERD [10].

D. C. Kunkel (✉)
University of California San Diego, Department of Medicine Gastroenterology,
La Jolla, CA, USA
e-mail: dkunkel@ucsd.edu

© Springer Nature Switzerland AG 2020

27

S. Horgan, K.-H. Fuchs (eds.), *Management of Gastroesophageal Reflux Disease*,
https://doi.org/10.1007/978-3-030-48009-7_3

Endoscopy

Esophago-gastro-duodenoscopy is a well-established diagnostic technique and can provide a precise assessment of the mucosal damage and also the anatomical changes of the esophagogastric junction, which is involved in the characteristics of GERD. In addition, histologic evaluation is possible with endoscopy and also in some cases necessary to identify Barrett's esophagus or other tissue changes [10–12].

Two major classifications exist in endoscopy for the description of GERD changes in the esophagus [11, 12]. The Savary and Miller classification has been established several decades ago and is still used by many endoscopists [11].

Endoscopic classification of esophagitis by Savary and Miller:

- Grade 1: Single areas of redness or single erosions in the distal esophagus
- Grade 2: Stripes of erosions in the distal esophagus, nonconfluent
- Grade 3: Confluent, circular erosions in the esophagus
- Grade 4: Presence of complications of a massive esophagitis such as ulcers, strictures, and/or Barrett's esophagus

Endoscopic Los Angeles classification of esophagitis (Figs. 3.1 and 3.2):

- Grade A: Mucosal lesions of maximum 5 mm diameter
- Grade B: Mucosal lesions >5 mm, not circumferential
- Grade C: Confluent mucosal lesions, less than 75% of the circumference
- Grade D: Confluent mucosal lesions, more than 75% of the circumference

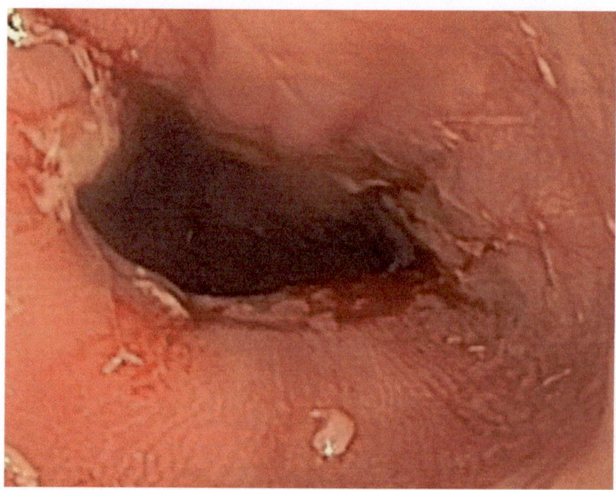

Fig. 3.1 Endoscopic visible Los Angeles Grade C esophagitis

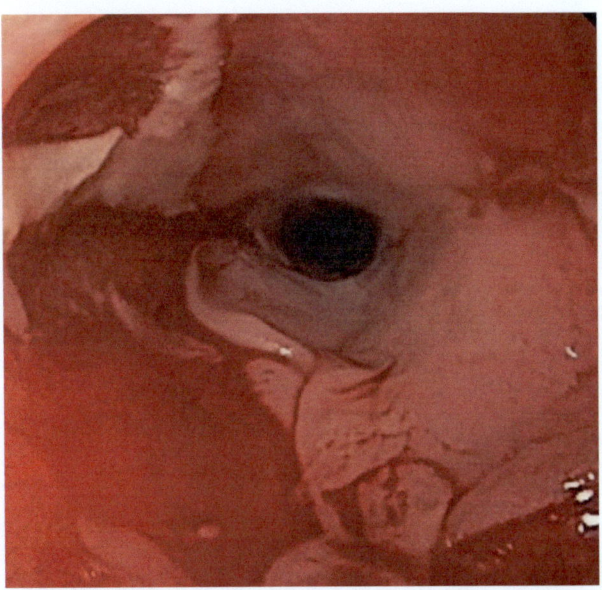

Fig. 3.2 Endoscopic visible Los Angeles Grade D esophagitis with stricture

Radiographic Investigations

Today, radiographic investigations in GERD are often used for the typing of large hiatal hernias, or they are used as dynamic investigations, for example, as dynamic barium-burger or barium-sandwich swallowing tests, to verify problems in the passage of a solid or semisolid bolus. These tests are very helpful in the identification of functional and/or mechanical problems in the esophageal passage of a bolus [10, 11, 13] (Fig. 3.3). The advantage is a better diagnostic value for these findings. Furthermore, this investigation can also be used for the evaluation of the subsequent gastric emptying process [10, 11, 13] (Figs. 3.4 and 3.5).

Impedance-pH Monitoring

It is essential to differentiate between the investigations necessary to establish the diagnosis of GERD and those necessary to establish the indication for surgery or any other invasive therapy. The most important diagnostic investigations to prove GERD are endoscopy and long-term impedance-pH monitoring [10, 14–17]. For accurate placement of the impedance-pH probe, manometry measurements are recommended. The test should be performed after adequate discontinuation for about 10–14 days of PPI or other antisecretory drugs prior to the test.

The dual technology of impedance-pH – monitoring allows for recording of the intraluminal pH – value as well as the impedance within the esophageal lumen (Fig. 3.6). This provides the identification of all intraluminal fluid and gas movements and their direction of flow associated with their pH. With this acid reflux

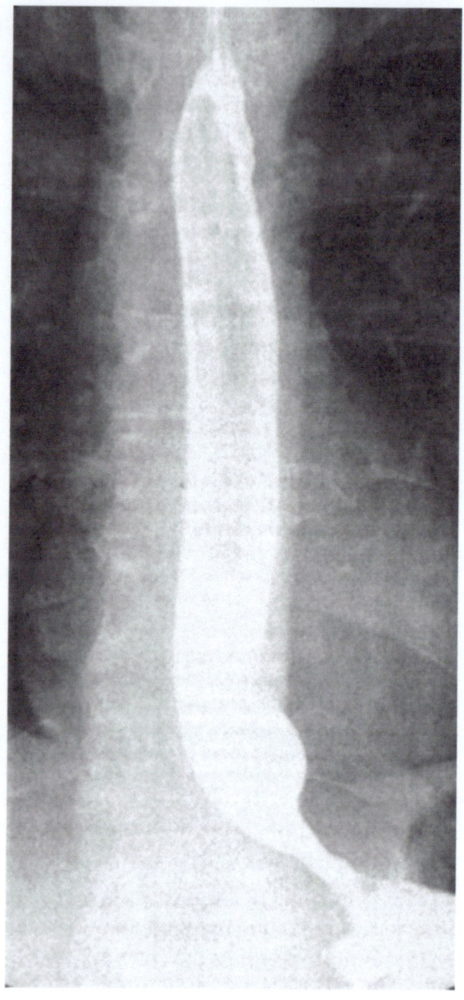

Fig. 3.3 Barium-sandwich of a person with a normal esophageal motility and anatomy

episode (pH < 4), weak acid reflux episodes (pH 4–7) as well as nonacid reflux episodes can be individually identified and correlated with symptoms, if the latter are also recorded, allowing for a determination of the Symptom Association Probability (SAP) [14–17].

The most important investigation is pH monitoring/impedance-pH monitoring, which is obligatory to objectively document pathologic acid exposure and/or other pathologic reflux activities. Impedance-pH monitoring increases the diagnostic value of these functional studies by quantifying acid and nonacid reflux as well as by providing correlation between symptoms and documented reflux episodes [10, 14–17].

The position, pressure, and length of the lower esophageal sphincter were determined with esophageal manometry, using these measurements for the correct

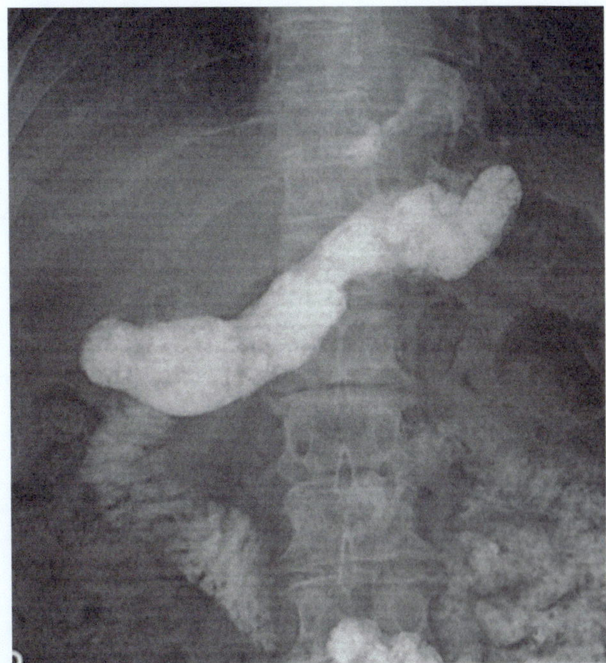

Fig. 3.4 Barium-sandwich initially after ingestion with regular gastric filling

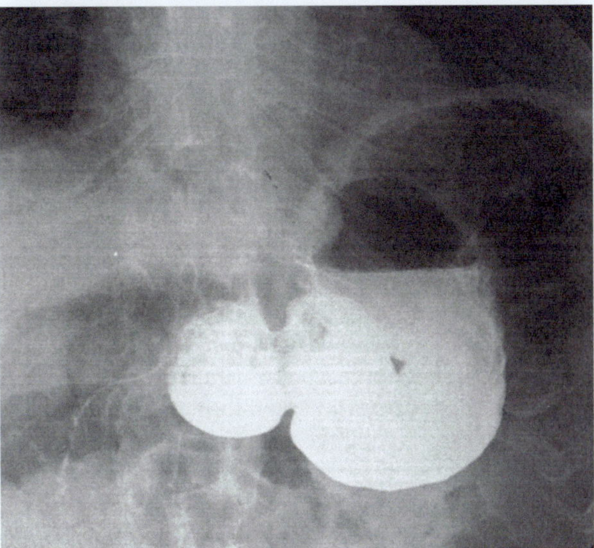

Fig. 3.5 Barium-sandwich after 4 h in a patient with massive gastroparesis

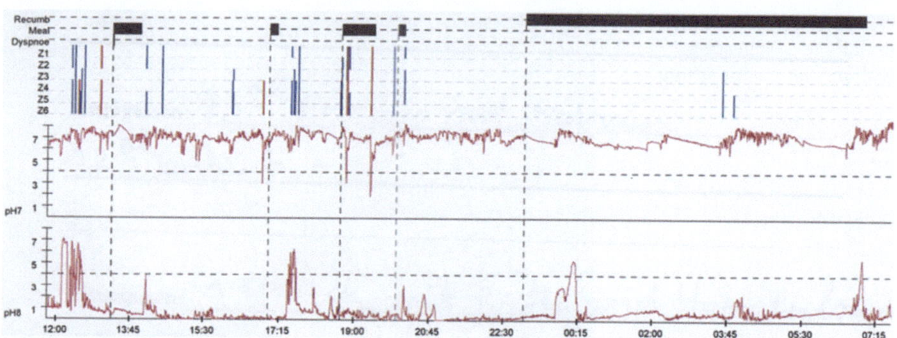

Fig. 3.6 A 24-h impedance-pH monitoring of esophagus and stomach of a normal healthy person with no pathologic reflux

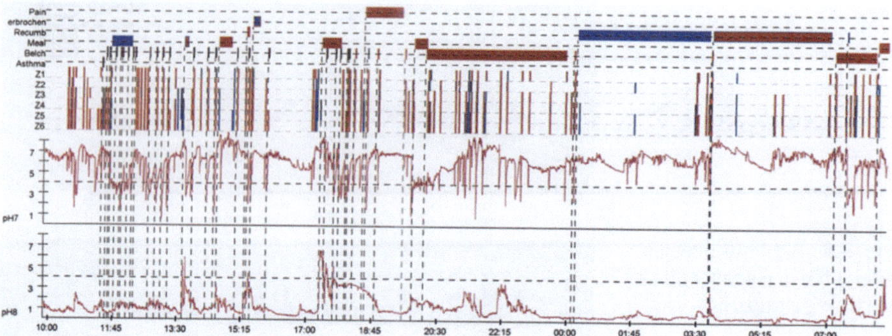

Fig. 3.7 A 24-h impedance-pH monitoring of esophagus and stomach of a patient with moderate pathologic gastroesophageal reflux (DeMeester score 26.5; normal <14.7)

positioning of the pH probes 5 cm above the upper border of the lower esophageal sphincter. pH monitoring or later impedance-pH monitoring was performed in a standard technique using, for analysis, the DeMeester reflux score criteria [14]. This implemented a borderline between physiologic and pathologic esophageal acid exposure, if the score reached a value of 14.7.

A 24-h (impedance-)pH monitoring is considered to be the gold standard investigation for the quantitative evaluation of acid exposure in the distal esophagus [10, 15] (Figs. 3.7 and 3.8). Most gastroenterologists prefer pH monitoring only in the absence of esophagitis. Since esophagitis can also be due to ulcers by medication and since many studies and surgical literature show the value of pH monitoring in the detection of the presence of the disease, preoperative workup should include impedance-pH monitoring [10, 18–20].

The more atypical symptoms are present in a given patient, the more detailed diagnostic assessment should be performed prior to surgery to detect all functional defects. When extra-esophageal symptoms are present or especially are the chief

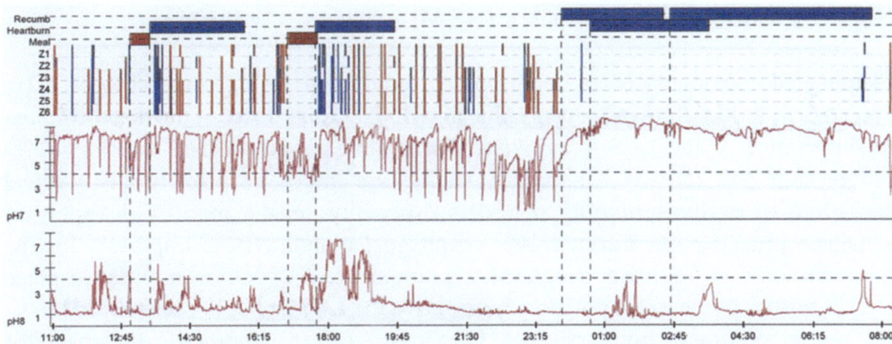

Fig. 3.8 A 24-h-impedance-pH monitoring of esophagus and stomach of a patient with GERD and a pathologic gastroesophageal reflux (DeMeester score 41.8). The visual analysis shows that most reflux episodes occur during daytime in this patient

Table 3.1 Normal data for 24-h impedance-pH monitoring as published by Shay et al. [16]

Median/95th percentile	Total reflux	Acid reflux pH < 4	Weakly acid pH 4–7
Total	30/73	18/55	9/26
Upright	27/67	17/52	8/24
Supine	1/7	0/5	0/4

complaints, it is extremely important to correlate the atypical symptoms with the reflux episodes to justify invasive antireflux therapies [10, 18–20].

Results of 24-h pH monitoring can be expressed in different ways. One option is the expression as percentage of pH < 4 during the measured time period. A borderline has been determined between 4.5% and even as high as 6% for the pathologic range above these values [14–17, 21].

Another option is the well-established DeMeester score with a borderline between normal and pathologic at 14.7 score value [14, 15]. Other criteria have been tried but have not been used very often. For the impedance evaluation, Table 3.1 shows the available data. Shay et al. have analyzed 60 individuals to gain normal values [16].

The median acid exposure in the distal esophagus (percentage acid exposure) was in this analysis for the total time of measurement 1.6% (95th percentile: 5%). In upright position, these data were 1.5% (6.2%) and supine 0.1% (5.3%).

As transnasal probes can be quite uncomfortable for the patients, wireless probes and detection systems were developed such as the BRAVO™ system. The probe is placed in the esophagus above the endoscopic visible Z-line or by measuring the distance by manometry or by pH change, which would be less accurate. The advantage of the system is the measurement only on one spot of the esophagus and only acid assessment. The disadvantage is that the probe is not able to measure impedance, which misses the weak acid and nonacid reflux episodes.

High-Resolution Manometry (HRM)

Esophageal manometry is not important in establishing the diagnosis of GERD [10, 15, 22–26]. It does, however, have value as a marker of severity of the disease in that incompetence of the LES is associated with more severe disease and long-term progression [10, 15, 23]. Manometry studies are important prior to any surgical procedure to evaluate motility disorders especially spastic motility disorders or achalasia [10, 18, 19]. Furthermore, esophageal manometry is important for the measurements of the lower esophageal sphincter (LES) position in order to place the pH probes at the exact position 5 cm above the LES upper border [10, 15].

High-resolution manometry (HRM) has improved the manometric diagnostic for the esophagus substantially, since it is more easy for the patient and esophageal motility can be classified in a more differentiated way [19] (Fig. 3.9).

The indications for HRM are discussed sometimes controversially, since some follow the idea that manometry is necessary for identifying the correct position of the LES for pH probe placement, while others think this is not necessary and could be done by pullback of the pH probe and wait for the pH change from intragastric acidic values to esophageal levels. In most guidelines, it is requested or suggested to perform an esophageal manometry before pH monitoring [10].

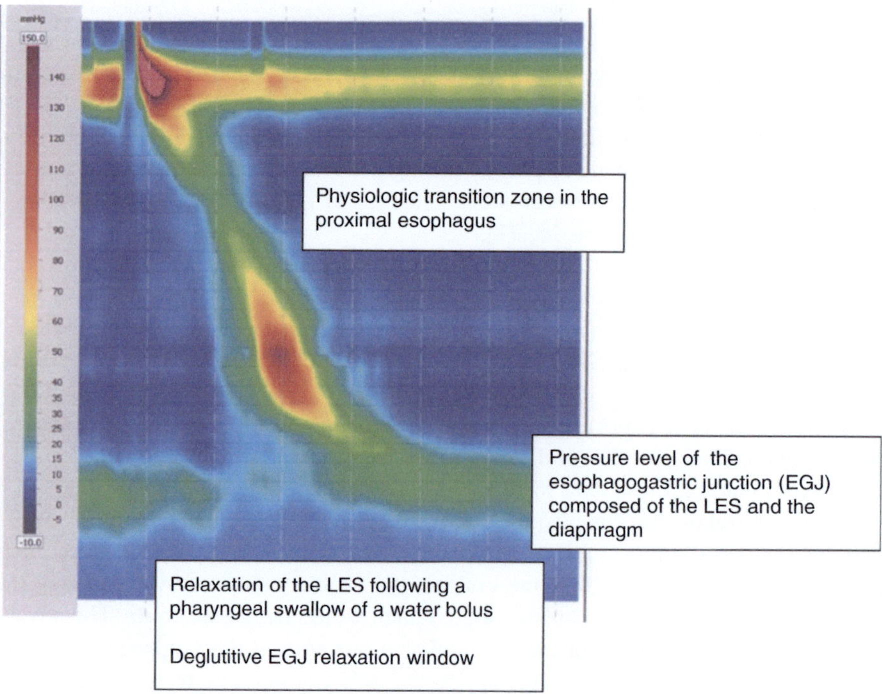

Fig. 3.9 Demonstration of a physiologic esophageal response to a swallow with normal peristalsis and relaxation of the LES for a symptom-free passage of the bolus

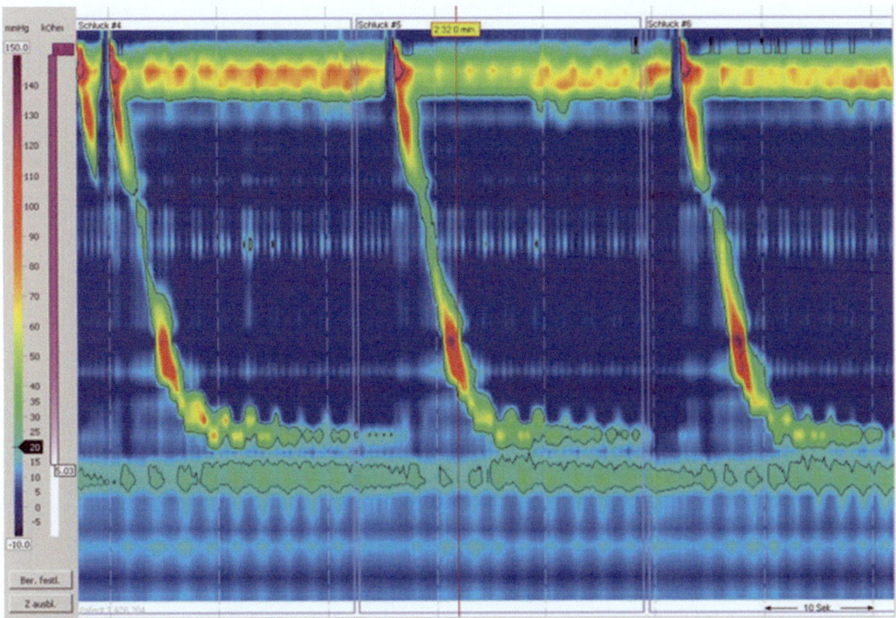

Fig. 3.10 HRM of a patient with GERD and hiatal hernia. The separation between LES and the diaphragm is clearly demonstrated indicating also the weakness of the LES and the anatomical alteration by the growing hiatal hernia

Another important indication for HRM is the verification or exclusion of esophageal motility disorders in GERD patients (Figs. 3.10 and 3.11). This information is especially important prior to interventional therapy and antireflux surgery [10, 18, 19].

Conclusion

Further diagnostic investigations may be needed to verify functional abnormalities and establish the indication for surgery or other invasive therapies. Investigations that can evaluate the status of esophageal and gastric function include high-resolution manometry.

HRM facilitates the procedure for the patients. Dynamic barium-sandwich videography is important to evaluate patients with dysphagia. In large hernias, a barium study can provide information about the possibility of a short esophagus. In GERD patients with nausea and vomiting as major complaint, gastric emptying studies and duodeno-gastroesophageal reflux assessment should be done to evaluate the presence of a gastroduodenal motility disorder such as delayed gastric emptying.

Endoscopy is especially important in exclusion of malignant disease and in the presence of alarm symptoms such as dysphagia, retrosternal pain, and bleeding. With endoscopy, it is possible to establish the diagnosis of GERD and its grade of

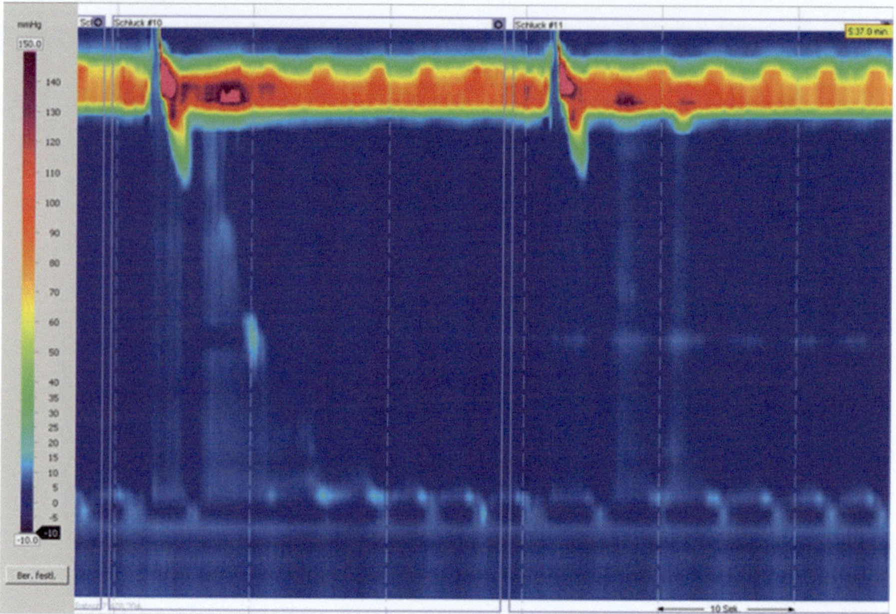

Fig. 3.11 HRM study of a patient with GERD, an absent LES, and a severe esophageal motility problem indicating a possible presence of scleroderma

severity, if reflux esophagitis is present. If esophagitis is excluded, the presence of NERD must be established using functional studies.

For diagnostic workup prior to surgery, endoscopy, 24-h pH monitoring, and manometry are important for the optimal selection for patients. For the surgical relevant pathophysiologic background, it is important to determine either the LES incompetence by esophageal manometry or the increased incidence of transient sphincter relaxations by sleeve manometry. Manometry prior to surgery is important in order to exclude spastic esophageal motility disorders.

References

1. Bradley LA, Richter JE, Pulliam TJ, et al. The relationship between stress and symptoms of gastroesophageal reflux: the influence of psychological factors. Am J Gastroenterol. 1993;88(1):11–9.
2. Johnston BT, Lewis SA, Love AH. Stress, personality and social support in gastro-oesophageal reflux disease. J Psychosom Res. 1995;39(2):221–6.
3. Tack J, Caenepeel P, Arts J, Lee KJ, Sifrim D, Janssens J. Prevalence of acid reflux functional dyspepsia and its association with symptom profile. Gut. 2005;54(10):1370–6.
4. Savarino E, Pohl D, Zentilin P, Dulbecco P, Sammito G, Sconfienza L, Vigneri S, Camerini G, Tutuian R, Savarino V. Functional heartburn has more in common with functional dyspepsia than with non-erosive reflux disease. Gut. 2009;58(9):1185–91.

5. Kahrilas PJ, Jonsson A, Denison H, Wernerson B, Hughes N, Howden CW. Concomitant symptoms itemized in the Reflux Disease Questionnaire are associated with attenuated heartburn response to acid suppression. Am J Gastroenterol. 2012;107(9):1354–60.
6. Fuchs KH, Musial F, Ulbricht F, Breithaupt W, Reinisch A, Schulz T, Babic B, Fuchs HF, Varga G. Foregut symptoms, somatoform tendencies, and the selection of patients for antireflux surgery. Dis Esophagus. 2017;30:1–10.
7. Broderick R, Fuchs KH, Breithaupt W, Varga G, Schulz T, Babic B, Lee A, Musial F, Horgan S. Clinical presentation of GERD: a prospective study on symptom diversity and modification of questionnaire application. Dig Dis. 2019;12:1–8. https://doi.org/10.1159/000502796.
8. Vakil N, van Zanten SV, Kahrilas PJ, Dent J, Jones R, The Global Consensus Group. The Montreal definition and classification of GERD: a global evidence-based consensus. Am J Gastroenterol. 2006;101:1900–20.
9. Costantini M, Crookes PF, Bremner RM, Hoeft SF, Ehsan A, Peters JH, Bremner CG, DeMeester TR. Value of physiologic assessment of foregut symptoms in a surgical practice. Surgery. 1993;114(4):780–6.
10. Jobe BA, Richter JE, Hoppo T, Peters JH, Bell R, Dengler WC, DeVault K, Fass R, Gyawali CP, Kahrilas PJ, Lacy BE, Pandolfino JE, Patti MG, Swanstrom LL, Kurian AA, Vela MF, Vaezi M, DeMeester TR. Preoperative diagnostic workup before antireflux surgery: an evidence and experience-based consensus of the Esophageal Diagnostic Advisory Panel. J Am Coll Surg. 2013;217(4):586–97. https://doi.org/10.1016/j.jamcollsurg.2013.05.023.
11. Genta RM, Spechler SJ, Kielhorn AF. The Los Angeles and Savary-Miller systems for grading esophagitis: utilization and correlation with histology. Dis Esophagus. 2011;24(1):10–7. https://doi.org/10.1111/j.1442-2050.2010.01092.x.
12. Lundell LR, Dent J, Bennett JR, Blum AL, Armstrong D, Galmiche JP, Johnson F, Hongo M, Richter JE, Spechler SJ, Tytgat GN, Wallin L. Endoscopic assessment of oesophagitis: clinical and functional correlates and further validation of the Los Angeles classification. Gut. 1999;45(2):172–80.
13. Raskin HF. Barium-burger roentgen study for unrecognized, clinically significant, gastric retention. South Med J. 1971;64(10):1227–35. PMID 5097797
14. Johnson LF, DeMeester TR. Twenty-four-hour pH monitoring of the distal esophagus. A quantitative measure of gastroesophageal reflux. Am J Gastroenterol. 1974;62:325–32.
15. DeMeester TR. Etiology and natural history of gastroesophageal reflux disease and predictors of progressive disease. In: Yeo CJ, DeMeester SR, Mc Fadden DW, editors. Shackelford's surgery of the alimentary tract. 8th ed. Philadelphia: Elsevier; 2019. p. 204–20.
16. Shay S. Esophageal impedance monitoring: the ups and downs of a new test. Am J Gastroenterol. 2004;99(6):1020–2.
17. Zerbib F, des Varannes SB, Roman S, Pouderoux P, Artigue F, Chaput U, Mion F, Caillol F, Verin E, Bommelaer G, Ducrotte P, Galmiche JP, Sifrim D. Normal values and day-to-day variability of 24-h ambulatory oesophageal impedance-pH monitoring in a Belgian French cohort of healthy subjects. Aliment Pharmacol Ther. 2005;22(10):1011–21.
18. Stefanidis D, Hope WW, Kohn GP, Reardon PR, Richardson WS, Fanelli RD, SAGES Guideline Committee. Guidelines for surgical treatment of GERD. Surg Endosc. 2010;24(11):2647–69.
19. Fuchs KH, Babic B, Breithaupt W, Dallemagne B, Fingerhut A, Furnee E, Granderath F, Horvath OP, Kardos P, Pointner R, Savarino E, Van Herwarden-Lindeboom M, Zaninotto G. EAES recommendations for the management of gastroesophageal reflux disease. Surg Endosc. 2014;28:1753–73.
20. Gyawali CP, Fass R. Management of gastroesophageal reflux disease. Gastroenterology. 2018;154(2):302–18. https://doi.org/10.1053/j.gastro.2017.07.049.
21. Gyawali CP, Kahrilas PJ, Savarino E, Zerbib F, Mion F, Smout AJPM, Vaezi M, Sifrim D, Fox MR, Vela MP, Tutuian R, Tack J, Bredenoord AJ, Pandolfino J, Roman S. Modern diagnosis of GERD: the Lyon Consensus. Gut. 2018;67(7):1351–62.
22. Dent J, Holloway RH, Toouli J, Dodds WJ. Mechanisms of lower oesophageal sphincter incompetence in patients with symptomatic gastro-oesophageal reflux. Gut. 1988;29:1020–8.

23. Kuster E, Ros E, Toledo-Pimentel V, Pujol A, Bordas JM, Grande IC. Predictive factors of the long term outcome in gastro-oesophageal reflux disease: six year follow up of 107 patients. Gut. 1994;35(1):8–14.
24. Mittal RK, Holloway RH, Penagini R, Blackshaw A, Dent J. Transient lower esophageal sphincter relaxations. Gastroenterology. 1995;109:601–10.
25. Kahrilas PJ, Sifrim D. High-resolution manometry and impedance-pH/manometry: valuable tools in clinical and investigational esophagology. Gastroenterology. 2008;135(3):756–69.
26. Mittal RK, Holloway R, Dent J. Effect of atropine on the frequency of reflux and transient lower esophageal sphincter relaxation in normal subjects. Gastroenterology. 1995;109:1547.

Medical Therapy of GERD

4

Karima Farrag and Jürgen Stein

Introduction

In Western industrial societies, it is estimated that 10–15% of the population suffers from gastroesophageal reflux disease (GERD) [1–3]. Over the past three decades, medical therapies have developed to the point where an overwhelming majority of patients with mild to moderate symptoms of GERD can be quite successfully treated [2, 4]. With a view to therapeutic decision-making, however, diagnosis may in some cases be hindered by the wide diversity of symptoms associated with GERD [2, 5–7].

The Montréal definition and classification of GERD describes and categorizes different types of symptoms of GERD [2]. While heartburn and regurgitation are specific symptoms of the disease that characterize the reflux event quite clearly, other symptoms such as nausea, vomiting, dysphagia, and chest pain, extraesophageal symptoms such as cough or hoarseness, and other respiratory symptoms are more difficult to relate to reflux events [2]. Furthermore, the Montréal classification differentiates symptoms into groups, such as the typical "reflux syndrome" with esophageal lesions, strictures, and reflux or "reflux and chest pain syndrome" or "extraesophageal symptoms" such as laryngitis, cough syndrome, and even dental erosions, possibly in association with pulmonary fibrosis, pharyngitis, and sinusitis.

Medical therapy can be applied in all these conditions. However, different syndromes respond differently and may therefore require a more differentiated therapeutic approach [2, 4].

K. Farrag · J. Stein (✉)
Department of Gastroenterology, Krankenhaus Sachsenhausen, Frankfurt am Main, Germany
e-mail: J.Stein@em.uni-Frankfurt.de

© Springer Nature Switzerland AG 2020
S. Horgan, K.-H. Fuchs (eds.), *Management of Gastroesophageal Reflux Disease*,
https://doi.org/10.1007/978-3-030-48009-7_4

Lifestyle Intervention in GERD

Ingestion of alcohol has been shown to exacerbate reflux symptoms by decreasing the pressure of the lower esophageal sphincter (LES), increasing acid secretion through gastrin stimulation, and decreasing esophageal motility [8, 9].

Furthermore, nonalcoholic carbonated beverages such as carbonated water and caffeinated or caffeine-free cola have been shown to cause a short-term reduction in the intraesophageal pH and a transient decrease in LES basal pressure and to increase gastric acid secretion. In some cases, therefore, it may be beneficial for the patient to reduce or avoid their consumption [9, 10].

While tea and especially coffee consumption have previously been reported to be associated with GERD, two recent meta-analyses failed to show a significant relationship between tea and/or coffee consumption and the overall risk of GERD [11, 12].

Along with diet, an important lifestyle component of GERD symptoms is the timing of meals in relation to sleep. Dinner within 2–3 hours of bedtime and snacking after dinner were strongly associated with increased reflux symptoms [8, 9, 13]. In order to reduce reflux during sleep, it has been recommended to raise the head end of the bed. Sleeping with a bedhead elevation achieved using 28 cm blocks was associated with faster acid clearing and fewer and shorter reflux episodes. Moreover, sleeping with a wedge pillow has also been associated with decreased esophageal acid exposure. Such a strategy may be especially beneficial in patients with late evening or nocturnal GERD [8, 9].

Accumulating epidemiological data clearly suggest obesity to be among the root causes of the GERD epidemic of the twenty-first century. Not only does obesity affect esophageal motility, but in patients with obesity, an increase in abdominal pressure frequently causes the disruption of the gastroesophageal junction [13]. Both of these effects have sparked debate on obesity as a likely causative factor for GERD. Not surprisingly, a weight loss of 10% was demonstrated to be associated with significantly decreased reflux symptoms, i.e., heartburn, regurgitation, and noncardiac chest pain. Therefore, the improvement or normalization of BMI is considered a first step toward lifestyle modification in patients with obesity-related GERD [8, 9].

As smoking has been shown to be implicated in the exacerbation of reflux symptoms, cessation of smoking should also be recommended. Last but not least, patients should be instructed to exercise regularly in order to strengthen the striated muscle in the diaphragmatic crura, resulting in a stronger antireflux barrier [8, 9].

Medical Therapy

While in the last century antacids were over many decades the best medical options that were available, H2 blockers in the 1970s and the development of proton pump inhibitors (PPI) in the 1980s have advanced the therapeutic success of medical therapy substantially. The effectivity of PPIs compared to other medical agents has been shown in many randomized trials showing the healing of reflux esophagitis and reducing the major symptom of heartburn, when taken in adequate dosage and sequence [2, 4, 14, 15]. The latter seems very important, and one cannot emphasize this point enough for a successful therapy. Since GERD is a disease with a multifactorial background and a number of pathophysiologic components involved, it is not surprising that the therapeutic response may vary from patient to patient. In addition, there may be different therapeutic responses among patients depending on different PPIs on the market as well as with different concepts of dosage [2, 4, 15].

PPI therapy in the acute situation is a very effective treatment to compensate and reduce the acute symptoms, mainly epigastric and thoracic pain and heartburn. There is in this situation no role for any surgical treatment. There are many studies showing the effect of PPIs in improving the patient's symptoms and healing reflux-based esophagitis [2, 4, 15–20]. PPIs are the first-line treatment. Dosage and duration of treatment can be individualized and depends on the patient's status and problems. PPIs are more effective than all the other available medical options [2, 15, 18–20]. The aim of the treatment is usually the reduction of reflux esophagitis and the reduction/stopping of the major symptoms such as heartburn, chest pain, or epigastric pain.

There is a substantial discussion about that time of the first endoscopy to verify the diagnosis [2, 4, 15, 18–20]. According to most of the current guidelines, it is suggested that an initial treatment of PPI can be administered in patients with this suspicion for GERD and typical symptoms [2, 4, 11–15]. Especially if the initial PPI therapy is successful, no urgent endoscopy or other diagnostics are needed. However, in case of "alarm symptoms" such as bleeding or dysphagia, earlier diagnostic intervention is absolutely necessary [2, 4, 18–20].

The response to PPI therapy may differ depending on the individual patient and also depending on differences in the status of GERD in a given patient. Several factors may play a role such as the degree of failure of the antireflux barrier, a possible failure of esophageal motility, and also a disorder in gastric emptying. Table 4.1 demonstrates the overview on the acute therapy of GERD. Several guidelines have expressed these actions to treat patients in the acute situation [2, 4, 18–20].

Long-term therapy of GERD is often necessary, since GERD is a chronic disease [2, 18–22]. Frequently, patients are treated over more than 5 or 10 years. This is done in clinical practice despite the fact that the drug's use is recommended usually only for months. Since every day millions of patients take PPIs against symptoms in the upper gastrointestinal tract, there should be, from the medical standpoint, some strong influence to push the evidence from guidelines for the indications for PPI therapy [20]. Furthermore, GERD may have a mild to moderate clinical course, and there is a clinical form of a progressive disease, causing functional and anatomical alterations that will limit the success of medical therapy [21, 22].

PPIs are very successful for the majority of patients with GERD as a long-term treatment, which has been shown by many large trials [2, 4, 16–18]. In randomized controlled trials, this success of PPI therapy in adequate dosage is shown that typical reflux symptoms can be stopped in 50–70% [2, 4, 16–18]. However,

Table 4.1 Therapy of GERD in the acute situation

Indication	Drugs	Dosage	Duration
Reflux symptoms: Heartburn Regurgitation	Antacids PPI ± alginate	Standard dosage: Omeprazole 20 mg Lansoprazole 30 mg Rabeprazole 20 mg Pantoprazole 40 mg Esomeprazole 40 mg	4 weeks
NERD	PPI ± alginate Antacids H_2-blockers	Standard dosages	4 weeks
Esophagitis Los Angeles A, B	PPI	Standard dosage	4–6 weeks
Esophagitis Los Angeles C, D	PPI	Standard dosage Up to double 1-0-1	Minimum 8 weeks Often long term
Esophageal stricture	PPI	Double standard dosage 1-0-1	Long term
Chest pain and reflux	PPI	Double standard dosage 1-0-1	Testing 2 weeks 8 weeks
Extraesophageal symptoms	PPI + alginate	Double standard dosage 1-0-1	4 weeks
Barrett's esophagus	PPI	Depending on esophagitis and present symptoms	Depending on esophagitis and present symptoms

approximately 30% of patients under long-term PPI therapy were not completely satisfied with their therapeutic result [16–18, 22]. These patients need diagnostic workup to evaluate possibilities of a progressive form of disease which may be better off with surgical therapy.

Table 4.2 demonstrates the effect of long-term treatment with PPI therapy applying adequate dosage and intake of the medication. A systematic analysis of the literature shows that healing of a mild-to-moderate reflux esophagitis is almost always successful by PPI therapy [2, 4, 16–20]. Healing rates in patients with severe reflux esophagitis are more limited, and a control of symptoms in these cases may be only up to 75% success rate. Symptom control by PPI therapy in patients with extraesophageal symptoms may be even worse [23–29].

Therefore, a differentiated diagnostic analysis of the precise background of the disease in a given patient is important [30–34]. A limited success of PPI therapy is very often due to an insufficient intake in sequence and dosage of the patient. Patient's compliance plays a major role in the insufficiency of PPI therapy [2, 18]. As a consequence, this should be checked initially, when the patient complains about insufficient treatment by PPI therapy, whether he or she follows the correct instructions of intake.

Another reason for insufficient treatment and insufficient effect of PPI therapy can be the multifactorial background and pathophysiology of GERD [4, 19–22, 35–38]. In a patient with severe mechanical incompetence of the lower esophageal sphincter or in patients with severe alterations of esophageal and/or gastric motility, a medical therapy may be limited [19–22, 35].

Table 4.2 Long-term therapy for maintenance in GERD

Indication	Drugs	Dosage	Suggestions
Reflux symptoms less than three times a week: Heartburn Regurgitation	Antacids Alginate	Standard	Endoscopy scheduled Follow-up after 6 months
NERD	PPI Alginate Antacids	Standard dosage	If response not sufficient or recurrence, diagnostics necessary
Esophagitis Los Angeles A, B	PPI	Standard dosage	If response not sufficient or recurrence, diagnostics necessary
Esophagitis Los Angeles C, D Stricture	PPI	Double standard dosage 1-0-1	Long-term
Sleeping disorder	PPI + nighttime alginate	Standard dosage	Individual
Extraesophageal symptoms	PPI Alginate	Individual	Individual

Safety of PPI Therapy

Therapeutic use of PPI in GERD has a very good safety record over the years [4, 14–18]. However, in the last 5 years, several reports have emerged about the association of PPI therapy with osteoporosis and other side effects [36–38]. Considering the worldwide use of PPI therapy on a daily basis, many millions of persons around the world have been exposed to PPI therapy, and therefore, it seems not to be surprising that some severe side effects have been reported [2]. In contrast, in randomized and controlled trials, no specific side effects or severe adverse events related to PPI therapy have been reported in a substantial amount [15–18]. Furthermore, it must also be emphasized that many of the PPI users are elderly patients with several risk factors and concomitant diseases, who may have per se a higher risk of problems and adverse event [38].

Patients are usually irritated by information about potential side effects and complications of PPI therapy such as osteoporosis. Their reach for safety may lead to more general caution and irritation. At this point, it must be emphasized that a general caution about drug treatment is reasonable, but the evidence is quite overwhelming that PPI therapy is a safe treatment option for millions of patients with GERD. Regarding long-term PPI therapy, the therapeutic concept should be evaluated critically after the initial therapy and a certain time interval to assess other therapeutic options if applicable.

Problems with PPI Therapy

Occasional problems during long-term PPI therapy are persisting reflux symptoms and/or persisting or recurrent reflux esophagitis [15–18]. The reasons for an insufficient effect of PPI therapy are multifactorial. Therefore, a first initiative is the deeper analysis of the symptoms that are persisting. It should be explored whether other reasons may be found and why PPI therapy and acid reduction do not influence the symptoms [39].

If an endoscopy has not been performed before, it is now the time to explore the upper gastrointestinal tract and look for additional information and explanations such as a more severe grade of esophagitis or any presence of complications such as strictures, Barrett's esophagus, and/or ulcers, which may explain the limited success of PPI therapy [18, 39]. The latter may require an adaptation of the dosage. It is also important to check on the compliance of the patients.

If these options are explored and no explanation is found, a change in therapeutic concept may be advisable. A first possibility could be the choice for a different PPI, which may be a simple and effective solution. Another therapeutic option could be the combination of a PPI with an alginate [40–45]. Recent evidence has shown that shortly after a meal, an acid collection can emerge in the proximate stomach below the cardia [46–48]. The therapeutic control of the acid pocket by a combination of PPI and alginate seems to be a promising alternative [40–45].

A persisting reflux esophagitis may be quite troublesome and frustrating both for the patient and the therapist. If the limited response to a correct PPI dosage and intake persists, a more extensive diagnostic workup is needed to verify the correct diagnosis and possibly also the underlying pathophysiologic agents that contribute to the individual patient's disease.

The mainstay of conservative management of GERD remains PPI therapy, which can be successful used in many patients and which has a satisfying safety record.

References

1. Dent J, El-Serag HB, Wallander MA. Epidemiology of gastroesophageal reflux disease: a systematic review. Gut. 2005;54:710.
2. Vakil N, van Zanten SV, Kahrilas PJ, Dent J, Jones R, The Global Consensus Group. The Montreal definition and classification of GERD: a global evidence-based consensus. Am J Gastroenterol. 2006;101:1900–20.
3. El-Serag HB, Sweet S, Winchester CC, Dent J. Update on the epidemiology of gastro-oesophageal reflux disease: a systematic review. Gut. 2014;63:871–80.
4. Boeckxstaens G, El-Serag HB, Smout AJPM, Kahrilas PJ. Symptomatic reflux disease: the present, the past and the future. Gut. 2014;63:1185–93.
5. Costantini M, Crookes PF, Bremner RM, Hoeft SF, Ehsan A, Peters JH, Bremner CG, DeMeester TR. Value of physiologic assessment of foregut symptoms in a surgical practice. Surgery. 1993;114(4):780–6.
6. Tack J, Caenepeel P, Arts J, Lee KJ, Sifrim D, Janssens J. Prevalence of acid reflux functional dyspepsia and its association with symptom profile. Gut. 2005;54(10):1370–6.

7. Broderick R, Fuchs KH, Breithaupt W, Varga G, Schulz T, Babic B, Lee A, Musial F, Horgan S. Clinical presentation of GERD: a prospective study on symptom diversity and modification of questionnaire application. Dig Dis. 2019;12:1–8. https://doi.org/10.1159/000502796.

8. Ness-Jensen E, Hveem K, El-Serag H, et al. Lifestyle intervention in gastroesophageal reflux disease. Clin Gastroenterol Hepatol. 2016;14:175182.

9. Sethi S, Richter JE. Diet and gastroesophageal reflux disease: role in pathogenesis and management. Curr Opin Gastroenterol. 2017;33:107–11.

10. Fiorentino E. The consumption of snacks and soft drinks between meals may contribute to the development and to persistence of gastro-esophageal reflux disease. Med Hypotheses. 2019;125:84–8.

11. Kim J, Oh SW, Myung SK, et al. Association between coffee intake and gastroesophageal reflux disease: a meta-analysis. Dis Esophagus. 2014;27:311–7.

12. Cao H, Huang X, Zhi X, Han C, Li L, Li Y. Association between tea consumption and gastro-esophageal reflux disease: a meta-analysis. Medicine (Baltimore). 2019;98:e14173.

13. Ness-Jensen E, Lindam A, Lagergren J, Hyeem K. Weight loss and reduction in gastroesophageal reflux. A prospective population-based cohort study: the HUNT study. Am J Gastroenterol. 2013;108:376–82.

14. Lindow SW, Regnéll P, Sykes J, Little S. An open-label, multicentre study to assess the safety and efficacy of a novel reflux suppressant (Gaviscon Advance) in the treatment of heartburn during pregnancy. Int J Clin Pract. 2003;57:175–9.

15. El-Serag H, Becher A, Jones R. Systematic review: persistent reflux symptoms on proton pump inhibitor therapy in primary care and community studies. Aliment Pharmacol Ther. 2010;32:720–37.

16. Galmiche JP, Hatlebakk J, Attwood S, et al. Laparoscopic antireflux surgery vs esomeprazole treatment for chronic GERD: the LOTUS randomized clinical trial. JAMA. 2011;305:1969–77.

17. Malfertheiner P, Nocon M, Vieth M, et al. Evolution of gastro-oesophageal reflux disease over 5 years under routine medical care – the ProGERD study. Aliment Pharmacol Ther. 2012;35:154–64.

18. Gyawali CP, Fass R. Management of gastroesophageal reflux disease. Gastroenterology. 2018;154(2):302–18. https://doi.org/10.1053/j.gastro.2017.07.049.

19. Stefanidis D, Hope WW, Kohn GP, Reardon PR, Richardson WS, Fanelli RD, SAGES Guideline Committee. Guidelines for surgical treatment of GERD. Surg Endosc. 2010;24(11):2647–69.

20. Fuchs KH, Babic B, Breithaupt W, Dallemagne B, Fingerhut A, Furnee E, Granderath F, Horvath OP, Kardos P, Pointner R, Savarino E, Van Herwarden-Lindeboom M, Zaninotto G. EAES recommendations for the management of gastroesophageal reflux disease. Surg Endosc. 2014;28:1753–73.

21. DeMeester TR. Etiology and natural history of gastroesophageal reflux disease and predictors of progressive disease. In: Yeo CJ, DeMeester SR, Mc Fadden DW, editors. Shackelford's surgery of the alimentary tract. 8th ed. Philadelphia: Elsevier; 2019. p. 204–20.

22. Labenz J, Chandrasoma PT, Knapp LJ, DeMeester TR. Proposed approach to the challenging management of progressive gastroesophageal reflux disease. World J Gastrointest Endosc. 2018;10(9):175–83. https://doi.org/10.4253/wjge.v10.i9.175.

23. Jaspersen D, Kulig M, Labenz J. Prevalence of extra-oesophageal manifestations in gastro-oesophageal reflux disease: an analysis based on the ProGERD study. Aliment Pharmacol Ther. 2003;17:1215–20.

24. Vertigan AE, Theodoros DG, Winkworth AL, et al. Chronic cough: a tutorial for speech-language pathologists. J Med Speech Lang Pathol. 2007;15(3):189–206.

25. Adcock JJ. TRPV1 receptors in sensitisation of cough and pain reflexes. Pulm Pharmacol Ther. 2009;22:65–70.

26. Labenz J. Facts and fantasies in extra-oesophageal symptoms in GORD. Best Pract Res Clin Gastroenterol. 2010;24:893–904.

27. Morice AH. The cough hypersensitivity syndrome: a novel paradigm for understanding cough. Lung. 2010;188(Suppl 1):S87–90.

28. Desjardin M, Roman S, des Varannes SB, et al. Pharyngeal pH alone is not reliable for the detection of pharyngeal reflux events: a study with oesophageal and pharyngeal pH-impedance monitoring. United European Gastroenterol J. 2014;1:438–44.
29. Gibson PG, Vertigan AE. Management of chronic refractory cough. Br Med J. 2015;351:h5590.
30. Dent J, Holloway RH, Toouli J, Dodds WJ. Mechanisms of lower oesophageal sphincter incompetence in patients with symptomatic gastro-oesophageal reflux. Gut. 1988;29:1020–8.
31. Kuster E, Ros E, Toledo-Pimentel V, Pujol A, Bordas JM, Grande IC. Predictive factors of the long term outcome in gastro-oesophageal reflux disease: six year follow up of 107 patients. Gut. 1994;35(1):8–14.
32. Mittal RK, Holloway RH, Penagini R, Blackshaw A, Dent J. Transient lower esophageal sphincter relaxations. Gastroenterology. 1995;109:601–10.
33. Mittal RK, Holloway R, Dent J. Effect of atropine on the frequency of reflux and transient lower esophageal sphincter relaxation in normal subjects. Gastroenterology. 1995;109:1547.
34. Kahrilas PJ, Sifrim D. High-resolution manometry and impedance-pH/manometry: valuable tools in clinical and investigational esophagology. Gastroenterology. 2008;135(3):756–69.
35. Lord RVN, DeMeester SR, Peters JH, Hagen JA, Elyssnia D, Sheth CT, DeMeester TR. Hiatal hernia, lower esophageal sphincter incompetence, and effectiveness of Nissen fundoplication in the spectrum of gastroesophageal reflux disease. J Gastrointest Surg. 2009;13:602–10.
36. Jackson MA, Goodrich JK, Maxan ME, et al. Proton pump inhibitors alter the composition of the gut microbiota. Gut. 2016;65:749–56.
37. Vaezi MF, Yang YX, Howden CW. Complications of proton pump inhibitor therapy. Gastroenterology. 2017;153:35–48.
38. Xie Y, Bowe B, Li T, Xian H, Yan Y, Al-Ay Z. Risk of death among users of proton pump inhibitors: a longitudinal observational cohort study of United States veterans. BMJ Open. 2017;7:e015735. https://doi.org/10.1136/bmjopen-2016-015735.
39. Kahrilas PJ, Keefer L, Pandolfino JE. Patients with refractory reflux symptoms: what do they have and how should they be managed? Neurogastroenterol Motil. 2015;27:1195–201.
40. Thomas E, Wade E, Crawford G, et al. Randomised clinical trial: relief of upper gastrointestinal symptoms by an acid pocket-targeting alginate-antacid (Gaviscon Double Action) – a double-blind, placebo-controlled, pilot study in gastro-oesophageal reflux disease. Aliment Pharmacol Ther. 2014;39:595–602.
41. Lai I-R, Wu M-S, Lin J-T. Prospective, randomized, and active controlled study of the efficacy of alginic acid and antacid in the treatment of patients with endoscopy-negative reflux disease. World J Gastroenterol. 2006;12:747–54.
42. Pouchain D, Bigard MA, Liard F, et al. Gaviscon® vs. omeprazole in symptomatic treatment of moderate gastroesophageal reflux. a direct comparative randomised trial. BMC Gastroenterol. 2012;23:12–8.
43. Schey R, Dickman R, Parthasarathy S, et al. Sleep deprivation is hyperalgesic in patients with gastroesophageal reflux disease. Gastroenterology. 2007;133:1787–95.
44. Manabe N, Haruma K, Ito M, et al. Efficacy of adding sodium alginate to omeprazole in patients with nonerosive reflux disease: a randomized clinical trial. Dis Esophagus. 2012;25:373–80.
45. Reimer C, Lodrup AB, Smith G, et al. Randomised clinical trial: alginate (Gaviscon Advance) vs. placebo as add-on therapy in reflux patients with inadequate response to a once daily proton pump inhibitor. Aliment Pharmacol Ther. 2016;43(8):899–909. https://doi.org/10.1111/apt.13567.
46. Fletscher J, Wirz A, Young J, et al. Unbuffered highly acidic gastric juice exists at the gastro-esophageal junction after a meal. Gastroenterology. 2001;121:775–83.
47. Clarke AT, Wirz AA, Seenan JP, Manning JJ, Gillen D, McColl KE. Paradox of gastric cardia: it becomes more acidic following meals while the rest of stomach becomes less acidic. Gut. 2009;58:904–9.
48. Beaument H, Benninck RJ, de Jong J, Boeckxstaens GE. The position of the acid pocket as a major risk factor for acidic reflux in healthy subjects and patients with GORD. Gut. 2010;59:441–51.

Indications for Interventional and Surgical Therapy in GERD

5

Hans Friedrich Fuchs

Basic Considerations for Alternative Options to Medical Therapy

Reflecting the multifactorial background of gastroesophageal reflux disease (GERD) and the large variation in it's clinical presentation, it is not surprising that "one therapeutic option would fit all patients with GERD" seems to be rather unrealistic [1–5]. Since 30 years, proton pump inhibitor (PPI) therapy has been very successful as medical therapy [1]. Since the advent of PPI therapy, for many years, gastroenterologists propagated that no further therapeutic options are necessary because this powerful drug proides sufficient therapeutic effect [6]. Over the years, however, it became evident that a certain portion of GERD patients continued having troublesome symptoms despite PPI therapy and also despite an increasing dosage of PPI therapy [1, 7–9].

At the same time with the rising success of minimally invasive surgery, laparoscopic fundoplication emerged as a very successful operation for long-term problems with GERD [10–14]. Unfortunately, gastroenterologists and surgeons spent unnecessary time to argue against each other about what is the better option, PPI therapy or antireflux surgery. Several randomized trials have been performed comparing these two treatment options showing controversial results [7, 15–17]. The results can hardly be used as a general guideline for therapeutic decision-making. After many studies showing the effectivity of PPI therapy and several randomized trials showing a rather close race in the investigated populations regarding the long-term results with PPI therapy versus laparoscopic antireflux surgery, it became evident that the investigated populations may be quite different in their selection and difficult to compare [3–5, 7, 15–17]. First, GERD patients differ in many parameters within different populations that were investigated. In some studies, the severity of

H. F. Fuchs (✉)
Department of General, GI- and Tumor Surgery, University of Cologne, Cologne, Germany
e-mail: Hans.Fuchs@uk-koeln.de

© Springer Nature Switzerland AG 2020
S. Horgan, K.-H. Fuchs (eds.), *Management of Gastroesophageal Reflux Disease*,
https://doi.org/10.1007/978-3-030-48009-7_5

47

the disease as expressed by the presence of esophagitis is, for example, below 40%, and in another study, it is above 60% or 70% [7, 10–14]. Data from populations with different selection criteria should not be compared.

As a consequence, extracting data and knowledge from literature regarding therapeutic decision-making requires a critical view for the composition of the involved patient populations and especially regarding indications for surgery. If symptoms are used to define the indications for surgery, there is always a risk for wrong decisions, since the variety and intensity of symptoms are large [18–24]. GERD may present with several different symptoms, which can overlap with other diseases and other disorders presenting with reflux-like symptoms [19–24]. In addition, the severity of the disease in a given patient may be judged differently by different authors especially if no clear defined criteria are used. Objective findings can be obtained by an adequate diagnostic workup [1]. Overlapping symptoms may be caused by other esophageal and gastric disorders, which may not surface in superficially investigated patients with reflux-like symptoms in dyspepsia and somatoform disorders and other motility disorders of the GI tract [19–24].

Therefore, the most important initial issue, when facing a patient who needs a decision regarding an indication for endoscopic or surgical therapy, is a precise diagnostic workup including an upper GI endoscopy, impedance-pH monitoring, high-resolution manometry, and, in cases of dysphagia or signs of delayed gastric emptying, additional radiographic and scintigraphic investigations [25–32].

The diagnostic workup to prove the presence of the GERD may differ from the diagnostic workup to help in the decision-making for surgical therapy [5]. In the first case, one has to decide whether to establish a conservative PPI therapy, which will not have the risks and consequences of an operation, if the decision turns out to be wrong. Therefore, if therapeutic decision-making regarding an indication for surgery has to be made, all of the abovementioned investigations should be considered to clarify with the highest possible accuracy the presence of the disease and its pathophysiologic background in this individual patient [5]. Furthermore, in patients with extra-esophageal symptoms, this is of utmost importance, because in these cases, overlap with other conditions occurs even more frequently than in "regular" GERD patients [5].

PPI therapy is very effective, and it remains the standard treatment for acute symptoms of GERD [3, 5, 7, 9]. There is no place for surgical therapy as an acute therapeutic option [5]. In addition, it must be emphasized that PPI therapy is the most frequent form of long-term therapy in GERD patients and shows a good safety profile [3, 5, 7, 9]. Having stated this, it needs also to be emphasized that the current discussion about possible long-term side effects of PPI therapy is rather exaggerated [33]. This has to be assessed accurately, but no hysteria is necessary in informing the patient about an acute danger of osteoporosis or dementia. There is certain evidence that in some patients these risks are present after long-term treatment, and therefore, the current measures of precaution have to be taken as mentioned in the chapter of conservative therapy. Surgical therapy bears definitely a risk of complications during and after the procedure [4, 5, 10–16]. This risk is in the acute situation higher than medical therapy. Therefore, any indication for surgical therapy must be critically assessed and reflected in every case.

It must be emphasized that an uncritical yearlong continuation of medical therapy despite persistent reflux and esophagitis can lead to progressive disease with ulcerations and the development of Barrett's esophagus, the development of a short esophagus after years due to inflammatory reactions in the esophageal wall, and especially scarring and shortening of the esophagus with an increase in the size of the hiatal hernia, until the development of respiratory symptoms and chronic aspiration develops [1, 30, 34–36]. Especially chronic aspiration in GERD patients without adequate therapy may lead to mortality [34]. This is a similar, severe mistake as an uncritical indication for surgical therapy in patients who may have just reflux-like symptoms from another disorder or who may have only a mild form of GERD [5].

The worst component in waiting for many years to establish a justified indication for antireflux surgery is the fact that after unnecessary waiting, the chances for being able to correct effectively the anatomical and functional changes in such a patient are decreasing, if this decision is postponed too long [1, 5, 30]. If the hiatal hernia has developed too large and the esophagus has shortened too much, there will be no possibility in reconstructing the normal anatomy again, and also it will be impossible to normalize esophageal and gastric function again [1, 30].

Therefore, it is important to start diagnostic activities at the right time to assess the functional and anatomic status of the patient and determine what the nature of her/his GERD is in order to gain objective findings for therapeutic decision-making [5].

Indication for Antireflux Surgery

The aim of antireflux surgery is the prevention of reflux by the correction of the defective antireflux barrier. For an optimal patient selection for surgery, only those patients should be selected, who have a high probability of having a sufficient benefit from the surgical procedure compared to PPI therapy.

As a consequence, no patient should have an antireflux surgery without a previous long-term PPI therapy prior to thinking about the indication for surgery [3–5]. With this concept, patient and physician know clearly what an optimal PPI therapy can do for this individual patient. This question can only be answered after an optimal PPI therapy with adequate dosage and adequate information to the patient about the details of intake.

An antireflux surgery has a chance to be superior to PPI therapy, if the patient's quality of life is still restricted despite adequate PPI therapy by nonacid-associated symptoms such as fluid and food regurgitation from hiatal hernias and the mechanical defective cardia [5, 7, 10–16]. In these patients, PPIs may have successfully stopped the acid-associated symptoms, but the remaining symptoms persist and the disease may be progressing despite PPI therapy [5].

The decision for medical therapy or surgical therapy has been studied by several randomized trials [7, 15, 16]. In the largest trial, esomeprazole was compared to laparoscopic Nissen fundoplication in the short floppy form [7]. After 3 years, the therapeutic effect was very good in both groups [7]. After 5 years, the results show that laparoscopic Nissen fundoplication developed more failures because of the development of persisting dysphagia and other side effects, while the reflux control was better in the surgical group compared to esomeprazole [7]. Other case-control studies have shown that the therapeutic success of laparoscopic Nissen fundoplication is around 90% in esophageal centers with a high expertise for this operation [10–14]. The success is based on a strict selection of patients after extensive diagnostic workup selecting only those patients with proven disease and severe course [10–14, 37, 38].

Laparoscopic fundoplication is successful, if the indications are correctly established and the procedure is performed based on the technical principles, which are published since many years [5, 37]. The selection criteria for the indication of antireflux surgery are published in several guidelines [3–5]. Table 5.1 shows the criteria for this selection, which should be worked up in each patient to perform a correct indication. An example for an optimal patient selection is a patient with all the following signs: a yearlong history of GERD, with typical reflux symptoms (heartburn and regurgitation of food and fluid); the endoscopic, visible presence of esophagitis especially grade LA B, C, and D; an anatomical alteration of the esophagogastric junction by a hiatal hernia; an improvement of acid-associated symptoms under PPI therapy; an incompetent lower esophageal sphincter on high-resolution manometry; a positive impedance-pH monitoring test with a positive symptom-reflux-episode correlation (Symptom Association Probability [SAP] 95%); a persistence of non-acid symptoms under adequate PPI therapy; a dosage escalation; and a reduced quality of life over years.

If not all of these criteria are fulfilled in the diagnostic workup and/or cannot be detected, then one should reflect critical over the results. If most of these criteria are fulfilled, it could be an individual decision to perform antireflux procedure. If the diagnostic results do not match together and questions rise as to the nature of the

Table 5.1 List of indication criteria for laparoscopic antireflux surgery [5]

Criterion	Investigation
Typical symptoms (heartburn, regurgitation)	History
Long duration of symptoms	History
Presence of a hiatal hernia	Endoscopy, radiography, high-resolution manometry
Esophagitis	Endoscopy
LES incompetence	Manometry
Pathologic esophageal acid exposure	Impedance-pH monitoring
Positive reflux-symptom correlation	Impedance-pH monitoring +SAP
Positive PPI response	History
PPI dose escalation	History
Reduced quality of life (lebensqualität)	Validated questionnaire GIQLI

findings, again a critical assessment of the findings has to be performed and the diagnostic workup may have to be repeated. It is always wise to put the patient on another episode of conservative therapy, until the findings match together. One should complete the picture and be sure of the presence of an advanced and progressive GERD in a patient, in whom we plan an antireflux procedure.

Indications for Antireflux Surgery in Special Circumstances

Indication for Surgery in the Elderly

An antireflux procedure can be performed in patients older than 70 or 80 years, if they match with the indication criteria as mentioned above [5, 39]. In several studies, the success of this procedure has been shown also in the elderly [39, 40]. In patients with risk factors, which can be more frequently present in elderly patients, one has to critically judge between the risk for possible complications due to risk factors and the age of the patient against the possible success for this patient regarding the Nissen fundoplication. One study showed that the morbidity rate in the elderly was not significantly different from those in younger age, and the functional result of the antireflux procedure was similarly good in both groups 5 years after surgery [39].

Indication for Antireflux Surgery in Patients with NERD (Nonerosive Reflux Disease)

There are patients with GERD who have no erosive esophagitis (NERD) [3]. In recent years, it has become more difficult to differentiate between a true NERD patient and patients with initial esophagitis, who has been treated by early PPI therapy prior to their first endoscopy. As a result, the initial esophagitis may have healed, and there is no possibility to differentiate later on between these two entities, because PPI therapy may have covered the initial existing esophagitis. Therefore, many so-called NERD patients are really patients with limited esophagitis. Evidence has shown that NERD patients can be successfully treated with antireflux surgery, but very accurate diagnostic workup has to be performed [40]. These patients must undergo impedance-pH monitoring with the symptom-reflux correlation to prove the presence of GERD in each case prior to surgery.

Indication for Antireflux Surgery in Patients with Extra-Esophageal Symptoms

Patients with extra-esophageal symptoms require an extensive diagnostic workup to prove the presence of GERD [41–45]. Extra-esophageal symptoms such as cough, sore throat, hoarseness, sore, and aspiration have its origin in pathologic acid reflux from the stomach; however, this often may have other causes [5]. The important question is the accurate identification of origin of these symptoms. They may be caused by esophago-pharyngo-laryngeal reflux leading to chronic aspiration and extra-esophageal symptoms. Often, these patients with these symptoms are referred to ENT colleagues, who call this reflux laryngopharyngeal reflux (LPR) even though it originates from the esophagus and furthermore from gastric fluids. The ENT colleagues use the Restech system to monitor the presence of acid in the pharynx. The limitation of this test is that the measurement is only measured at one point, which may be not enough to have an accurate assessment of true gastroesophageal acid reflux reaching up into the pharynx. In addition, the reflux episodes should be correlated to the symptoms, which is usually not performed. Recently, there are some critical reports in literature [46–48].

There is some controversial discussion between ENT colleagues and gastroenterologists as well as GI surgeons about this issue. For an accurate diagnosis of gastroesophageal acid reflux causing further up an esophago-pharyngo-laryngeal reflux with subsequent extra-esophageal symptoms, we need a proof of combined reflux episodes of gastroesophageal and esophago-pharyngeal reflux correlating with extra-esophageal symptoms. There is evidence that antireflux surgery is successful, if patient selection is correctly performed [4, 5]. It is important in these patients to invest an enormous effort in the diagnostic workup before establishing the indication for antireflux surgery, because many of these patients do not have gastroesophageal reflux disease despite their symptomatic appearance [5].

Indication for Antireflux Surgery in Patients with Delayed Gastric Emptying

Patients with altered gastric motility and delayed gastric emptying may have reflux problems due to the obstruction of fluid and food in the stomach [49, 50]. In these patients, it is also of importance to perform a precise diagnostic workup to detect these additional functional problems that are more located in the stomach than in the esophagogastric junction. In cases with the combination of GERD and other mild delayed gastric emptying, a fundoplication has a positive effect on the emptying [51, 52].

In severe gastroparesis, these patients do not need an antireflux surgery, but possibly some gastric surgery or initially medical therapy to solve the issue of delayed gastric emptying [49, 50]. The worst thing that can happen is that in these patients, who may have as chief complaint of regurgitation or heartburn as well as nausea and vomiting, a quick decision may be established to undergo a fundoplication, which may worsen the symptoms dramatically and may furthermore hide the original cause of their problem. There are other cases usually with more severe delayed gastric emptying and full gastroparesis that show a severe aggravation of the symptoms after an unjustified fundoplication.

In summary, the decision for an indication for antireflux surgery or other interventional therapies in GERD is a critical step in the patient's "carriere." Since antireflux surgery can also cause side effects or cause damage to the esophagogastric function, which may end up in persisting symptoms and may not be able to be corrected in the future such as vagal damage, it is very important for every single patient to undergo adequate investigations prior to surgery. Optimal information about the background of the disease can only be obtained by extensive diagnostic testing of the individual situation of the disease and its pathophysiologic causes.

References

1. DeMeester TR. Etiology and natural history of gastroesophageal reflux disease and predictors of progressive disease. In: Yeo CJ, DeMeester SR, Mc Fadden DW, editors. Shackelford's surgery of the alimentary tract. 8th ed. Philadelphia: Elsevier; 2019. p. 204–20.
2. Fuchs KH, Freys SM, Heimbucher J, Fein M, Thiede A. Pathophysiologic spectrum in patients with gastroesophageal reflux disease in a surgical GI function laboratory. Dis Esophagus. 1995;8:211–7.
3. Vakil N, van Zanten SV, Kahrilas PJ, Dent J, Jones R, The Global Consensus Group. The Montreal definition and classification of GERD: a global evidence-based consensus. Am J Gastroenterol. 2006;101:1900–20.
4. Stefanidis D, Hope WW, Kohn GP, Reardon PR, Richardson WS, Fanelli RD, SAGES Guideline Committee. Guidelines for surgical treatment of GERD. Surg Endosc. 2010;24(11):2647–69.
5. Fuchs KH, Babic B, Breithaupt W, Dallemagne B, Fingerhut A, Furnee E, Granderath F, Horvath OP, Kardos P, Pointner R, Savarino E, Van Herwarden-Lindeboom M, Zaninotto G. EAES recommendations for the management of gastroesophageal reflux disease. Surg Endosc. 2014;28:1753–73.
6. Klinkenberg-Knol EC, Nelis F, Dent J, Snel P, Mitchell B, Prichard P, Lloyd D, Havu N, Frame MH, Romàn J, Walan A, Long-Term Study Group. Long-term omeprazole treatment in resistant gastroesophageal reflux disease: efficacy, safety, and influence on gastric mucosa. Gastroenterology. 2000;118(4):661–9.
7. Galmiche J-P, Hatlebakk J, Attwood S, Ell C, Fiocca R, Eklund S, Langstrom G, Lind T, Lundell L. Laparoscopic antireflux surgery vs esomeprazole treatment for chronic GERD: the LOTUS randomized clinical trial. JAMA. 2011;305:1969–77.
8. Malfertheiner P, Nocon M, Vieth M, Stolte M, Jaspersen D, Koelz HR, Labenz J, Leodolter A, Lind T, Richter K, Willich SN. Evolution of gastro-oesophageal reflux disease over 5 years under routine medical care – the ProGERD study. Aliment Pharmacol Ther. 2012;35(1):154–64.
9. Leodolter A, Nocon M, Vieth M, Lind T, Jaspersen D, Richter K, Willich S, Stolte M, Malfertheiner P, Labenz J. Progression of specialized intestinal metaplasia at the cardia to macroscopically evident Barrett's esophagus: an entity of concern in the ProGERD study. Scand J Gastroenterol. 2012;47(12):1429–35. https://doi.org/10.3109/00365521.2012.733952.
10. Dallemagne B, Weertz J, Markiewicz S, Dewandre JM, Wahlen C, Monami B, Jehaes C. Clinical results of laparoscopic fundoplication ten years after surgery. Surg Endosc. 2006;20:159–65.
11. Peters JH, DeMeester TR, Crookes P, Oberg S, de Vos Shoop M, Hagen JA, Bremner CG. The treatment of gastroesophageal reflux disease with laparoscopic Nissen fundoplication. Ann Surg. 1998;228(1):40–50.
12. Kamolz T, Granderath F, Pointner R. Laparoscopic antireflux surgery: disease-related quality of life assessment before and after surgery in GERD patients with and without Barrett's esophagus. Surg Endosc. 2003;17:880–5.
13. Patti MG, Robinson T, Galvani C, Gorodner MV, Fisichella PM, Way LW. Total fundoplication is superior to partial fundoplication even when esophageal peristalsis is weak. J Am Coll Surg. 2004;198:863–9.
14. Fuchs KH, Breithaupt W, Fein M, Maroske J, Hammer I. Laparoscopic Nissen repair: indications, techniques and long term benefits. Langenbecks Arch Surg. 2005;390:197–202.

15. Metha S, Bennett J, Mahon D, Rhodes M. Prospective trial of laparoscopic Nissen fundoplication versus proton pump inhibitor therapy für gastroesophageal reflux disease: seven-year follow up. J Gastrointest Surg. 2006;10(9):1312–7.
16. Anvari M, Allen C, Marshall J, Armstrong D, Goree R, Ungar W, Goldsmith C. A randomized controlled trial of laparoscopic Nissen fundoplication versus proton pump inhibitors for the treatment of patients with chronic gastrooesophageal reflux disease (GERD): 3 year outcomes. Surg Endosc. 2011;25(8):2547–54.
17. Faria R, Bojke L, Epstein D, Corbacho B, Sculpher M, REFLUX Trial Group. Cost effectiveness of laparoscopic fundoplication versus continued medical management for the treatment of GERD based on long-term follow-up of the REFLUX trial. Br J Surg. 2013;100:1205–13.
18. Klauser AG, Schindlbeck NE, Müller-Lissner SA. Symptoms in gastro-esophageal reflux disease. Lancet. 1990;335:205–8.
19. Costantini M, Crookes PF, Bremner RM, Hoeft SF, Ehsan A, Peters JH, Bremner CG, DeMeester TR. Value of physiologic assessment of foregut symptoms in a surgical practice. Surgery. 1993;114(4):780–6.
20. Bradley LA, Richter JE, Pulliam TJ, et al. The relationship between stress and symptoms of gastroesophageal reflux: the influence of psychological factors. Am J Gastroenterol. 1993;88(1):11–9.
21. Tack J, Caenepeel P, Arts J, Lee KJ, Sifrim D, Janssens J. Prevalence of acid reflux functional dyspepsia and its association with symptom profile. Gut. 2005;54(10):1370–6.
22. Savarino E, Pohl D, Zentilin P, Dulbecco P, Sammito G, Sconfienza L, Vigneri S, Camerini G, Tutuian R, Savarino V. Functional heartburn has more in common with functional dyspepsia than with non-erosive reflux disease. Gut. 2009;58(9):1185–91.
23. Kavitt RT, Higginbotham T, Slaughter JC, et al. Symptom reports are not reliable during ambulatory reflux monitoring. Am J Gastroenterol. 2012;107:1826–32.
24. Fuchs KH, Musial F, Ulbricht F, Breithaupt W, Reinisch A, Schulz T, Babic B, Fuchs HF, Varga G. Foregut symptoms, somatoform tendencies, and the selection of patients for antireflux surgery. Dis Esophagus. 2017;30:1–10.
25. Lundell LR, Dent J, Bennett JR, Blum AL, Armstrong D, Galmiche JP, Johnson F, Hongo M, Richter JE, Spechler SJ, et al. Endoscopic assessment of oesophagitis: clinical and functional correlates and further validation of the Los Angeles classification. Gut. 1999;45:172–80.
26. Zerbib F, Roman S, Ropert A, des Varannes SB, Pouderoux P, Chaput U, Mion F, Vérin E, Galmiche JP, Sifrim D. Esophageal pH-impedance monitoring and symptom analysis in GERD: a study in patients off and on therapy. Am J Gastroenterol. 2006;101(9):1956–63.
27. Savarino E, Tutuian R, Zentilin P, Dulbecco P, Pohl D, Marabotto E, Parodi A, Sammito G, Gemignani L, Bodini G, Savarino V. Characteristics of reflux episodes and symptom association in patients with erosive esophagitis and nonerosive reflux disease: study using combined impedance-pH off therapy. Am J Gastroenterol. 2010;105:1053–61.
28. Lord RVN, DeMeester SR, Peters JH, Hagen JA, Elyssnia D, Sheth CT, DeMeester TR. Hiatal hernia, lower esophageal sphincter incompetence, and effectiveness of Nissen fundoplication in the spectrum of gastroesophageal reflux disease. J Gastrointest Surg. 2009;13:602–10.
29. Fein M, Ritter M, DeMeester TR, Oberg S, Peters JH, Hagen JA, Bremner CG. Role of lower esophageal sphincter and hiatal hernia in the pathogenesis of GERD. J Gastrointest Surg. 1999;3(4):405–10.
30. Mattioli S, Lugaresi ML, Costantini M, Del Genio A, Di Martino N, Fei L, Fumagalli U, Maffettone V, Monaco L, Morino M, Rebecchi F, Rosati R, Rossi M, Sant S, Trapani V, Zaninotto G. The short esophagus: intraoperative assessment of esophageal length. J Thorac Cardiovasc Surg. 2008;136:1610.
31. Wayman J, Myers JC, Jamieson GG. Preoperative gastric emptying and patterns of reflux as predictors of outcome after laparoscopic fundoplication. Br J Surg. 2007;94(5):592–8.
32. Chan WW, Haroian LR, Gyawali CP. Value of preoperative esophageal function studies before laparoscopic antireflux surgery. Surg Endosc. 2011;25:2943–9.
33. Haastrup PF, Thompson W, Søndergaard J, Jarbøl DE. Side effects of long-term proton pump inhibitor use: a review. Basic Clin Pharmacol Toxicol. 2018;123(2):114–21. https://doi.org/10.1111/bcpt.13023.

34. Rantanen TK, Salo JA. GERD as a cause of death: analysis of fatal cases under conservative therapy. Scand J Gastroenterol. 1999;34(3):229–33.
35. Labenz J, Chandrasoma PT, Knapp LJ, DeMeester TR. Proposed approach to the challenging management of progressive gastroesophageal reflux disease. World J Gastrointest Endosc. 2018;10(9):175–83. https://doi.org/10.4253/wjge.v10.i9.175.
36. Maret-Ouda J, Wahlin K, Artama M, Brusselaers N, Färkkilä M, Lynge E, Mattsson F, Pukkala E, Romundstad P, Tryggvadóttir L, von Euler-Chelpin M, Lagergren J. Risk of esophageal adenocarcinoma after antireflux surgery in patients with gastroesophageal reflux disease in the Nordic countries. JAMA Oncol. 2018;4(11):1576–82. https://doi.org/10.1001/jamaoncol.2018.3054.
37. DeMeester TR, Bonavina L, Abertucci M. Nissen fundoplication for gastroesophageal reflux disease. Evaluation of primary repair in 100 consecutive patients. Ann Surg. 1986;204:19.
38. Fein M, Bueter M, Thalheimer A, Pachmayer V, Heimbucher J, Freys SM, Fuchs KH. Ten year outcome of laparoscopic antireflux procedures. J Gastrointest Surg. 2008;12:1893–9.
39. Brehant O, Pessaux P, Arnaud JP, Delattre JF, Meyer C, Baulieux J, Mosnier H. Long-term outcome of laparoscopic antireflux surgery in the elderly. J Gastrointest Surg. 2006;10(3):439–44.
40. Grotenhuis BA, Wijnhoven BP, Bessell JR, Watson DI. Laparoscopic antireflux surgery in the elderly. Surg Endosc. 2008;22(8):1807–12.
41. Broeders JA, Draaisma WA, Bredenoord AJ, Smout AJ, Broeders IA, Gooszen HG. Long-term outcome of Nissen fundoplication in non-erosive and erosive gastro-oesophageal reflux disease. Br J Surg. 2010;97:845–52.
42. Kaufmann JA, Houghland JE, Quiroga E, Cahill M, Pellegrini CA, Oelschlager BK. Long-term outcomes of laparoscopic antireflux surgery for gastroesophageal reflux disease (GERD)-related airway disorder. Surg Endosc. 2006;20:1824–30.
43. Catania RA, Kavic Stephen M, Roth S, Lee TH, Meyer T, Fantry GT, Castellanos PF, Park A. Laparoscopic Nissen fundoplication effectively relieves symptoms in patient with laryngopharyngeal reflux. J Gastrointest Surg. 2007;11:1579–88.
44. Salminen P, Sala E, Koskenvuo J, Karvonen J, Ovaska J. Reflux laryngitis: a feasible indication for laparoscopic antireflux surgery. Surg Laparosc Endosc Percutan Tech. 2007;17:73–8.
45. Barry DW, Vaezi MF. Laryngopharyngeal reflux: more questions than answers. Cleve Clin J Med. 2010;77:337–4.
46. Wilhelm D, Jell A, Feussner H, Schmid RM, Bajbouj M, Becker V. Pharyngeal pH monitoring in gastrectomy patients – what do we really measure? United European Gastroenterol J. 2016;4(4):541–5. https://doi.org/10.1177/2050640615617637.
47. Nennstiel S, Andrea M, Abdelhafez M, Haller B, Schmid RM, Bajbouj M, Becker V. pH/multichannel impedance monitoring in patients with laryngo-pharyngeal reflux symptoms – prediction of therapy response in long-term follow-up. Arab J Gastroenterol. 2016;17(3):113–6. https://doi.org/10.1016/j.ajg.2016.08.007.
48. Fuchs HF, Muller DT, Berlth F, et al. Simultaneous laryngopharyngeal pH monitoring (Restech) and conventional esophageal pH monitoring-correlation using a large patient cohort of more than 100 patients with suspected gastroesophageal reflux disease. Dis Esophagus. 2018;31(10) https://doi.org/10.1093/dote/doy018.
49. Tack J, Van den Houte K, Carbone F. Gastroduodenal motility disorders. Curr Opin Gastroenterol. 2018;34(6):428–35. https://doi.org/10.1097/MOG.0000000000000473.
50. Zehetner J, Ravari F, Ayazi S, Skibba A, Iarehzereshki A, Pelipad D, Mason RJ, Katkhouda N, Lipham JC. Minimally invasive surgical approach for the treatment of gastroparesis. Surg Endosc. 2013;27:61–6.
51. Maddern GJ, Jamieson GG. Fundoplication enhances gastric emptying. Ann Surg. 1985;201:296–9.
52. Khajanchee YS, Dunst CM, Swanström LL. Outcomes of Nissen fundoplication in patients with gastroesophageal reflux disease and delayed gastric emptying. Arch Surg. 2009;144(9):823–8.

Endoscopic Therapy for GERD

Andreas Wannhoff and Karel Caca

Introduction

Proton pump inhibitors (PPIs) form the backbone of treatment for gastroesophageal reflux disease (GERD). They are well evaluated and effective, and serious side effects are very rare even during long-term treatment. Nevertheless, some patients have refractory symptoms despite acid suppression therapy, and few patients complain about side effects that lead to discontinuation of medical therapy. As alternative to medical treatment and surgical fundoplication, endoscopic treatments for GERD have been developed and are available for selected patients.

Indications and Contraindications

Endoscopic anti-reflux therapy (EART) can be evaluated after failure of treatment with PPI. This mainly includes patients with persistent symptoms and acid reflux despite high-dose PPI therapy. In rare circumstances, patients who do not tolerate a PPI therapy because of side effects may be candidates for EART as well. In some cases, the patient's refusal to take long-term PPI therapy might be a further indication for EART.

Mandatory examinations prior to EART include an upper GI endoscopy, a 24-hour pH monitoring, and a high-resolution manometry of the esophagus. The pH monitoring is done to verify the presence of gastroesophageal reflux and especially to document the ongoing acid reflux despite usage of high-dose PPI. The further aim of these examinations is to exclude the presence of a large hiatal hernia or the presence of Barrett's esophagus and to exclude esophageal motility disorders [1].

A. Wannhoff · K. Caca (✉)
Department of Gastroenterology, Hospital Ludwigsburg, Ludwigsburg, Germany
e-mail: Karel.Caca@rkh-kliniken.de

© Springer Nature Switzerland AG 2020
S. Horgan, K.-H. Fuchs (eds.), *Management of Gastroesophageal Reflux Disease*,
https://doi.org/10.1007/978-3-030-48009-7_6

Careful patient selection is of paramount importance, especially with regard to the presence of a large (>2–3 cm) hiatal hernia. These patients do not profit from EART and should preferentially be referred to surgery. It is important to inform the patient prior to EART that approximately one-third of patients will need long-term PPI treatment or a surgical therapy during follow-up.

Technical Aspects of Currently Available EART

The currently available EARTs are based upon either full-thickness tissue plication at the gastroesophageal junction (GEJ), radiofrequency ablation, or endoscopic mucosal resection and are summarized in Table 6.1 [2].

The Enteryx procedure (Boston Scientific Corp., Marlborough, MA, USA) was based upon endoscopic injection of a copolymer compound into the lower esophageal sphincter (LES). The device, however, was taken off the market after several occurrences of severe adverse events (including mediastinitis and mediastinal abscess) were reported and a warning by the Food and Drug Administration was issued [1].

Endoscopic Full-Thickness Plication

An endoscopic full-thickness plication with serosa-to-serosa apposition at the GEJ is the endoscopic technique that comes closest to surgical fundoplication. Different systems to perform the endoscopic full-thickness plication are currently available.

Table 6.1 Overview of different endoscopic anti-reflux therapies

Method	Device	Manufacturer	Comments
Tissue plication	GERDX	G-Surg GmbH, Seeon-Seebruck, Germany	Same mechanism as Plicator (NDO Surgical Inc., Mansfield, USA) Good evidence
	MUSE	Medigus, Omer, Israel	Only few data available
	EsophyX	EndoGastric Solutions Inc., Redmond, USA	Long-term efficacy questionable
	EndoCinch		Not available anymore Mucosal plication only, no full-thickness plication
Radiofrequency ablation	Stretta	Mederi Therapeutics Inc., Norwalk, USA	Insufficient long-term efficacy
Injection	Enteryx		Withdrawn from market due to serious adverse events
Mucosal resection			New procedure Based upon EMR/ESD, no specialized device necessary

Overview of the different modalities of endoscopic anti-reflux therapy and the commercially available devices

These are the GERDX device (G-Surg GmbH, Seeon-Seebruck, Germany), the MUSE system (Medigus, Omer, Israel), and the EsophyX device (EndoGastric Solutions Inc., Redmond, WA, USA) (Fig. 6.1). The GERDX device used the same technology as its predecessor Plicator (NDO Surgical Inc., Mansfield, USA), which is not available anymore. Not available anymore as well is the EndoCinch device (Bard Medical, Covington, GA, USA), which in contrast to the previous mentioned devices only facilitated a mucosal plication and no full-thickness plication.

The single steps of endoscopic full-thickness plication with the GERDX device are shown in Fig. 6.2.

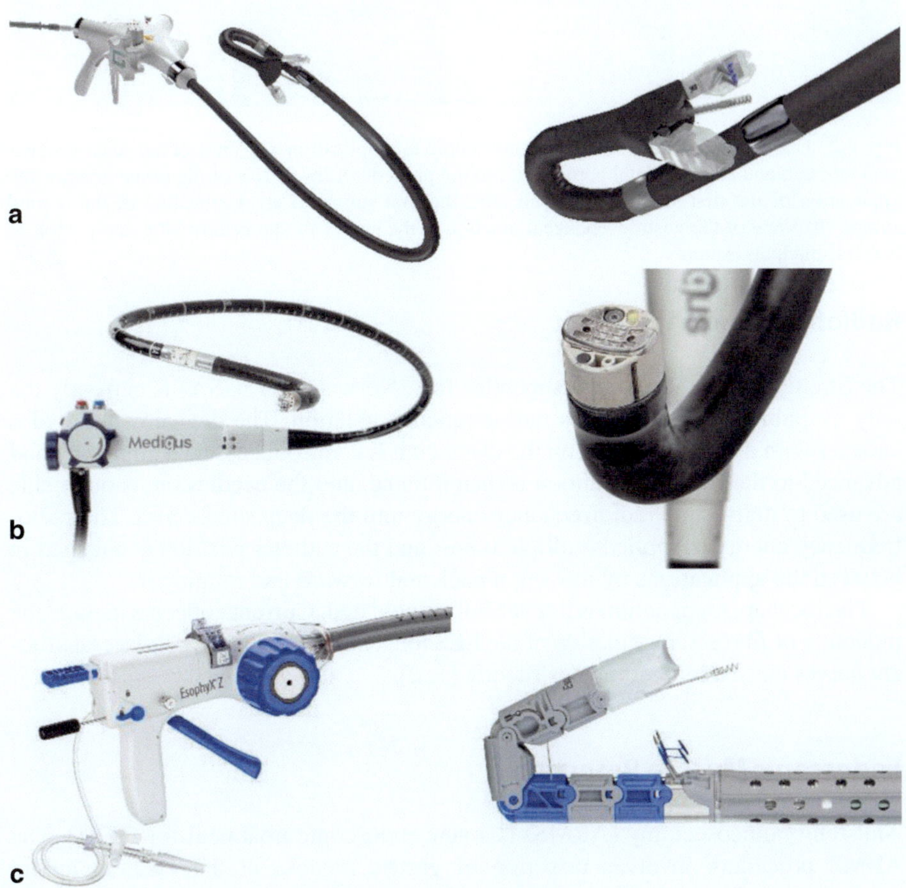

Fig. 6.1 Devices for full-thickness tissue plication. (**a**) GERDX device (G-Surg GmbH, Germany). (**b**) MUSE device (Medigus, Israel). (**c**) EsophyX device (EndoGastric Solutions Inc., USA)

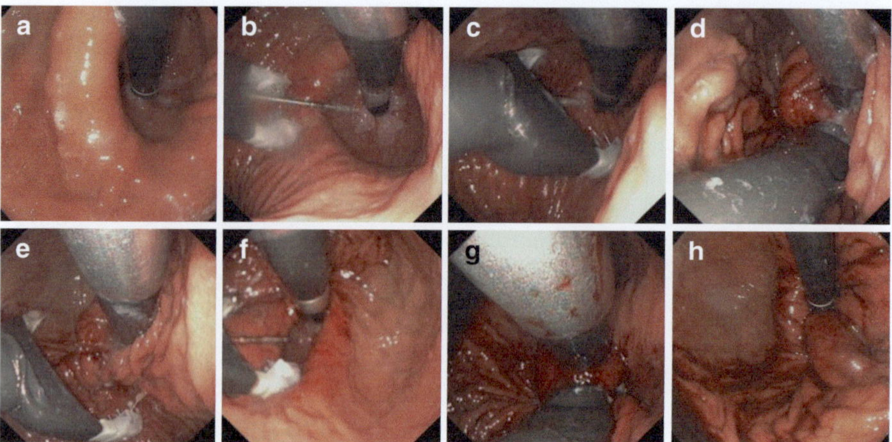

Fig. 6.2 Use of the GERDX device for endoscopic fundoplication. (**a**) View of the gastroesophageal junction and a small hiatal hernia prior to the procedure. (**b–d**) Use of the tissue grasper and application of the first suture. (**e**) Result after the first suture. (**f–g**) Application of the second suture. (**h**) View of the gastroesophageal junction at the end of the procedure after application of two full-thickness sutures

Radiofrequency Ablation

The Stretta device (Mederi Therapeutics Inc., Norwalk, CT, USA) is currently the only available system that uses radiofrequency ablation. The device consists of a catheter with a needle balloon on the distal end. It is introduced via a guidewire and advanced to the LES. The balloon is then inflated, and the needles on its outer side are used to deliver the radiofrequency energy into the deep submucosa. The radiofrequency energy is applied multiple times, and the catheter position is changed in between the applications by moving it back and forward and rotating it.

The mechanism of action is not yet fully elucidated. Current concepts include the induction of fibrosis, modulation of the LES tone, and an influence on visceral afferent nerves caused by thermic destruction [1, 2].

Endoscopic Mucosa Resection

Anti-reflux mucosectomy (ARMS) is a new endoscopic treatment for GERD. The ARMS procedure involves resection of gastric mucosa at the GEJ, including approximately 2 cm of gastric mucosa and 1 cm of esophageal mucosa. This results in scarring with shrinking and remodeling of the GEJ and creation of a flap valve, which causes an improvement of the Hill grade (Fig. 6.3). In the first two reported cases, a circumferential resection was done, which resulted in stricture formation and the need for dilation therapy. Thus, in later cases, a mucosal bridge of approximately twice the scope's diameter was left at the greater curvature and no stricture formation was observed [3].

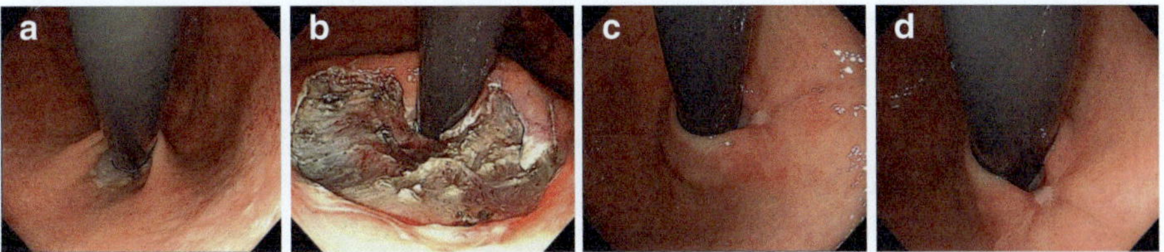

Fig. 6.3 Endoscopic anti-reflux mucosectomy. (**a**) Finding before the procedure. (**b**) Endoscopic mucosa resection. (**c**, **d**) Improvement of Hill grade after the procedure due to scarring. (From Inoue et al. [3])

Table 6.2 Long-term outcome of EART with the Plicator/GERDX device

Study	Patients (*n*)	Follow-up (months)	GERD-HRQL	PPI-free (%)
Pleskow et al. (2007) [17]	29	36	6 vs. 19∗	41
Birk et al. (2009) [18]	81	12	12 vs. 26.6∗	24
Von Renteln et al. (2008) [19]	41	12	11.0 vs. 26	39
Antoniou et al. (2012) [8]	29	12	(96.3 vs. 119.2∗)[a]	89

Summarized are the results of controlled studies that reported on long-term outcome and PPI usage with the Plicator/GERXD device

GERD-HRQL GERD-health related quality of life

[a]A different score to assess quality of life was used in that study

∗Significant change ($p < 0.05$)

The resection is done using endoscopic mucosal resection (EMR) or endoscopic submucosal dissection (ESD) techniques. Regarding EMR technique, cap-assisted EMR and a ligate-and-snare EMR technique were recently used successfully as well [4, 5].

Clinical Evidence for EART

Endoscopic Fundoplication

Good data is currently available for the Plicator and GERDX device (Table 6.2). A prospective and placebo-controlled trial showed a significant higher number of patients in the treatment group (56%) that experienced a significant improvement of GERD-related quality of life (defined as improvement of at least 50%) compared to patients in the control group (18.5%). In that study, esophageal acid exposure and PPI usage were significantly lower in the treatment group compared to the control group as well [6]. A further study showed that the improvement in quality of life was associated with improvement of objective measures, such as the DeMeester score or the absolute number of acid reflux episodes on 24-hour pH monitoring [7]. Information on the long-term outcome (>12 months) after full-thickness plication is available from noncontrolled studies only. Compared to surgical fundoplication, a randomized trial showed similar quality of life after 12 months in the group treated with endoscopic full-thickness plication compared to the group that underwent surgical fundoplication [8]. Further analysis revealed that patients after surgical fundoplication experienced less symptoms, while more patients after EART discontinued PPI therapy (89% vs. 48%).

The MUSE system has so far been only evaluated in noncontrolled trials. A significant improvement in quality of life was found after 6 months in a large multicenter trial, which as well showed significant improved results for 24-hour pH monitoring. Therapy with PPI could be discontinued in two-thirds of the patients [9]. These encouraging results could be confirmed in a long-term follow-up after 4 years [10]. Similar results were found in a small cohort of 13 patients that were followed for 5 years. At the end of the study, 7 of the 13 patients (64%) were off PPI therapy [11]. The main disadvantages of the MUSE device are related to the procedure itself. These are the complexity of the device as well as the need for endotracheal intubation and muscle relaxation.

The EsophyX device has so far been evaluated in multiple trials, including randomized and placebo-controlled studies. Recently, a meta-analysis was published that summarized the findings and revealed a significant higher response rate – defined as improvement of GERD-related quality of life >50% – compared to the control group [12]. This meta-analysis, however, also showed that the response rate dropped from approx. 70% to approx. 40% after a follow-up of 4–6 years (Fig. 6.4). The latter finding is most likely explained by an only temporary remodeling of the gastroesophageal junction. As soon as 12 months after the intervention, Hill grade had worsened again and almost reached the level prior to EART [13]. In our opinion, this reduced long-term efficacy is most likely due to a reduced stability of the used fasteners. Contrary to this, a recently published study on the long-term outcome after 1, 3, and 5 years revealed a persistent improvement of symptoms, yet approximately one-third of patients was still on daily PPI therapy after 5 years. Unfortunately, no data on pH monitoring results were presented [14]. Similar results were reported in a long-term follow-up study on 50 patients. After 6 years, 35.7% of the patients had stopped PPI therapy, 50.0% of the patients had halved the PPI dose, and the remaining 14.3% of the patients continued PPI therapy as before [15]. A network meta-analysis comparing the EsophyX procedure to surgical fundoplication showed significantly better results regarding findings of 24-hour pH monitoring for surgery compared to the endoscopic approach with the EsophyX [16].

Radiofrequency Ablation

The most important limitation of the Stretta system is its insufficient long-term efficacy. The first small and noncontrolled studies reported promising results for the device. More recent placebo-controlled trials could, however, not confirm these findings (Table 6.3). Taken together, the three studies found an improvement of symptoms, but objective parameters such as results of pH monitoring and need for

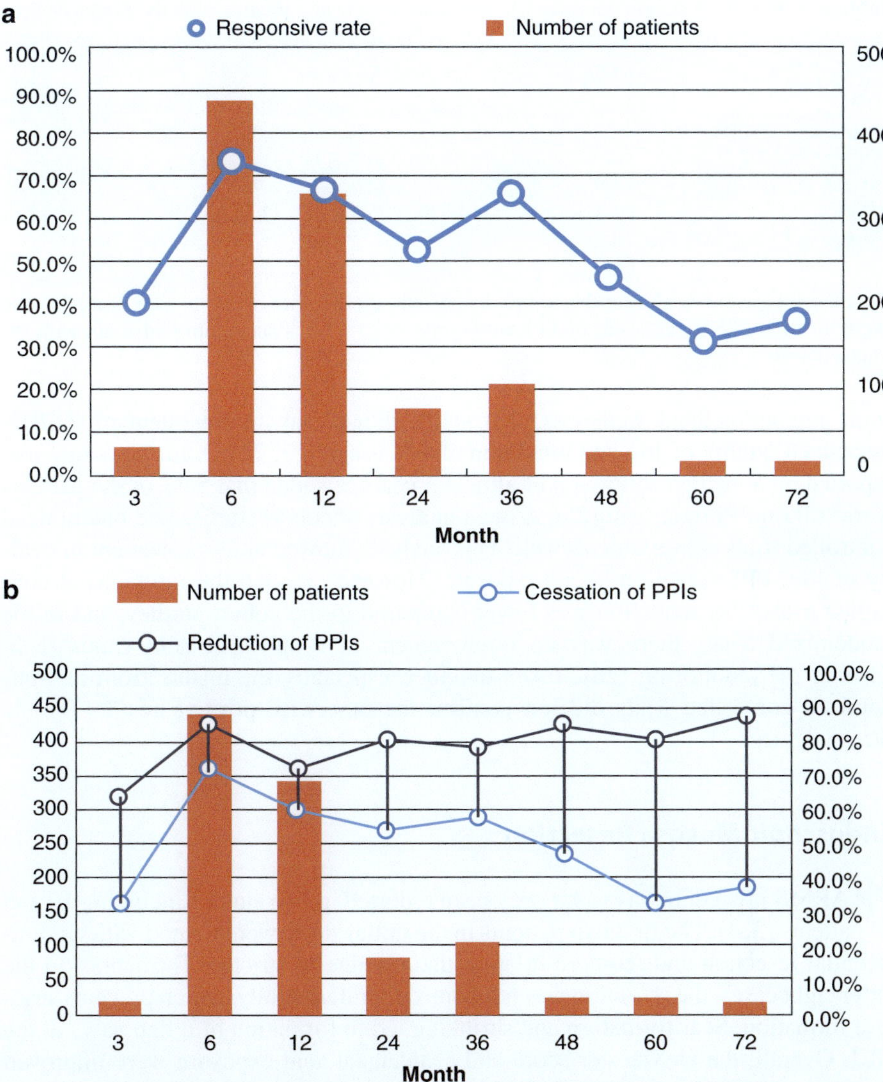

Fig. 6.4 Long-term results after treatment with the EsophyX device. (**a**) Response rate during short- and long-term follow-up. (**b**) Use of PPI during follow-up after the EsophyX procedure. (From Huang et al. [12])

PPI therapy showed no difference between baseline and end of the study in two of the three studies [20, 21]. Only the third study, which allowed the use of two sequential sessions with the Stretta device in a third arm, showed a reduction of PPI usage in that particular treatment arm [22]. The three studies, however, were limited to a follow-up of not more than 12 months. With regard to long-term outcome after radiofrequency ablation, there is data from a noncontrolled cohort study. Despite

Table 6.3 Results of sham-controlled trials for radiofreqeuency ablation with the Stretta device

Study	LES tone		AET (%)		PPI withdrawal (%)	
	Control	Stretta	Control	Stretta	Control	Stretta
Corley et al. (2003) [20]	18 (14.8–22.5)	16.2 (10.6–23)	10.7 (5.9–13)	9.9 (4–14.7)	52	58
Aziz et al. (2010) [22]	15.9 (+/− 3.2)	16.2 (+/− 4.5)	8.2 (3.1)	6.7 (2.8)	0	15
Arts et al. (2012) [21]	13.3 (+/− 2)	16.3 (+/− 2)	9	15	0	16

Summarized are the results for the control and Stretta groups with regard to LES tone, the acid exposure time (AET), and rate of PPI withdrawal from three sham-controlled trials with the Stretta device

some methodological weakness, that study showed an improvement of GERD-associated quality of life and reduction of PPI usage [23, 24]. A further study that reported on a median follow-up of almost 2 years revealed that 54% of the patients were still on PPI treatment [25]. A meta-analysis of cohort studies and randomized controlled trials is available as well. This analysis showed an improvement in quality of life, PPI usage, and acid exposure. However, among the randomized controlled trials, PPI reduction was lower compared to the cohort studies, and in the randomized trials, there was no improvement of esophageal acid exposure in 24-hour pH monitoring [26]. Taken together, especially the results from the randomized controlled trials did not confirm the otherwise positive results for the Stretta device.

Endoscopic Mucosa Resection

The ARMS procedure has so far only been reported in two studies including 10 and 33 patients [3, 4]. The first two patients in the initial study were treated with circumferential resection and required dilation therapy due to stricture formation. In the latter eight cases, the resection was not done circumferentially, which prevents stricture formation. Scar formation and shrinking led to formation of a flap valve at the GEJ. Overall, the DeMeester score and esophageal acid exposure were improved 2 months after the procedure. Further, PPI therapy could be discontinued in all eight patients [3]. The second study used cap-assisted EMR and included 33 patients. After 6 months, there was a significant improvement of GERD-related symptoms, the DeMeester score, and acid exposure time. Approximately two-thirds of patients were free of PPI after 6 months; however, their baseline DeMeester score was only 3.6, which is well within the range of normal and was significantly lower compared to patients that still needed PPI after 6 months [4]. Due to the lack of long-term results and controlled studies, it is still too early to make a final conclusion about this procedure. The first results nevertheless seem promising.

Table 6.4 Complications

Device	Self-limiting complications	Serious complications	Unpublished complications (MAUDE database)
Plicator/ GERDX	Sore throat (+) Chest pain(+) Shoulder pain Hemorrhage	Pneumoperitoneum Pneumothorax	Diaphragm injury Pneumoperitoneum Pneumothorax Perforation
EsophyX	Abdominal pain Shoulder pain Hemorrhage Dysphagia	Hemorrhage Shoulder pain Esophageal perforation	Perforation Pleural effusion Hemorrhage
Stretta	Chest pain (+) Fever (+) Esophagitis/ulcer Nausea	Gastroparesis Pancreatitis	Esophageal perforation Gastroparesis

Overview of the reported self-limiting and serious complications for the Plicator/GERDX device, the EsophyX device, and the Stretta device according to published data. Further included are complications reported in the MAUDE (Manufacturer and User Facility Device Experience) database (based upon Pandolfino et al. [1])
(+): >10 cases

Complications

The currently available EARTs are in general safe procedures. Serious adverse events occur in rare instances only (Table 6.4). With regard to the post-procedural management of these patients, it is however important to be aware of the more common and mostly self-limiting side effects of the different procedures. These are mainly chest, abdominal, or shoulder pain as well as dysphagia and a sore throat. Symptomatic treatment, especially adequate pain therapy, is required in these cases [1].

Summary

For carefully chosen patients, EART is an alternative to medical or surgical treatment of GERD. Careful selection of patients as well as the endoscopic procedure is of high importance for treatment success. Patients with refractory symptoms and proven acid reflux despite high-dose PPI therapy might be evaluated for EART. Among these patients, those with a large hiatal hernia should preferentially be referred to surgery and not undergo EART. For all available endoscopic treatment options, the best evidence currently exists for endoscopic full-thickness plication of the gastroesophageal junction. ARMS could become an alternative for selected patients. To summarize the results of EART: In one-third of patients, acid suppression therapy can be discontinued after EART; in one-third, an on-demand therapy is sufficient; and the last third will require either long-term medical treatment or surgery due to persistent acid reflux and symptoms.

References

1. Pandolfino JE, Krishnan K. Do endoscopic antireflux procedures fit in the current treatment paradigm of gastroesophageal reflux disease? Clin Gastroenterol Hepatol. 2014;12(4):544–54. https://doi.org/10.1016/j.cgh.2013.06.012.
2. Nabi Z, Reddy DN. Endoscopic management of gastroesophageal reflux disease: revisited. Clin Endosc. 2016;49(5):408–16. https://doi.org/10.5946/ce.2016.133.
3. Inoue H, Ito H, Ikeda H, Sato C, Sato H, Phalanusitthepha C, et al. Anti-reflux mucosectomy for gastroesophageal reflux disease in the absence of hiatus hernia: a pilot study. Ann Gastroenterol. 2014;27(4):346–51.
4. Yoo IK, Ko WJ, Kim HS, Kim HK, Kim JH, Kim WH, et al. Anti-reflux mucosectomy using a cap-assisted endoscopic mucosal resection method for refractory gastroesophageal disease: a prospective feasibility study. Surg Endosc. 2020;34(3):1124–31. https://doi.org/10.1007/s00464-019-06859-y.
5. Monino L, Gonzalez JM, Vitton V, Barthet M. Anti-reflux mucosectomy with band ligation in the treatment of refractory gastroesophageal reflux disease. Endoscopy. 2019;51(8):E215–E6. https://doi.org/10.1055/a-0875-3479.
6. Rothstein R, Filipi C, Caca K, Pruitt R, Mergener K, Torquati A, et al. Endoscopic full-thickness plication for the treatment of gastroesophageal reflux disease: a randomized, sham-controlled trial. Gastroenterology. 2006;131(3):704–12. https://doi.org/10.1053/j.gastro.2006.07.004.
7. Koch OO, Kaindlstorfer A, Antoniou SA, Spaun G, Pointner R, Swanstrom LL. Subjective and objective data on esophageal manometry and impedance pH monitoring 1 year after endoscopic full-thickness plication for the treatment of GERD by using multiple plication implants. Gastrointest Endosc. 2013;77(1):7–14. https://doi.org/10.1016/j.gie.2012.07.033.
8. Antoniou SA, Koch OO, Kaindlstorfer A, Asche KU, Berger J, Granderath FA, et al. Endoscopic full-thickness plication versus laparoscopic fundoplication: a prospective study on quality of life and symptom control. Surg Endosc. 2012;26(4):1063–8. https://doi.org/10.1007/s00464-011-1999-0.
9. Zacherl J, Roy-Shapira A, Bonavina L, Bapaye A, Kiesslich R, Schoppmann SF, et al. Endoscopic anterior fundoplication with the Medigus Ultrasonic Surgical Endostapler (MUSE) for gastroesophageal reflux disease: 6-month results from a multi-center prospective trial. Surg Endosc. 2015;29(1):220–9. https://doi.org/10.1007/s00464-014-3731-3.
10. Kim HJ, Kwon CI, Kessler WR, Selzer DJ, McNulty G, Bapaye A, et al. Long-term follow-up results of endoscopic treatment of gastroesophageal reflux disease with the MUSE endoscopic stapling device. Surg Endosc. 2016;30(8):3402–8. https://doi.org/10.1007/s00464-015-4622-y.
11. Roy-Shapira A, Bapaye A, Date S, Pujari R, Dorwat S. Trans-oral anterior fundoplication: 5-year follow-up of pilot study. Surg Endosc. 2015;29(12):3717–21. https://doi.org/10.1007/s00464-015-4142-9.
12. Huang X, Chen S, Zhao H, Zeng X, Lian J, Tseng Y, et al. Efficacy of transoral incisionless fundoplication (TIF) for the treatment of GERD: a systematic review with meta-analysis. Surg Endosc. 2017;31(3):1032–44. https://doi.org/10.1007/s00464-016-5111-7.
13. Witteman BP, Conchillo JM, Rinsma NF, Betzel B, Peeters A, Koek GH, et al. Randomized controlled trial of transoral incisionless fundoplication vs. proton pump inhibitors for treatment of gastroesophageal reflux disease. Am J Gastroenterol. 2015;110(4):531–42. https://doi.org/10.1038/ajg.2015.28.
14. Trad KS, Barnes WE, Prevou ER, Simoni G, Steffen JA, Shughoury AB, et al. The TEMPO trial at 5 years: transoral fundoplication (TIF 2.0) is safe, durable, and cost-effective. Surg Innov. 2018;25(2):149–57. https://doi.org/10.1177/1553350618755214.
15. Testoni PA, Testoni S, Mazzoleni G, Vailati C, Passaretti S. Long-term efficacy of transoral incisionless fundoplication with Esophyx (TIF 2.0) and factors affecting outcomes in GERD patients followed for up to 6 years: a prospective single-center study. Surg Endosc. 2015;29(9):2770–80. https://doi.org/10.1007/s00464-014-4008-6.

16. Richter JE, Kumar A, Lipka S, Miladinovic B, Velanovich V. Efficacy of laparoscopic Nissen fundoplication vs transoral incisionless fundoplication or proton pump inhibitors in patients with gastroesophageal reflux disease: a systematic review and network meta-analysis. Gastroenterology. 2018;154(5):1298–1308.e7. https://doi.org/10.1053/j.gastro.2017.12.021.
17. Pleskow D, Rothstein R, Kozarek R, Haber G, Gostout C, Lembo A. Endoscopic full-thickness plication for the treatment of GERD: long-term multicenter results. Surg Endosc. 2007;21(3):439–44. https://doi.org/10.1007/s00464-006-9121-8.
18. Birk J, Pruitt R, Haber G, Raijman I, Baluyut A, Meiselman M, et al. The Plicator procedure for the treatment of gastroesophageal reflux disease: a registry study. Surg Endosc. 2009;23(2):423–31. https://doi.org/10.1007/s00464-008-0109-4.
19. von Renteln D, Schiefke I, Fuchs KH, Raczynski S, Philipper M, Breithaupt W, et al. Endoscopic full-thickness plication for the treatment of GERD by application of multiple Plicator implants: a multicenter study (with video). Gastrointest Endosc. 2008;68(5):833–44. https://doi.org/10.1016/j.gie.2008.02.010.
20. Corley DA, Katz P, Wo JM, Stefan A, Patti M, Rothstein R, et al. Improvement of gastroesophageal reflux symptoms after radiofrequency energy: a randomized, sham-controlled trial. Gastroenterology. 2003;125(3):668–76.
21. Arts J, Bisschops R, Blondeau K, Farre R, Vos R, Holvoet L, et al. A double-blind sham-controlled study of the effect of radiofrequency energy on symptoms and distensibility of the gastro-esophageal junction in GERD. Am J Gastroenterol. 2012;107(2):222–30. https://doi.org/10.1038/ajg.2011.395.
22. Aziz AM, El-Khayat HR, Sadek A, Mattar SG, McNulty G, Kongkam P, et al. A prospective randomized trial of sham, single-dose Stretta, and double-dose Stretta for the treatment of gastroesophageal reflux disease. Surg Endosc. 2010;24(4):818–25. https://doi.org/10.1007/s00464-009-0671-4.
23. Noar M, Squires P, Noar E, Lee M. Long-term maintenance effect of radiofrequency energy delivery for refractory GERD: a decade later. Surg Endosc. 2014;28(8):2323–33. https://doi.org/10.1007/s00464-014-3461-6.
24. Pandolfino JE, Krishnan K. Reply: To PMID 23811248. Clin Gastroenterol Hepatol. 2015;13(2):407–8. https://doi.org/10.1016/j.cgh.2014.10.001.
25. Viswanath Y, Maguire N, Obuobi RB, Dhar A, Punnoose S. Endoscopic day case antireflux radiofrequency (Stretta) therapy improves quality of life and reduce proton pump inhibitor (PPI) dependency in patients with gastro-oesophageal reflux disease: a prospective study from a UK tertiary centre. Frontline Gastroenterol. 2019;10(2):113–9. https://doi.org/10.1136/flgastro-2018-101028.
26. Fass R, Cahn F, Scotti DJ, Gregory DA. Systematic review and meta-analysis of controlled and prospective cohort efficacy studies of endoscopic radiofrequency for treatment of gastroesophageal reflux disease. Surg Endosc. 2017;31(12):4865–82. https://doi.org/10.1007/s00464-017-5431-2.

Surgical Management of Gastroesophageal Reflux Disease

7

Sean M. Flynn, Ryan C. Broderick, and Santiago Horgan

Indications

Gastroesophageal reflux disease (GERD) affects up to 40% of the US adult population [1]. The cornerstone of GERD symptom management includes lifestyle modification and medical therapy. Acid-suppressing medications, such as proton pump inhibitors (PPIs), have shown great efficacy in achieving satisfactory symptom control for most patients and are the only treatment that the majority of patients will require [2, 3]. However, for a certain number of patients, lifestyle modification and acid suppression are insufficient to adequately control their symptoms and sequelae of GERD, and surgical options should be considered.

Failure of medical therapy can be divided into noncompliance with daily medication dosing or progression of GERD symptoms and complications despite adequate medical therapy. Noncompliance with medical therapy can stem from patient's unwillingness to take lifelong medical therapy or an inability to, which occurs for a number of reasons. Lifelong PPI therapy is a significant financial cost for a number of patients [4]. While highly effective, PPIs are also not without their own adverse effects and risks. Studies have shown that long-term PPI therapy can cause increased risk of gastrointestinal infections, especially *Clostridium difficile* [5]. Patients on long-term PPI therapy are also at risk of developing vitamin malabsorption and

S. M. Flynn · R. C. Broderick (✉) · S. Horgan
Division of Minimally Invasive Surgery, Department of Surgery,
University of California San Diego, La Jolla, CA, USA
e-mail: rbroderick@ucsd.edu

© Springer Nature Switzerland AG 2020
S. Horgan, K.-H. Fuchs (eds.), *Management of Gastroesophageal Reflux Disease*,
https://doi.org/10.1007/978-3-030-48009-7_7

deficiencies from long-term acid suppression. Deficiencies in magnesium, calcium, vitamin B12, and iron have all been reported. Rarely, PPI use has also been associated with acute interstitial nephritis and drug-induced lupus.

Development of complicated GERD while on appropriate medical therapy is another common indication for anti-reflux surgery. Complicated GERD includes the spectrum of esophageal changes incurred from persistent exposure to an acidic environment. Patients may develop esophageal strictures, ulcers, or esophagitis. All of which can negatively impact patient's quality of life. Barrett's esophagus can also be associated with GERD, and anti-reflux surgery has shown equivalent 5-year remission rates as esomeprazole and thus may be another indication for surgery in select patients [6]. DeMeester also performed a literature review in which Barrett's regressed in a significant proportion of patients who underwent anti-reflux surgery [7]. He notes that Barrett's should be considered end-stage reflux disease and that patients with disease progression on medical therapy should be offered surgical attempt at controlling their disease [7].

Patients with anatomic pathologies also often fail medical therapy and are good surgical candidates. Hiatal hernias are the most common anatomic pathology that can lead to GERD. Hiatal hernias result in intrathoracic migration of the lower esophageal sphincter, which disrupts its normal physiologic function. Up to 84% of patients with reflux esophagitis are found to have a concomitant hiatal hernia [8]. Anti-reflux procedures performed in these patients must include repair of the hiatal hernia or else will almost invariably fail. Likewise, obesity is closely linked to GERD. In this special patient population, bariatric surgical procedures can provide significant improvement in reflux symptoms and should be strongly considered.

Preoperative Evaluation

Preoperative evaluation should include a thorough extensive symptom history, preferably with free-form questionnaires followed by evaluation of the esophageal function, any esophageal pathophysiology, esophageal length, and any potentially contributing anatomic defects, such as a hiatal hernia. We typically begin with upper endoscopy to evaluate the esophageal and gastric mucosa to detect any evidence of Barrett's esophagus, esophageal strictures, or malignancies, which may change operative planning or surveillance. Impedance-pH monitoring probes are placed at the time of EGD, and 96 hours off-PPI acid exposure and symptom correlation are used to objectively quantify GERD. An upper gastrointestinal (UGI) contrast study is useful to evaluate esophageal length and presence of a hiatal hernia, which may also alter surgical planning. Finally, esophageal manometry can provide insight into any underlying esophageal pathophysiology, which can significantly change the planned procedure, or reveal contraindications to anti-reflux surgery.

Operative Procedures

Anti-reflux procedures can be broken down into either gastric wraps, sphincter augmentation, endoscopic interventions, or gastric bypass. A practicing foregut surgeon should be able to provide a variety of options for anti-reflux surgery and tailor treatment for each individual patient.

Nissen Fundoplication

The Nissen fundoplication was first described in 1956 by Rudolf Nissen and has become one of the most commonly performed anti-reflux procedures to date. It involves wrapping the fundus 360 degrees around the intra-abdominal portion of the esophagus to bolster the LES. When wrapped in this manner, gastric muscle contractions, which previously may have increased the intragastric pressure and esophageal reflux, now help maintain the LES. Detailed operative steps of a laparoscopic Nissen fundoplication are further discussed in Chap. 8.

Partial Fundoplication

Complete 360-degree fundoplication should be avoided in patients with esophageal motility disorders as it can lead to severe dysphagia. This has led to the modification of the Nissen fundoplication to partial fundoplications, which in their own right have seen great success as anti-reflux procedures. The Dor and Toupet fundoplications are the two most commonly utilized partial fundoplications. Dor fundoplication involves a 180-degree anterior fundal wrap, while the Toupet fundoplication involves at 270-degree posterior fundal wrap. The Dor fundoplication has also found great use after esophageal (Heller) myotomy to both buttress tissue over the divided muscle fibers, as well as a means of preventing severe reflux after this procedure. Detailed description of Toupet fundoplication can be found in a later chapter.

Belsey Mark IV Fundoplication

The Belsey Mark IV fundoplication is another partial fundoplication, but it is performed from a transthoracic approach. This technique involves a 240-degree anterior partial fundoplication, with associated crural plication to narrow the esophageal hiatus and provide extra support of the LES [9].

Magnetic Sphincter Augmentation

Magnetic sphincter augmentation involves placement of a magnetic prosthesis around the distal esophagus to bolster the LES. The device used is the LINX Reflux Management System, which gained FDA approval in 2012. This device includes a ring of magnets that sit around the distal esophagus. The magnetic force serves to bolster the LES resting pressure [10] while still allowing passage of swallowed food and liquids, as well as regurgitation of gas. Detailed description of MSA placement and indications can be found in a later chapter.

Endoscopic Methods

Endoscopic techniques are the newest developments in anti-reflux surgery, and their efficacy and long-term durability are still being validated. The Stretta procedure is one of the most commonly used and studied endoscopic methods. This procedure involves endoscopic radiofrequency ablation of the LES fibers, which results in scarring and hypertrophy of the muscle fibers, with a subsequent increase in LES strength and resting pressure. Transoral incisionless fundoplication (TIF) is a newer technique. It utilizes endoscopically placed full-thickness sutures to complete a partial gastric fundoplication, though evaluation of short- and long-term outcomes is still needed.

Gastric Bypass

GERD disproportionately affects obese patients, with prevalence rates as high as 37–72% [11, 12]. Reflux in the obese is due to a number of anatomic and physiologic factors, such as increased intra-abdominal pressure which disrupts the normal physiology of the LES. Roux-en-Y gastric bypass (RYGB) has shown positive results in ameliorating obesity-related GERD. Seventy percent of patients were found to have improvement or resolution of GERD symptoms at 1 year postoperative [13]. This is especially notable as obese patients typically have higher rates of failure for other standard anti-reflux procedures, such as fundoplication [14]. The relationship between GERD and sleeve gastrectomy is discussed in greater detail in a later chapter.

Comparative Outcomes

Outcomes of surgical anti-reflux procedures in comparison to best medical therapy with PPIs are generally mixed, but when performed by experienced surgeons, fundoplication appears to be at least comparable to PPI therapy and may be superior in the short term. All fundoplication procedures show excellent results, regardless of the approach or wrap used. A randomized controlled trial by Grant et al. showed that patients undergoing posterior fundoplication of any type had better 5-year reported reflux scores, and only 44% of patients in the surgical arm required ongoing medical therapy, compared to 82% of the medically managed patients [15]. Adverse effects of surgery were rare (3%) and typically occurred only in the early postoperative period. When performed by experience surgeons, anti-reflux procedures are safe and effective in providing sustainable long-term results.

Anterior and posterior partial wraps are not equivalent in their outcomes. A 2010 meta-analysis by Broeders et al. found that posterior wraps resulted in decreased esophageal acid exposure time, decreased heartburn symptoms, and decreased long-term PPI use when compared to anterior wraps. Anterior wraps were also associated with higher rates of reoperation, primarily for these recurrent GERD symptoms. In the short term, posterior wraps had higher rates of associated dysphagia, though this difference resolved in the long term. There was no significant difference in patient satisfaction between anterior and posterior wraps. However, given the objectively superior outcomes seen above, posterior wraps should be the partial fundoplication of choice when being performed purely for GERD [16].

Total and partial posterior wraps appear to be comparable in their overall outcomes. In a randomized trial, Mardani et al. found no significant difference between total and partial posterior fundoplication with regard to long-term heartburn and acid regurgitation symptoms [17]. Likewise, other trials have found no significant difference in the rates of recurrent GERD symptoms after total fundoplication or posterior fundoplication (5% vs. 6%) at 3 years [18]. Total fundoplication is often noted to have higher rates of short-term mechanical issues, such as dysphagia and gas bloating, though these differences disappear in long-term follow-up [17].

Outcomes between fundoplication and newer techniques, such as magnetic sphincter augmentation or endoscopic procedures, have not yet been extensively studied. One comparison of fundoplication and magnetic sphincter augmentation did find similar results in objective control of GERD. Both DeMeester scores and percentage of time of esophageal pH was less than four normalized in the two groups, though fundoplication resulted in significantly lower overall scores. However, magnetic sphincter augmentation was associated with significantly shorter operative time and decreased rates of bloating and inability to belch [19]. Further studies will be needed in the future to reach more definitive conclusions on their comparative outcomes and efficacies. Currently, MSA placement is safe and effective and results in lower operative times than fundoplication. Outcomes are still being studied, but MSA offers another option for anti-reflux surgery with good outcomes.

Conclusion

Anti-reflux procedures are safe and effective in relieving GERD. Medical therapy remains the gold standard of reflux management, but in the select group of patients who fail medical therapy or are unable/unwilling to adhere to lifelong medical therapy, surgical anti-reflux therapy is indicated. One surgical procedure is not markedly superior when comparing long-term outcomes as all operations show favorable results with improvement in symptoms and evidence of Barrett's stabilization or regression. It is important for the practicing foregut surgeon to have multiple tools in their surgical toolbox in order to treat GERD, so each operation may be tailored to the patient's specific needs for best outcomes.

References

1. Nebel OT, Fornes MF, Castell DO. Symptomatic gastroesophageal reflux: incidence and precipitating factors. Am J Dig Dis. 1976;21(11):953–6. https://doi.org/10.1007/BF01071906.
2. Sigterman KE, van Pinxteren B, Bonis PA, Lau J, Numans ME. Short-term treatment with proton pump inhibitors, H2-receptor antagonists and prokinetics for gastro-oesophageal reflux disease-like symptoms and endoscopy negative reflux disease. Cochrane Database Syst Rev. 2013;2013(5):CD002095. https://doi.org/10.1002/14651858.CD002095.pub5.
3. Chiba N, De Gara CJ, Wilkinson JM, Hunt RH. Speed of healing and symptom relief in grade II to IV gastroesophageal reflux disease: a meta-analysis. Gastroenterology. 1997;112(6):1798–810. https://doi.org/10.1053/gast.1997.v112.pm9178669.
4. Gerson LB, Robbins AS, Garber A, Hornberger J, Triadafilopoulos G. A cost-effectiveness analysis of prescribing strategies in the management of gastroesophageal reflux disease. Am J Gastroenterol. 2000;95(2):395–407.
5. Kwok CS, Arthur AK, Anibueze CI, Singh S, Cavallazzi R, Loke YK. Risk of Clostridium difficile infection with acid suppressing drugs and antibiotics: meta-analysis. Am J Gastroenterol. 2012;107(7):1011–9.
6. Galmiche J-P, Hatlebakk J, Attwood S, et al. Laparoscopic antireflux surgery vs esomeprazole treatment for chronic GERD: the LOTUS randomized clinical trial. JAMA. 2011;305(19):1969–77. https://doi.org/10.1001/jama.2011.626.
7. Demeester SR. Barrett's oesophagus: treatment with surgery. Best Pract Res Clin Gastroenterol. 2015;29(1):211–7. https://doi.org/10.1016/j.bpg.2014.12.004.
8. Wright RA, Hurwitz AL. Relationship of hiatal hernia to endoscopically proved reflux esophagitis. Dig Dis Sci. 1979;24(4):311–3. https://doi.org/10.1007/BF01296546.
9. Cooke DT. Belsey mark IV repair. Oper Tech Thorac Cardiovasc Surg. 2013;18(3):215–29. https://doi.org/10.1053/j.optechstcvs.2013.10.001.
10. Warren HF, Louie BE, Farivar AS, Wilshire C, Aye RW. Manometric changes to the lower esophageal sphincter after magnetic sphincter augmentation in patients with chronic gastro-esophageal reflux disease. Ann Surg. 2017;266(1):99–104.
11. Lundell L, Ruth M, Sandberg N, Bove-Nielsen M. Does massive obesity promote abnormal gastroesophageal reflux? Dig Dis Sci. 1995;40(8):1632–5. https://doi.org/10.1007/BF02212682.
12. Anand G, Katz PO. Gastroesophageal reflux disease and obesity. Rev Gastroenterol Disord. 2008;8(4):233–9.
13. Hutter MM, Schirmer BD, Jones DB, et al. First report from the American College of Surgeons Bariatric Surgery Center Network. Ann Surg. 2011;254(3):410–22. https://doi.org/10.1097/sla.0b013e31822c9dac.
14. Perez AR, Moncure AC, Rattner DW. Obesity adversely affects the outcome of antireflux operations. Surg Endosc. 2001;15(9):986–9. https://doi.org/10.1007/s004640000392.
15. Grant AM, Cotton SC, Boachie C, et al. Minimal access surgery compared with medical management for gastro-oesophageal reflux disease: five year follow-up of a randomised controlled trial (REFLUX). BMJ. 2013;346(7905):1–11. https://doi.org/10.1136/bmj.f1908.
16. Broeders JA, Roks DJ, Ahmed Ali U, Draaisma WA, Smout AJ, Hazebroek EJ. Laparoscopic anterior versus posterior fundoplication for gastroesophageal reflux disease: systematic review and meta-analysis of randomized clinical trials. Ann Surg. 2011;254(1):39–47.

17. Mardani J, Lundell L, Engström C. Total or posterior partial fundoplication in the treatment of GERD: results of a randomized trial after 2 decades of follow-up. Ann Surg. 2011;253(5):875–8.
18. Lundell L, Abrahamsson H, Ruth M, Rydberg L, Lönroth H, Olbe L. Long-term results of a prospective randomized comparison of total fundic wrap (Nissen-Rossetti) or semifundoplication (Toupet) for gastro-oesophageal reflux. Br J Surg. 1996;83(6):830–5. https://doi.org/10.1002/bjs.1800830633.
19. Louie BE, Farivar AS, Shultz D, Brennan C, Vallières E, Aye RW. Short-term outcomes using magnetic sphincter augmentation versus Nissen fundoplication for medically resistant gastroesophageal reflux disease. Ann Thorac Surg. 2014;98(2):498–505. https://doi.org/10.1016/J.ATHORACSUR.2014.04.074.

The Nissen Fundoplication

8

Karl-Hermann Fuchs, Wolfram Breithaupt, and Gabor Varga

Introduction

The "Nissen fundoplication" was first published in 1956 by Rudolf Nissen, a surgeon from Basel, Switzerland [1]. He created the first mechanical effective plication of the gastric fundus around the distal esophagus, which proved to be a true antireflux procedure in the subsequent years with its augmentation effect on the lower esophageal sphincter (LES). With increasing understanding of gastroesophageal reflux disease (GERD) as a distinct entity, this paralleled the development of surgery as a treatment option [2–5]. The history of antireflux surgery in the twentieth century is initially characterized by a reconstruction of the anatomical alterations after the development of a hiatal hernia [1–7]. Especially Allison initiated and propagated the first step in antireflux surgery with an anatomical reconstruction of the hiatus and a gastric fixation by a pexy [2, 3]. However, over the 1950s and 1960s, it became quite evident from clinical experience that only an anatomical reconstruction was not sufficient enough to effectively treat pathologic reflux [4–7]. Allison himself published at the end of his career a summary of his experience with the pexy technique showing a recurrence rate of around 50% [5]. As a consequence, it could be concluded from this era that the technical strategy of an isolated anatomical reconstruction and fixation is probably not sufficient enough to stop reflux for good, especially not in patients with advanced disease [5–7].

The Nissen fundoplication became a successful antireflux procedure during the 1960s and 1970s; however, the published side effects were substantial especially

K.-H. Fuchs (✉)
University of California San Diego, Center for the Future of Surgery, La Jolla, CA, USA

W. Breithaupt · G. Varga
Agaplesion Markus Krankenhaus, Department of General and GI-Surgery, Frankfurt am Main, Germany

© Springer Nature Switzerland AG 2020
S. Horgan, K.-H. Fuchs (eds.), *Management of Gastroesophageal Reflux Disease*,
https://doi.org/10.1007/978-3-030-48009-7_8

dysphagia [4, 7]. This led to searching for a better "fundoplication" and several other procedures like various forms of partial fundoplications such as the Belsey Mark IV procedure or the Lind operation [4, 7, 8]. Very few comparative studies were performed at that time, showing quite superior antireflux effect of the full 360° Nissen fundoplication [6].

In Chicago, a group of surgeons Donahoe, Bombeck, and DeMeester modified the technique to create the short floppy Nissen fundoplication [6, 9, 10]. This version of the Nissen fundoplication with documented fewer side effects as the original version became the most successful Nissen technique in the 1980s and 1990s. DeMeester et al. documented that by using a shorter wrap and a larger bougie during calibration and shaping of the wrap, one can reduce postoperative dysphagia and side effects substantially [10].

With the advent of minimal invasive surgery, the laparoscopic Nissen fundoplication became a "boom operation" [11]. Again, during the learning curve of laparoscopic Nissen fundoplication, the incidence of postoperative dysphagia was high, indicating the need for a very meticulous technique to shape and to suture the fundus around the weak LES [12–16]. Surgeons looking for an alternative with less side effects picked up the posterior hemifundoplication technique published by Toupet in the early 1960s [17]. In subsequent years, the laparoscopic Nissen fundoplication and the laparoscopic Toupet hemifundoplication became the most frequently used minimal invasive techniques [18–21].

Among surgeons, the discussion and the choice for one or the other technique, Nissen or Toupet, have continued with persisting engagement. A number of randomized trials have been performed to compare full and partial fundoplication techniques [18, 19, 22–33]. Several meta-analyses are available to judge over the two versions of fundoplication [34–39]. Based on the evidence in literature, the Toupet fundoplication bears less risk for postoperative dysphagia and side effects, as well as the Toupet has a lower rate of necessary reoperations for dysphagia [34–39]. The level of reoperations for Nissen in these randomized trials and meta-analysis is around 10–15% [22–39].

These results are in severe contrast to results from experienced centers with large case series with Nissen fundoplications, which show a much lower dysphagia rate and reoperation rate at the level of 5% [12–16, 37]. Many discussions have been performed also in several guideline committees about these controversies [40–42]. In addition, it has been discussed whether a partial Toupet fundoplication may have less durability than the Nissen fundoplication, where the posterior fundus is sutured to the anterior fundus wall and additionally to the esophagus, thus creating a possibly more dependable connection of tissue, compared to the fixation of the fundic wall only on the esophageal wall in the Toupet fundoplication [43, 44]. A consensus based on these controversial data was impossible. The guideline commissions have decided to suggest that the surgeons should make this decision based on their experience and their choice of procedure, Nissen or Toupet [40–42].

The Principle of Action of a Nissen Fundoplication

The major pathophysiologic background of GERD is the failure of the natural anti-reflux barrier and especially the mechanical and functional weakness of the LES as well as the anatomical alteration in that the sphincter is not anymore exposed to the abdominal pressure environment due to the development of a hiatal hernia [45]. As a consequence, these two major components have to be corrected by an effective antireflux procedure [10, 12, 45].

Therefore, a prerequisite for an optimal working action for a Nissen fundoplication is the mobilization of the esophagus out of the mediastinum in order to gain a sufficient intra-abdominal length of the sphincter. This anatomical reconstruction of the position of the cardia below the hiatus is important to regain the physiologic position of the sphincter within the abdominal pressure system [10, 12, 45]. Then the intra-abdominal pressure system can support the remaining sphincter pressure to close off the intra-abdominal segment of the LES, especially when intra-abdominal pressure or intragastric pressure rises. Figure 8.1 demonstrates the principle of action of a fundoplication. The symmetric wrap around the weakened LES after its correct positioning in the abdomen augments the cardia.

Prior to surgery, an increased intra-abdominal and/or an intragastric pressure will easily cause reflux through a mechanically weak LES because there is no resistance. After performing a technically correct fundoplication, an increased intragastric pressure will cause also a pressure increase within the fundic wrap. The wrap will

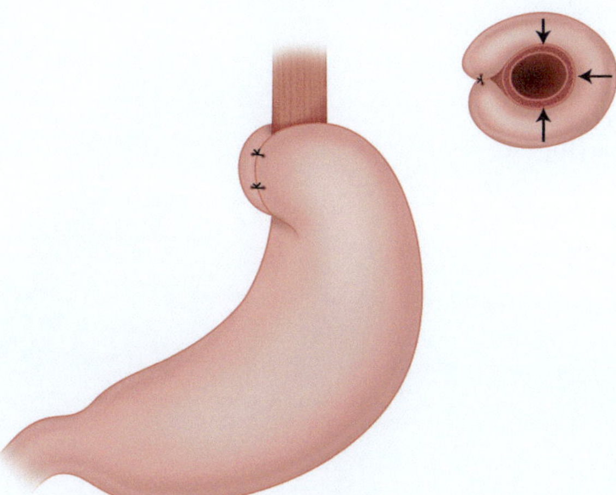

Fig. 8.1 Principle of action of the Nissen fundoplication: After anatomical reconstruction of the hiatus, the fundoplication remains in the abdominal pressure environment. The symmetric shape of the wrap will cause a mechanical augmentation of the weakened cardia. In addition, a rise in intra-gastric pressure will also cause a rise of the pressure inside the fundoplication, which will cause additional closure of the cardia. The latter will prevent excessive reflux, if the position of the wrap is secured intra-abdominally

have the ability to compress the distal esophagus helping to fulfill the task of an antireflux barrier. In addition, an increased intra-abdominal pressure will create the similar effect. Therefore, an important technical prerequisite for a good result after a Nissen procedure is the anatomical reconstruction to ensure an intra-abdominal position of the sphincter as well as the fundoplication.

Operative Technique

The Nissen fundoplication should consist of a few very important basic technical steps to have the highest probability for a successful operation besides a correct indication for surgery.

The first step is the dissection of the hiatus and the cardia. The second step is a sufficient mobilization of the esophagus in the mediastinum to position the LES in the abdominal pressure environment. The third step is the narrowing of the hiatus to an adequate width around the esophagus. The fourth important step is the shaping of the wrap. Each step is important in creating a functional good result with a long-lasting durability.

We have followed the "DeMeester School" in creating a short floppy Nissen fundoplication in the sandwich technique (Fig. 8.2) [10, 12]. The patient is placed in a French position and in a 30° anti-Trendelenburg situation. Five trocars are used for the laparoscopic fundoplication. Initially, the left liver lobe is retracted toward the right side of the patient to have an optimal exposure of the hiatal region. Especially

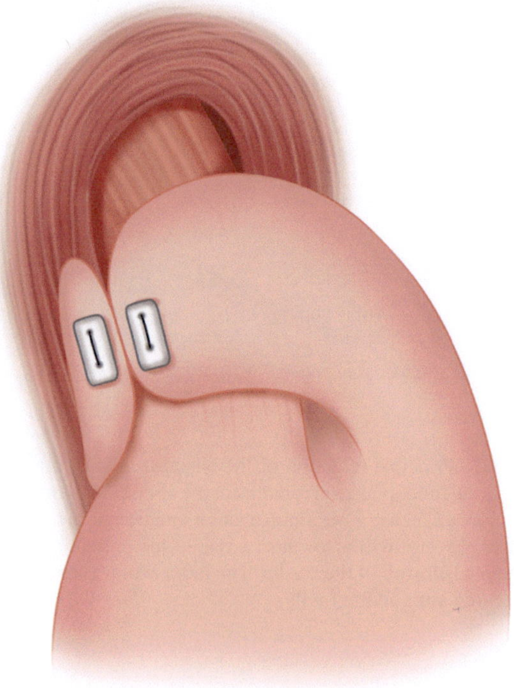

Fig. 8.2 Scheme of a short, floppy total fundoplication in the Nissen-DeMeester-sandwich technique [10]

in obese patients, the anti-Trendelenburg position will facilitate a sufficient exposure of the cardia, since gravity will pull fatty omentum and bowel downward. Initially, the size of the hiatal hernia and the width of the hiatus are evaluated to get an impression about the possibility of a short esophagus and the mobility of the esophagus.

For dissection, the stomach and especially the fundus are pulled downward, and the gastrosplenic ligament is exposed. With an energy instrument, the short gastric vessels are separated starting at the upper pole of the spleen in order to free the fundus. It is important to mobilize all tissue connections of the posterior fundus with the retroperitoneum, with the spleen, and with left hiatal crus. In addition, the left crus is completely dissected as an important landmark for later approximation with the right crus. Later, the posterior fundus will be pulled over to the right side of the patient. It is important that the fundus has space to move around in this area especially when the fundus will be filled with food and will need space for fundic accommodation. At the left crus, the hernia sac can be grasped and pulled downward in order to get in the tissue layer between the left crus and the hernia sac into the mediastinum. This is a very important step. It should be executed with caution. If this is done accurately in the correct tissue layer, the hernia sac can be dissected completely out of the mediastinum rather easily. An incision is carried out around the hiatal arch toward the right side of the patient, constantly pulling the hernia sac downward.

On the right side of the hiatus, the most upper part of pars flaccida is opened to visualize the right crus. This opening is kept limited in size to keep only a rather small window for the posterior flap of fundus. Many surgeons open the pars flaccida completely and divide all vagal branches toward the liver. We try to preserve these branches for their functional task and also to keep the opening small to have an abutment for the posterior fundic flap. A complete dissection of the smaller curvature would allow for an easy sliding of the fundoplication downward on the stomach, which would facilitate slipping. This can be prevented by keeping this opening small.

Once the hernia sac is completely mobilized out of the mediastinum, the aorta and the esophagus become nicely visible on the aorta (Fig. 8.3). If one has dissected these layers carefully with minimal bleeding, it is usually easy to identify the two vagal trunks around the esophagus. During further blunt dissection and mobilization

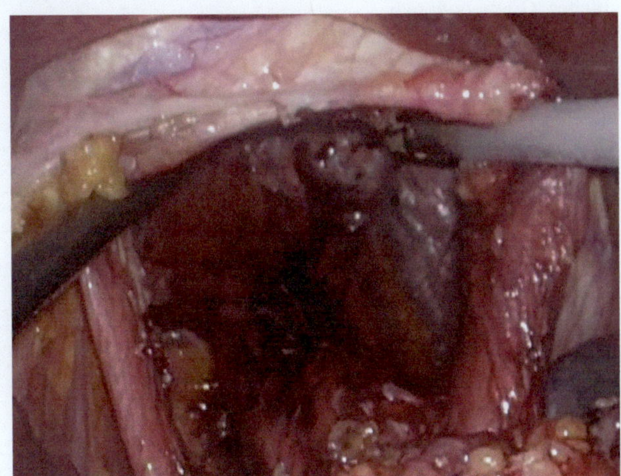

Fig. 8.3 View in the mediastinum after mobilization and resection of the hernia sac. Only these preparations will allow a sufficient anatomical assessment of the esophagus in the mediastinum and a full mobilization

of the esophagus in the mediastinum, it is advisable to keep those two trunks together with the esophagus as a package to avoid any lesions. The next step is the complete resection of the hernia sac and all fatty tissue around the esophagus, especially around the esophagogastric junction. The step requires extreme caution not to harm the vagal trunks. Care should be taken to avoid thermal damage to the vagus by energy devices. On the other hand, it is important to clean the cardia from any of this superfluous tissue. This will allow for a scar tissue development between the esophagus and the fundus. If fatty tissue remains around the cardia and/or this tissue is interposed between the muscle of the cardia and the stomach wall, it will create an easy sliding area for future recurrence of hiatal hernia.

Now, a Penrose drain is slung around the cardia, and the esophagus is pulled downward. It must be double-checked whether the length of the intra-abdominal segment of the LES is sufficient. If this is not the case, more mediastinal dissection is necessary to get a tension-free segment of the LES into the abdominal pressure environment. The resected hernia sac is removed through the largest trocar.

Now, the approximation of the crura is performed by crural hiatoplasty (Fig. 8.4). The esophagus is pulled toward the left side of the abdomen, and this allows for a sufficient view from the right side on the aorta and the hiatus. A figure-of-8 stitch is performed at the lower and posterior part of the crura above the arcuate ligament. Usually, a second figure-of-8 stitch with non-resorbable material size 0 is needed to achieve sufficient narrowing of the hiatus. If the hiatal opening is large and two sutures still leave a gap, more stitches may be needed. There is a danger in creating a posterior obstruction of the esophagus when placing too many posterior crural sutures because the esophagus may be indented by the crura. Such a situation must be avoided. A third suture or more can always be quite easily added in the anterior position of the hiatus ventral to the esophagus. These combined posterior and anterior hiatoplasty should be performed, adequately downsizing the hiatal opening [46]. If the hiatal narrowing cannot be performed sufficiently because the hiatus is

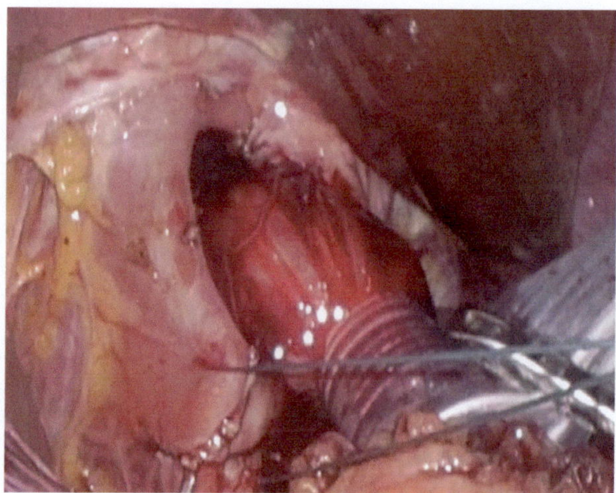

Fig. 8.4 Posterior hiatoplasty with figure-of-8 stitches. Often, only two stitches are sufficient. Otherwise, this can be completed with anterior hiatoplasty stitches

too wide and/or the crural material is too weak to carry a sufficient number of sutures and/or the tension is too large, the surgeon must consider the use of a mesh to complete the hiatal narrowing (see also Chap. 10). If the esophageal mobilization cannot be performed sufficiently because the esophagus is too short, an esophageal lengthening procedure must be added at this point (see Chap. 12).

After narrowing of the hiatus, attention is focused on the shaping and creation of the fundoplication. The mechanical effect of the fundoplication must prevent pathologic reflux in the future, and at the same time, passage of fluids and food must occur without dysphagia. As a consequence, time and care must be invested for this important step of the procedure. In addition, the shape of the wrap must leave enough volume and mobility of the fundus to allow for a postprandial enlargement and fundic accommodation without subsequent early satiety, postprandial epigastric pain, and other unpleasant postprandial symptoms.

To achieve this functional status for the shape of the wrap, an adequate part of the posterior fundic flap must be identified and grasped from the left side of the esophagus and pushed behind the esophagus toward the right side where it is taken over by another grasper to ensure its position. At the same time, the anterior fundic flap is also grasped at the future connection point and pulled over across the anterior aspect of the cardia toward the right side of the esophagus. In doing so, great care is taken to shape the wrap in symmetrical portions around the esophagus (Fig. 8.5). If this is done in the correct fashion, the greater curvature remains on the left side of the esophagus and allows for a sufficient postprandial fundic enlargement and fundic accommodation (Fig. 8.6).

These are very important steps of the procedure, and unfortunately, it is very often done incorrectly as can be seen in many revisional surgeries. An incorrect shaping of the wrap will result in unhappy patients with troublesome and annoying postprandial symptoms after the procedure. Therefore, it is worthwhile to spend time and attention for these maneuvers.

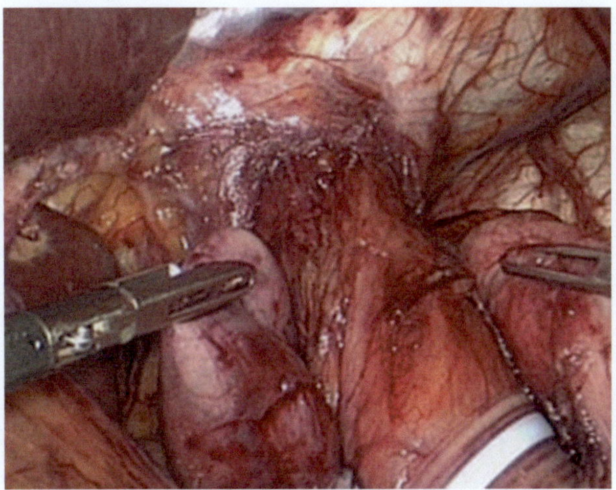

Fig. 8.5 The correct shaping of the Nissen fundoplication is very important for the postoperative long-term function. Care should be invested to shape the wrap short, symmetrical, and floppy to avoid side effects

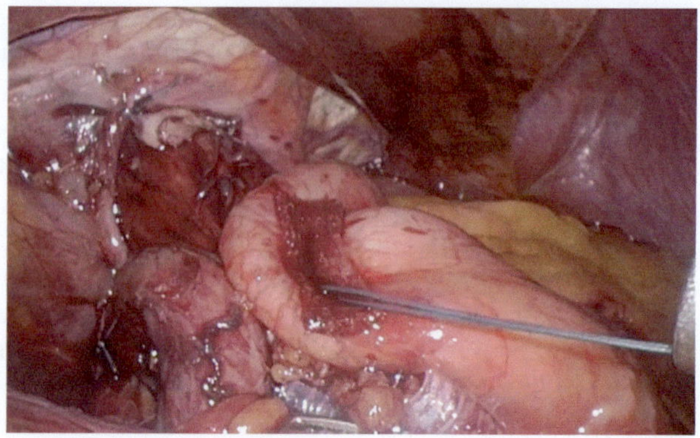

Fig. 8.6 The completed Nissen fundoplication with a short, floppy, and symmetrical-shaped fundic flaps, sutured together with only one U-shaped suture, enforced with pledgets and positioned at the right lateral aspect of the esophagus

To make sure that the wrap is not too tight, a 54 French bougie is placed through the esophagus in the antrum for calibrating the cardia to an optimal size. The advancement of the bougie is observed with great attention by both the anesthesiologist (or whoever person advances the bougie) and the surgeon to make sure that the advancement of the bougie corresponds with the expected intra-abdominal observations. For this procedure, a good communication between the anesthesiologist and the surgeon is very important. If the anesthesiologist pushes the bougie further down the esophagus into the stomach, and at the same time the surgeon cannot see this bougie advancement in the esophagus, there may have been already a perforation in the upper mediastinum or throat. Therefore, to avoid this catastrophe, the communication between these two therapists is essential for the safety of the patients. When the bougie is in its correct antral position, the shape of the wrap is rechecked. Usually, the size of the bougie (54 French) creates an additional tension on the wrap, and it may need some reshaping. This is very important because the fundoplication should be still floppy with the bougie in place [10, 47]. If the tension is too big on the previously shaped fundic flaps after the bougie is placed, the surgeon has to take everything down and reshape the fundic flaps again in order to create a less tight wrap.

When shape and position of the wrap is again double-checked and confirmed to be correct, the wrap is completed and fixed with the typical "DeMeester-sandwich-suture technique" using one U-shaped suture. The suture material (size 0 non-resorbable) is armed with pledgets (Ethisorb™ size 4 × 10 mm). The U-stitch includes the anterior flap of the fundus and then the right lateral aspect of the esophageal wall (on the right side to the anterior vagus) and the posterior fundus followed by another set of pledgets. Then the needle is driven back through the same layers to complete the U-stitch (Fig. 8.6). The suture is tied and the position is secured. The fundoplication is secured by two additional sutures on the fundic flaps. These sutures should not enlarge the fundoplication but just create more suture safety.

After the procedure, the patients may drink fluids in the afternoon after surgery. Since there is quite some edema due to the manipulation and the suturing at the wrap, all patients will have dysphagia directly postoperatively. This is not worrisome. In order to provide time for the edema to resolve on the first postoperative day, only fluids may be given to prevent dysphagia, choking, and vomiting, which may endanger the operative result. On the second postoperative day, usually the edema is reduced, and the patients can have more fluids and semisolid food. Usually, they have very little epigastric pain. On the third postoperative day, the patients eat semisolid food.

Any alteration from this general pathway such as heavy pain should create special attention from the surgeon and nursing staff because that would be unusual and could mean problems may be developing. Patients after primary fundoplications do rarely have severe pain after the first postoperative day. They usually improve their general condition within the first 48 hours remarkably, and any deviation from that should draw attention to it. Some authors start giving patients very early solid food, which is of course also a possibility. Our experience showed that this may be often tolerated. However, with the risk of dysphagia, choking, and vomiting, the latter could be a reason for a high pressure and strain on the sutures and the tissue, followed by an early weakening of the suture situation and also the risk for early migration. Therefore, we decided to stay for 2 days with fluids and liquid nutrition in the early phase.

Special Issues

Vagal lesions can occur during antireflux surgery because their location at the distal esophagus bears the risk of damage during dissection [48–50]. As a consequence, patients should be informed about this possibility for forensic reasons. There are quite some controversial opinions about actions to avoid such lesions. Some authors are convinced that it is not necessary to identify the vagal trunks at the distal esophagus when performing an antireflux surgery. We are convinced that it is of importance to dissect carefully the hiatus and focus during that section rather on the hiatus and then on the esophagus because after a clean dissection of the hiatus, the esophagus and the vagal trunks will remain unharmed in the middle between the crura and the hiatal arch. Afterward, the vagal trunks can be rather easily identified. In the subsequent maneuvers, damage can be prevented by leaving them on the esophageal package.

Vagal damage can result in some functional problems such as chronic diarrhea or increased dumping. However, it can also develop in a complete gastroparesis. The latter can emerge into a catastrophe for the patient because quality of life can be bad. Therefore, this complication should be prevented by all means. There are only few studies investigating the role of vagal lesions after antireflux surgery [50]. These studies show that it is important that the vagal branches should be identified and damage should be avoided [48, 50].

Patients with a large hiatal hernias may run the risk that their hiatus is too large to achieve a sufficient hiatal narrowing. This may require certain surgical steps such as an implantation of the mesh [51–57]. As shown and discussed in a special chapter, the implantation of a mesh can cause severe problems and complications and therefore should be considered carefully for its indication [58–61]. As has been shown in the past 10–15 years, surgeons entertain a controversial discussion about this subject [62–64]. While most surgeons favor only hiatal mesh implantation in selective cases, where an effective narrowing of the hiatus may not be possible with simple sutures, other surgeons like to implant a mesh as hiatal enforcement in every case.

The latter position is not supported by evidence from the last 5 years; however, especially in Europe, hiatal mesh enforcement during laparoscopic antireflux surgery is widespread. The problem is that this can cause severe side effects and complications leading repetitively to resections during the second or third reoperation [60–64] (see Chap. 10).

The term "short esophagus" is used for those cases, in which the esophagus cannot be sufficiently mobilized during an antireflux procedure to achieve a tension-free position of the LES 2–3 cm into the abdominal pressure environment. The incidence of this finding varies in literature remarkably between 1% and 20% [65–67]. A possible surgical solution is the esophageal lengthening procedures such as the Collis cardioplasty (see Chap. 12).

Results of Laparoscopic Nissen Fundoplication

The success rate of laparoscopic Nissen fundoplication has been around 90% good results in experienced esophageal centers in studies with a follow-up time of around 5 years [12–16]. Table 8.1 shows an overview of a selection of publications focusing on laparoscopic Nissen fundoplication. There are some studies available with long-term results of 10 years with a remaining success rate of 80–85% [12, 20, 21, 68–75]. It must be emphasized that at least half of the success for an antireflux surgery is created by an optimal selection of the right patients for surgery and the other half is created by the correct operative technique [41, 42]. As a consequence, only this combination of selection of patients based on extensive diagnostic preparation and well-experienced technique will create good results.

Since laparoscopic antireflux surgery is performed worldwide not only in esophageal centers but also in general surgery services, it may not be surprising that in some overviews, results may be less optimal than in those from esophageal centers. The morbidity of laparoscopic antireflux surgery can be assessed from the results of several randomized trials and large case-control series, which are also demonstrated in Table 8.1 [12, 20, 21, 68–75]. Complication rates may be elevated in the learning phase. Therefore, teaching these laparoscopic procedures is essential for quality and patient care [76–79]. The possible surgical complications can be esophageal and gastric perforations, bleeding, spleen lacerations, and infections as well as early signs of vagal lesions [50]. These complications occur in only 2–3%, while general complications (pneumonia, urinary infections) can be as high as 5–6%. There is evidence that in experienced centers with high caseload, morbidity is below 5% and the mortality below 0.2% [12, 20, 21, 68–75]. Several meta-analyses show a good success rate for laparoscopic antireflux surgery both for a Nissen fundoplication and a Toupet hemifundoplication (Table 8.2). In these studies, the morbidity is

Table 8.1 Overview on results of laparoscopic Nissen fundoplication

Author/year	n	Techniques	Morbidity (%)	Follow-up (months)	Good results (%)	Reflux recurrence (%)
Champault [68] 1994	940	Nissen Hill	5	4–10	92	2
Fuchs [69] 1997	221	Nissen	14	1–56	92	2.4
Peters [12] 1998	100	Nissen	6	8–60	95	2.1
Dallemagne [70] 1998	550	Nissen Toupet	2.3	16–44	96	2
Zaninotto [71] 2000	513	Nissen	15	1–25	91	8.5
Granderath [72] 2003	668	Nissen Toupet	7.6	3–94	93	7
Dallemagne [20] 2006	100	Nissen Toupet	–	60	89.5	6.7 18.2
Fein [21] 2008	120	Nissen Toupet/Dor	3	60	85	15 30/44
Gee [73] 2008	173	Nissen Toupet	–	60	88	10
Anvari [74] 2011 RCT	51	Nissen	–	36	88	11.8
Maret-Ouda [75] 2017	2655	Total + partial fundoplication	4.1	49	82	17.7

published at 0–13%, while the dysphagia rate (3–100%) is under controversial discussion depending on the definition [34, 36–39].

Gastroenterologists report sometimes on quite negative results [80]. The long-term results of antireflux surgery depend on the criteria used to define a failure. If the criteria are any symptoms and/or the use of PPI, the failure rate may be quite high. The latter is caused by the wide use of PPIs with any abdominal or upper GI symptoms occurring within the years after antireflux surgery [81–83]. As a consequence, this criterion is not very discriminative and should not be used. Better are well-established assessments of quality-of-life or objective measurements of the functional result, necessary to receive an in-depth assessment of antireflux surgery.

In upper GI surgery, the discussion around an optimal antireflux procedure is an ongoing process, since many surgeons are entertaining controversial opinions about the optimal technique such as a Nissen fundoplication or a partial fundoplication [34, 36–39]. New antireflux procedures have entered the market such as the LINX antireflux device or endoscopic antireflux procedures [84, 85]. Until decisive randomized comparative trials are finished, this discussion will go on.

Table 8.2 Overview on results of meta-analyses [34, 36–39]

Author/year	Comparison	n	Morbidity (%)	Dysphagia (%)	Reflux recurrence (%)	Redo surgery (%)
Catarci [34] 2004	Total vs. partial wrap	388 405	9.4 13.1	16.8 10.1	16.5 14.9	9.6 1.6
Davis [36] 2010	Total vs. partial wrap	1302	Major morbid 0–7 total 0–5 partial	17 8	7 9	
Broeders [38] 2010	Total vs. partial wrap	371 261	2.5 4.4	13.5 8.6	22.6 18.2	6.9 3.1
Fein [37] 2010	Total vs. partial wrap	1061	0–8 1–10	2–19 0–8	0.4–19.1 0–15.3	–
Tan [39] 2011	Total vs. partial wrap	478 461	Overall: ns (early compl. partial wrap $P < 0.04$)	16.4 6.9	13.1 13	–

Conclusion

Regarding the choice for a Nissen versus a partial fundoplication, the evidence-based data support a partial fundoplication, since the hemifundoplication provides lower reoperation rates and lower postoperative dysphagia than a Nissen fundoplication [34–39]. However, the rates of postoperative dysphagia and postoperative reoperation rate from these studies are at a level of 10–15% [29, 37–39]. In contrast, the levels of postoperative dysphagia and reoperation rate in large case-controlled series from esophageal centers with Nissen fundoplication are both below 5% [12–16, 20, 21]. As a consequence, despite evidence-based results, these experienced surgeons would not change from their standard Nissen procedure to a partial fundoplication because their results are even better than those in the reported trials. This sort of discussion occurred in several guideline committees, and as a conclusion, it was suggested that the surgeons familiar with Nissen or Toupet fundoplication should perform the technique, with which they have the largest experience [40–42].

The principle of mechanical augmentation of the cardia around the incompetent sphincter in GERD remains the best of concept to reconstruct a weak and deteriorated antireflux barrier. Until new data may emerge in the future, the Nissen fundoplication is the best surgical treatment for patients with advanced progressive GERD.

References

1. Nissen R. Eine einfache Operation zur Beeinflussung des Refluxösophagitis. Schweiz Med Wochenschr. 1956;86:590.
2. Allison PR. Peptic ulcer of the oesophagus. Thorax. 1948;3(1):20–42.
3. Allison PR. Reflux esophagitis, sliding hernia and the anatomy of repair. Surg Gynecol Obstet. 1951;92:419–31.

4. Skinner DB, Belsey RH. Surgical management of esophageal reflux and hiatus hernia. Long-term results with 1,030 patients. J Thorac Cardiovasc Surg. 1967;53(1):33–54.
5. Allison PR. Hiatus hernia; a 20 year retrospective survey. Ann Surg. 1973;178:273–6.
6. DeMeester TR, Johnson LF, Kent AH. Evaluation of current operations for the prevention of gastroesophageal reflux. Ann Surg. 1974;180:511–25.
7. Stylopoulos N, Rattner DW. The history of hiatal hernia surgery: from Bowditch to laparoscopy. Ann Surg. 2005;241(1):185–93.
8. Walker SJ, Holt S, Sanderson CJ, Stoddard CJ. Comparison of Nissen total and Lind partial transabdominal fundoplication in the treatment of gastro-oesophageal reflux. Br J Surg. 1992;79(5):410–4.
9. Donahue PE, Samelson S, Nyhus LM, Bombeck CT. The floppy Nissen fundoplication. Arch Surg. 1985;120:A1440.
10. DeMeester TR, Bonavina L, Abertucci M. Nissen fundoplication for gastro-esophageal reflux disease. Evaluation of primary repair in 100 consecutive patients. Ann Surg. 1986;204:19.
11. Dallemagne B, Weerts JM, Jehaes C, Markewicz S, Lombard R. Laparoscopic Nissen fundoplication: preliminary report. Surg Laparosc Endosc. 1991;1:138–43.
12. Peters JH, DeMeester TR, Crookes P, Oberg S, de Vos Shoop M, Hagen JA, Bremner CG. The treatment of gastroesophageal reflux disease with laparoscopic Nissen fundoplication. Ann Surg. 1998;228(1):40–50.
13. Kamolz T, Granderath F, Pointner R. Laparoscopic antireflux surgery: disease-related quality of life assessment before and after surgery in GERD patients with and without Barrett's esophagus. Surg Endosc. 2003;17:880–5.
14. Patti MG, Robinson T, Galvani C, Gorodner MV, Fisichella PM, Way LW. Total fundoplication is superior to partial fundoplication even when esophageal peristalsis is weak. J Am Coll Surg. 2004;198:863–9.
15. Fuchs KH. Conventional and minimally invasive surgical methods for gastro-esophageal reflux. Chirurg. 2005;76:370–8.
16. Fuchs KH, Breithaupt W, Fein M, Maroske J, Hammer I. Laparoscopic Nissen repair: indications, techniques and long term benefits. Langenbeck's Arch Surg. 2005;390:197–202.
17. Thor KB, Silander T. A long-term randomized prospective trial of the Nissen procedure versus a modified Toupet technique. Ann Surg. 1989;210(6):719–24.
18. Laws HL, Clements RH, Swillie CM. A randomized, prospective comparison of the Nissen fundoplication versus the Toupet fundoplication for gastroesophageal reflux disease. Ann Surg. 1997;225(6):647–53.
19. Fibbe C, Layer P, Keller J, Strate U, Emmermann A, Zornig C. Esophageal motility in reflux disease before and after fundoplication: a prospective, randomized, clinical, and manometric study. Gastroenterology. 2001;121:5–14.
20. Dallemagne B, Weertz J, Markiewicz S, Dewandre JM, Wahlen C, Monami B, Jehaes C. Clinical results of laparoscopic fundoplication ten years after surgery. Surg Endosc. 2006;20:159–65.
21. Fein M, Bueter M, Thalheimer A, Pachmayer V, Heimbucher J, Freys SM, Fuchs KH. Ten year outcome of laparoscopic antireflux procedures. J Gastrointest Surg. 2008;12:1893–9.
22. Watson DI, Jamieson GG, Pike GK, Davies N, Richardson M, Devitt PG. Prospective randomized double blind trial between laparoscopic Nissen fundoplication and anterior partial fundoplication. Br J Surg. 1999;86:123–30.
23. Watson DI, Jamieson GG, Ludemann R, Game PA, Devitt PG. Laparoscopic total versus anterior 180 degree fundoplication – Five year follow-up of a prospective randomised trial. Dis Esophagus. 2004;17(suppl 1):A 81,8.
24. Baigrie RJ, Cullis SNR, Ndhluni AJ, Cariem A. Randomized double-blind trial of laparoscopic Nissen fundoplication versus anterior partial fundoplication. Br J Surg. 2005;92:819–23.
25. Ludemann R, Watson DI, Jamieson GG, Game PA, Devitt PG. Five-year follow up of a randomized clinical trial of laparoscopic total versus anterior 180 degrees fundoplication. Br J Surg. 2005;92(2):240–3.

26. Spence GM, Watson DI, Jamieson GG, Lally CJ, Devitt PG. Single center prospective randomized trial of laparoscopic Nissen versus anterior 90 degrees fundoplication. J Gastrointest Surg. 2006;10:698–705.

27. Engström C, Lonroth H, Mardani J, Lundell L. An anterior or posterior approach to partial fundoplication? Long-term results of a randomized trial. World J Surg. 2007;3:1221–5.

28. Guerin E, Betroune K, Closset J, Mehdi A, Lefebre JC, Houben JJ, Gelin M, Vaneukem P, El Nakadi I. Nissen versus Toupet fundoplication: results of a randomized and multicenter trial. Surg Endosc. 2007;21:1985–90.

29. Strate U, Emmermann A, Fibbe C, Layer P, Zornig C. Laparoscopic fundoplication: Nissen versus Toupet two-year outcome of prospective randomized study of 200 patients regarding preoperative esophageal motility. Surg Endosc. 2008;22:21–30.

30. Antanas M, Žilvinas E, Mindaugas K, Laimas J, Limas K, Almantas M, Juzonas P. Influence of wrap length on the effectiveness of Nissen and Toupet fundoplication: a prospective randomized study. Surg Endosc. 2008;22:2269–76.

31. Booth MI, Stratfford J, Jones L, Dehn TC. Randomized clinical trial of laparoscopic Nissen versus posterior partial Toupet fundoplication for GERD based on preoperative manometry. Br J Surg. 2008;95:57–63.

32. Engström C, Lonroth H, Mardani J, Lundell L. An anterior or posterior approach to partial fundoplication? Long-term results of a randomized trial. World J Surg. 2007;31(6):1221–5.

33. Shaw JM, Bornmann PC, Callanan MD, Beckingahm IJ, Metz DC. Long-term outcome of laparoscopic Nissen and laparoscopic Toupet fundoplication for gastroesophageal reflux disease: a prospective, randomized trial. Surg Endosc. 2010;24:924–32.

34. Catarci M, Gentileschi P, Papi C, Carrara A, Marrese R, Gaspari AL, Grassi GB. Evidenced based appraisal of antireflux fundoplication. Ann Surg. 2004;239:325–37.

35. Neufeld M, Graham A. Levels of evidence available for techniques in antireflux surgery. Dis Esophagus. 2007;20:161–7.

36. Davis CS, Baldea A, Johns JR, Joehl RJ, Fisichella PM. The evolution and long-term results of laparoscopic antireflux surgery for the treatment of gastroesophageal reflux disease. JSLS. 2010;14(3):332–41.

37. Fein M, Seyfried F. Is there a role for anything other than a Nissen's operation? J Gastrointest Surg. 2010;14(suppl):S67–74.

38. Broeders JAJL, Mauritz FA, Ahmed Ali U, Draaisma WA, Ruurda JP, Gooszen HG, Smout AJPM, Broeders IAMJ, Hazebroek EJ. Systematic review and metaanalysis of laparoscopic Nissen versus Toupet fundoplication for gastro-esophageal reflux disease. Br J Surg. 2010;97:1318–30.

39. Tan G, Yang Z, Wang Z. Metaanalysis of laparoscopic total Nissen versus posterior Toupet fundoplication for GERD based on randomized clinical trials. ANZ J Surg. 2011;81:246–52.

40. Stefanidis D, Hope WW, Kohn GP, Reardon PR, Richardson WS, Fanelli RD, SAGES Guideline Committee. Guidelines for surgical treatment of GERD. Surg Endosc. 2010;24:2647–69.

41. Fuchs KH, Babic B, Breithaupt W, Dallemagne B, Fingerhut A, Furnee E, Granderath F, Horvath OP, Kardos P, Pointner R, Savarino E, Van Herwarden-Lindeboom M, Zaninotto G. EAES recommendations for the management of gastroesophageal reflux disease. Surg Endosc. 2014;28:1753–73.

42. Koop H, Fuchs KH, Labenz J, Lynen-Jansen P, Messmann H, Miehlke S, Schepp W, Wenzl TG, Mitarbeiter der Leitliniengruppe. S2k-Leitlinie: Gastroösophageale Refluxkrankheit unter der Federführung der DGVS; AWMF-Register Nr. 021013. Z Gastroenterol. 2014;52:1299–346.

43. Horvath KD, Jobe BA, Herron DM, Swanström LL. Laparoscopic Toupet fundoplication is an inadequate procedure for patients with severe reflux disease. J Gastrointest Surg. 1999;3:583–91.

44. Morgenthal CB, Shane MD, Stival A, Gletsu N, Milam G, Swafford S, Hunter JG, Smith CD. The durability of laparoscopic Nissen fundoplication: 11-yeat outcome. J Gastrointest Surg. 2007;11:693–700.

45. DeMeester TR. Etiology and natural history of gastroesophageal reflux disease and predictors of progressive disease. In: Yeo CJ, DeMeester SR, Fadden DWM, editors. Shackelford's surgery of the alimentary tract. 8th ed. Philadelphia: Elsevier; 2019. p. 204–20.
46. Chew CR, Jamieson GG, Devitt PG, Watson DI. Prospective randomized trial of laparoscopic Nissen fundoplication with anterior versus posterior hiatal repair: late outcomes. World J Surg. 2011;35:2038–44.
47. Patterson EJ, Herron DM, Hansen PD, Ramzi N, Standage BA, Swanstrom LL. Effect of an esophageal bougie on the incidence of dysphagia following Nissen fundoplication; a prospective, blinded, randomized clinical trial. Arch Surg. 2000;135(9):1055–61.
48. Peillon C, Manouvrier JL, Labreche J, Kaeffer N, Denis P, Testart J. Should be vagus nerves be isolated from the fundoplication wrap? A prospective study. Arch Surg. 1994;129(8):814–8.
49. Purdy M, Nykopp TK, Kainulainen S, Pääkkönen M. Division of the hepatic branch of the anterior vagus verve in fundoplication: effects on gallbladder function. Surg Endosc. 2009;23:2143–6.
50. Van Rijn S, Roebroek YGM, Conchillo JM, Bouvy ND, Masclee AAM. Effect of vagus nerve injury on the outcome of antireflux surgery: an extensive literature review. Dig Surg. 2016;33:230–9.
51. Frantzides CT, Madan AK, Carlson MA, Stavrpoulos GP. A prospective randomized trial of laparoscopic polytetrafluoroethylene (PTFE) patch repair vs simple cruroplasty for large hiatal hernia. Arch Surg. 2002;137(6):649–52.
52. Granderath FA, Schweiger UM, Kamolz T, Asche KU, Pointner R. Laparoscopic Nissen fundoplication with prosthetic hiatal closure reduces postoperative intrathoracic wrap herniation: preliminary results of a prospective randomized functional and clinical study. Arch Surg. 2005;140:40–8.
53. Rathore MA, Andrabi SIH, Bhatti MI, Najfi SMH, McMurray A. Metaanalysis of recurrence after laparoscopic repair of paraesophageal hernia. JSLS. 2007;11(4):456–60.
54. Soricelli E, Basso N, Genco A, Cipriano M. Long-term results of hiatal hernia mesh repair and antireflux laparoscopic surgery. Surg Endosc. 2009;23:2499–504.
55. Oelschlager BK, Pellegrini CA, Hunter JG, Brunt ML, Soper NJ, Sheppard BC, Polisaar NL, Neradilek MB, Mitsumori LM, Rohrmann CA, Swanstrom LL. Biologic prosthesis to prevent recurrence after laparoscopic paraesophageal hernia repair: long-term follow-up from a multicenter, prospective, randomized trial. J Am Coll Surg. 2011;213:461–8.
56. Watson DI, Thompson SK, Devitt PG, Smith L, Woods SD, Aly A, Gan S, Game PA, Jamieson GG. Laparoscopic repair of very large Hiatus hernia with sutures versus absorbable mesh versus nonabsorbable mesh: a randomized controlled trial. Ann Surg. 2015;261:282–9.
57. Müller-Stich BP, Kenngott HG, Gondan M, Stock C, Linke GR, Fritz F, Nickel F, Diener MK, Gutt CN, Wente M, Büchler MW, Fischer L. Use of mesh in laparoscopic paraesophageal hernia repair: a meta-analysis and risk-benefit analysis. PLoS One. 2015;10(10):eO139547.
58. Arendt T, Stuber E, Monig H, Folsch UR, Katsoulis S. Dysphagia due to transmural migration of surgical material into the esophagus nine years after Nissen fundoplication. Gastrointest Endosc. 2000;51:607–10.
59. Targarona EM, Bendahan G, Balague C, Garriga J, Trias M. Mesh in the hiatus a controversial issue. Arch Surg. 2004;139:1286–96.
60. Stadlhuber RJ, Sherif AE, Mittal SK, Fitzgibbons RJ, Brunt LM, Hunter JG, DeMeester TR, Swanstrom LL, Smith CD, Filipi CJ. Mesh complications after prosthetic reinforcement of hiatal closure: a 28-case series. Surg Endosc. 2009;23:1219–26.
61. Parker M, Bowers SP, Bray JM, Harris AS, Belli EV, Pfluke JM, Preissler S, Asbun HJ, Smith CD. Hiatal mesh is associated with major resection at revisional operation. Surg Endosc. 2010;24(12):3095–101.
62. Koetje JH, Oor JE, Roks DJ, Van Westreenen HL, Hazebroek EJ, Nieuwenhuijs VB. Equal patient satisfaction, quality of life and objective recurrence rate after laparoscopic hiatal hernia repair with and without mesh. Surg Endosc. 2017;31(9):3673–80. https://doi.org/10.1007/s00464-016-5405-9.

63. Zhang C, Liu D, Li F, Watson DI, Gao X, Koetje JH, Luo T, Yan C, Du X, Wang Z. Systematic review and metaanalysis of laparoscopic mesh versus suture repair of hiatus hernia: objective and subjective outcomes. Surg Endosc. 2017;31(12):4913–22. https://doi.org/10.1007/s00464-017-5586-x.

64. Oor JE, Roks DJ, Koetje JH, Broeders JA, van Westreenen HL, Nieuwenhuijs VB, Hazebroek EJ. Randomized clinical trial comparing laparoscopic hiatal hernia repair using sutures versus sutures reinforced with non-absorbable mesh. Surg Endosc. 2018;32(11):4579–89. https://doi.org/10.1007/s00464-018-6211-3.

65. Mattioli S, Lugaresi ML, Costantini M, Del Genio A, Di Martino N, Fei L, Fumagalli U, Maffettone V, Monaco L, Morino M, Rebecchi F, Rosati R, Rossi M, Sant S, Trapani V, Zaninotto G. The short esophagus: intraoperative assessment of esophageal length. J Thorac Cardiovasc Surg. 2008;136:1610.

66. Yano F, Stadlhuber K, Tsuboi J, Gerhard C, Filipi J, Mittal SK. Outcomes of surgical treatment of intrathoracic stomach. Dis Esophagus. 2009;22:284–8.

67. DeMeester SR. Laparoscopic paraesophageal hernia repair: critical steps and adjunct techniques to minimize recurrence. Surg Laparosc Endosc Percutan Tech. 2013;23(5):429–35. https://doi.org/10.1097/SLE.0b013e3182a12716.

68. Champault G. Gastroesophageal reflux treatment by laparoscopy in 940 cases – French experience. Ann Chir. 1994;48:159–64.

69. Fuchs KH, Feussner H, Bonavina L, Collard JM, Coosemans W. Current status and trends in laparoscopic antireflux surgery: results of a consensus meeting. The European Study Group dor Antireflux Surgery (ESGARS). Endoscopy. 1997;29:298–308.

70. Dallemagne B, Weerts JM, Jehaes C, Markiewicz S. Results of laparoscopic Nissen fundoplication. Hepato-Gastroenterology. 1998;45:1338–43.

71. Zaninotto G, Molena D, Ancona E. A prospective multicentre study on laparoscopic treatment of GERD in Italy: type of surgery, conversions, complications, and early results. Surg Endosc. 2000;14:282–8.

72. Granderath FA, Kamolz T, Schweiger UM, Pointner R. Laparoscopic antireflux surgery for GERD: experience with 668 laparoscopic antireflux procedures. Int J Color Dis. 2003;18:73–7.

73. Gee DW, Andreoli ABA, Rattner DW. Measuring the effectiveness of laparoscopic antireflux surgery. Arch Surg. 2008;143:482–7.

74. Anvari M, Allen C, Marshall J, Armstrong D, Goree R, Ungar W, Goldsmith C. A randomized controlled trial of laparoscopic Nissen fundoplication versus proton pump inhibitors for the treatment of patients with chronic gastrooesophageal reflux disease (GERD): 3 year outcomes. Surg Endosc. 2011;25(8):2547–54.

75. Maret-Ouda J, Wahlin K, El-Serag HB, Lagergren J. Association between laparoscopic antireflux surgery and recurrence of gastroesophageal reflux. JAMA. 2017;318:939–46.

76. Watson DI, Baigrie RJ, Jamieson GG. A learning curve for laparoscopic fundoplication: definable, avoidable, or a waste of time? Ann Surg. 1996;224:198–203.

77. Champault GG, Barrat C, Rozon RC, Rizk N, Catheline JM. The effect of the learning curve on the outcome of laparoscopic treatment for gastroesophageal reflux. Surg Laparosc Endosc Percutan Tech. 1999;9(6):375–81.

78. Salminen PTP, Hiekkanen HI, Laine H, Ovaska JT. Surgeons experience with laparoscopic fundoplication after early personal experience: does it have an impact on the outcome? Surg Endosc. 2007;21:1377–82.

79. Tsuboi K, Gazallo J, Yano F, Filipi CJ, Mittal SK. Good training allows excellent results for laparoscopic Nissen fundoplication even early in the surgeon's experience. Surg Endosc. 2010;24:2723–9.

80. Spechler SJ, Lee E, Ahnen D, Goyal RK, Hirano I, Ramirez F, Raufman JP, Sampliner R, Schnell T, Sontag S, Vlahcevic ZR, Young R, Williford W. Long-term outcome of medical and surgical therapies for gastroesophageal reflux disease: follow-up of a randomized controlled trial. JAMA. 2001;285(18):2331–8.

81. Bonatti H, Bammer T, Achem SR, Lukens F, DeVault KR, Klaus A, Hinder RA. Use of acid suppressive medications after laparoscopic antireflux surgery: prevalence and clinical indications. Dig Dis Sci. 2007;52:267–72.
82. Madan A, Minoch A. Despite high satisfaction, majority of gastro-esophageal reflux disease patients continue to use PPI after antireflux surgery. Aliment Pharmacol Ther. 2006;23(5):601–5.
83. Ciovica R, Riedl O, Neumayer C, Lechner W, Schwab GP, Gadenstätter M. The use of medication after laparoscopic antireflux surgery. Surg Endosc. 2009;23:1938–46.
84. Alicuben ET, Bell RCW, Jobe BA, Buckley FP 3rd, Daniel Smith C, Graybeal CJ, Lipham JC. Worldwide experience with erosion of the magnetic sphincter augmentation device. J Gastrointest Surg. 2018;22(8):1442–7. https://doi.org/10.1007/s11605-018-3775-0.
85. Aiolfi A, Asti E, Bernardi D, Bonitta G, Rausa E, Siboni S, Bonavina L. Early results of magnetic sphincter augmentation versus fundoplication for gastroesophageal reflux disease: Systematic review and meta-analysis. Int J Surg. 2018;52:82–8. https://doi.org/10.1016/j.ijsu.2018.02.041.

The Posterior Partial Toupet Hemifundoplication

9

Wolfram Breithaupt and Gabor Varga

Introduction

The history of antireflux surgery reflects on one hand the search for a stable mechanical augmentation of the weak lower esophageal sphincter (LES) as part of the antireflux barrier and on the other hand the search for a mechanical augmentation with only few side effects for the patients [1–6]. With the Nissen fundoplication, a full 360° wrap around the cardia, already in the early experience dysphagia and other side effects occurred and were reported [2]. For a long time, the pexy procedures were a competition to the Nissen fundoplication [1, 4]. Especially Allison favored his technique of gastropexy [1, 4]. However, during the 1960s, he realized that his pexy procedures were rather too weak to prevent long-term gastroesophageal reflux [4]. In North America and Western Europe, the Belsey Mark IV procedure was very popular in the 1960s and 1970s as partial fundoplication [3, 6, 7]. However, this technique suffered somewhat from the sequelae of the left thoracic approach with persisting thoracic pain. Other partial fundoplications were introduced such as the Thal, the Dor, and the Lind procedures, which had possibly less postoperative dysphagia and other side effects than the 360° Nissen fundoplication [8–10].

The posterior partial Toupet hemifundoplication was published in the early 1960s but was not used very frequently until it was reintroduced in the early 1990s with the advent of minimal invasive surgery [8, 11, 12]. The popular Belsey Mark IV procedure in the open transthoracic technique turned out to be very difficult to perform in the early days of thoracoscopic experience and therefore was abandoned. The laparoscopic technique of the Toupet procedure was introduced quite quickly because, on one hand, it was similar to the successful laparoscopic Nissen

W. Breithaupt (✉) · G. Varga
Agaplesion Markus Krankenhaus, Department of General and GI-Surgery, Frankfurt am Main, Germany
e-mail: wolfram.Breithaupt@fdk.info

© Springer Nature Switzerland AG 2020
S. Horgan, K.-H. Fuchs (eds.), *Management of Gastroesophageal Reflux Disease*,
https://doi.org/10.1007/978-3-030-48009-7_9

procedure and, at the other hand, it promised to have less side effects because of its partial shape [12].

Other partial fundoplications were also performed in the laparoscopic technique such as the Lind, the Watson, and the Dor procedure [9, 10]. A number of comparative studies and randomized trials were performed to evaluate the advantages of partial fundoplications [13–29]. The results of a selective group of studies are demonstrated in Table 9.1 [14–18, 20, 21].

The Toupet hemifundoplication was also used for the "tailored concept" by surgeons whose standard antireflux procedure was the Nissen fundoplication, but they were looking for a weaker augmentation of the cardia for patients with insufficient esophageal motility [5, 16, 28, 30]. The posterior partial Toupet hemifundoplication became one of the most successful laparoscopic antireflux procedures [20, 29].

Operative Technique

The patient is positioned in a steep anti-Trendelenburg position to gain a good exposure of the upper two abdominal quadrants and the hiatal region. The operation is started by introducing four or five trocars (3 × 10 mm and 2 × 5 mm). The left liver lobe can be retracted by a 5 mm instrument. The gastric fundus is pulled down and to the right with a grasper, exposing the left subphrenic area. Then the most cranial

Table 9.1 Overview on early results after laparoscopic posterior partial Toupet hemifundoplication

Author/year	Pt. n	Follow-up months	Good results (%)	Recurrence (%)	Dysphagia (%)	Morbidity (%)	Study
Cuschieri [14] 1993	36	13	86	11	0	3	Case control Toupet
Wetscher [16] 1997	32	15	97	3	3	13	Case control Toupet
McKernan [17] 1998	348	33	90	5.5	0	–	Case control Toupet
Lundell [15] 1998	72	60	90	5.5	3	–	RCT Ant. vs. post.
Rydberg [18] 1999	53	36	80	3.7	0	–	RCT Ant vs. post.
Freys [21] 2000	51	48	88	8	2	6	Case control
Zornig [20] 2001	100	12	90	10	6	–	RCT Nissen vs. Toupet

part of the fundus is dissected from the spleen by dividing the short gastric vessels with an energy instrument. The mobilization of the fundus especially in its posterior aspect is necessary in order to free the posterior part of the fundus to allow for a symmetric partial wrap. As a consequence, the fundic mobilization along the spleen and the separation of the short gastric vessels can be kept quite minimal to the most upper part.

The left crus is dissected, and the left lateral border of the hernia sac at the left crus is lifted with a grasper, allowing for a blunt dissection of the hernia sac in the lower mediastinum. This will eventually allow a view on the aorta and the distal esophagus. Now, the attention is focused on the right crus and its dissection. For this step, the upper part of the pars flaccida is opened. It must be emphasized that we like to leave the vagal branches in the pars flaccida toward the liver intact and keep the opening of the pars flaccida limited in order to preserve a support structure for the fundoplication to avoid migration.

Similar to the left crus, the lateral border of the hiatal sac at the right crus can be grasped, dissected, and pulled up to complete the mobilization of the hernia sac at the right side in the mediastinum. The hernia sac is resected completely under careful precautions and preservation of the vagal trunks. A full mobilization of the distal esophagus is added until the lower esophageal sphincter can be placed tension-free approximately 2–3 cm within the abdominal cavity. A loop is placed around the esophagus to pull on the distal esophagus while mobilizing the esophagus in the mediastinum.

After full dissection and mobilization of the esophagus, the crural narrowing can be performed using a standard technique with non-resorbable suture material (size 0). In a figure-of-8 stitch fashion, the crura are approximated and adapted just above the arcuate ligament. Usually, two figure-of-8 stitches are sufficient to adapt the crura posterior to the esophagus. In large hiatal openings, a third stitch and/or an additional anterior hiatoplasty may be added as needed. It must be ensured that there is still room for a 10 mm instrument between crural muscular border and the esophageal wall in order to avoid hiatal dysphagia.

Now, the shaping of the partial fundoplication is performed by identifying the posterior and the anterior aspect of the fundus. Then the posterior aspect of the fundus is grasped and pushed over from the left side to the right side of the esophagus. The hemifundoplication is shaped using a shoeshine maneuver as well as making sure that the fundus has a loose position to be able to enlarge in its volume postoperatively when food is filled into the stomach. For calibration, a 54 French bougie may be entered into the esophagus and stomach; however, it is probably less necessary than in total fundoplication.

The pulled-over posterior part of the fundus is fixed with two sutures on the right crus, and then the fundus flap is also fixed on the distal esophagus with three sutures. Care is taken not to harm the anterior vagus when placing the sutures for the posterior fundic flap on the right lateral side of the esophagus. This is followed by the fixation of the anterior fundic flap on the left lateral side of the esophagus by again three sutures of non-resorbable material (Fig. 9.1). Some authors also fix the anterior fundic flap to the left crus with a few stitches.

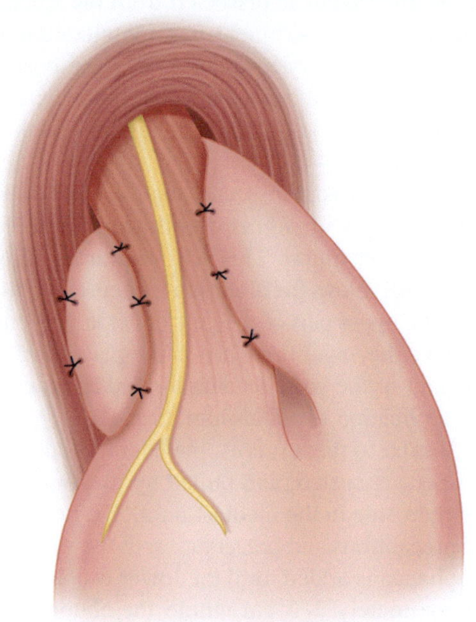

Fig. 9.1 Scheme of a laparoscopic Toupet hemifundoplication. Note the fixation of the posterior and anterior fundic flap on the right and respectively left side of the esophageal wall, leaving in the middle space for the anterior vagal nerve

Special Issues About the Partial Fundoplication

Evidence in literature has shown that partial fundoplications may have less mechanical effect of augmentation on the distal esophagus [16, 28, 30, 31]. This can be of advantage in patients with insufficient esophageal motility and sometimes impaired esophageal clearance in that a partial fundoplication would allow a dysphagia-free passage of food through a somewhat weaker wrap at the lower esophageal sphincter [32]. This effect was used in the tailored approach, which was popularized in the 1990s as a possible concept using the fundoplication with a 360° wrap as the standard procedure and the 240–270° partial fundoplication as a somewhat weaker wrap for patients with esophageal motility disorders [28, 30, 31]. This tailored approach required the preoperative assessment of the esophageal motility in order to make a therapeutic decision whether to perform a partial or full fundoplication. On the other hand, there was some evidence that a partial fundoplication may have less durability and worse long-term results than in Nissen fundoplication [5, 33, 34].

This data is discussed very controversially among surgeons [16, 20, 22, 30, 32–34]. Two randomized trials have shown that a tailored concept may be not justified since a Nissen fundoplication can also be used in esophageal motility disorder patients to a certain extent and furthermore that partial fundoplication may still have less side effects than a Nissen fundoplication [18–20]. Different conclusions were drawn from these results, and since some authors expanded their indication for a Nissen fundoplication to almost all GERD patients even with impaired esophageal motility, others would completely switch to hemifundoplications. Several randomized trials and meta-analyses have been performed for technical aspects of fundoplications [35–41]. It was demonstrated that there were increased rates of side effects with the Nissen fundoplication and a reduced revisional surgery rate for partial fundoplication [35–41].

These findings fueled the discussions even more since some authors decided to focus only on partial fundoplications and the majority of these favored the Toupet hemifundoplication [20, 32]. It must be emphasized that evidence shows that there is probably an increased risk for problems for inexperienced surgeons in the Nissen technique regarding dysphagia rate postoperatively [35, 36]. Therefore, it is advisable that surgeons with limited experience in antireflux surgery should definitely start with a Toupet fundoplication and prevent and avoid a full fundoplication in their initial experience [35, 36]. It must be further emphasized that the partial Toupet hemifundoplication is an ideal procedure for patients with gastroesophageal reflux and associated esophageal motility disorders with weak peristalsis [42–44]. This technique can even be used in patients with aperistalsis [44].

Results of Partial Toupet Hemifundoplication

A number of case-control series with laparoscopic Toupet fundoplication have been published in the 1990s, as well as several randomized trials have shown advantages for the posterior partial Toupet hemifundoplication. In Table 9.1, the early results of laparoscopic Toupet hemifundoplications are demonstrated as well as the results of randomized trials [14–18, 20]. The data show a recurrence rate of reflux in 4–6% and a dysphagia rate of 0–3%. In patients with severe and advanced GERD with higher grades of reflux esophagitis, defective lower esophageal sphincter, Barrett's esophagus, and strictures, the Toupet hemifundoplication may have a higher recurrence rate compared to Nissen fundoplication [33, 34].

It is interesting that esophageal motility may well partially recover after a partial fundoplication is used as antireflux therapy since some studies show an improved peristalsis sometimes after antireflux surgery [42–44].

Current evidence shows that the antireflux effect of laparoscopic Toupet hemifundoplication is comparable to the effect of a full wrap (Nissen fundoplication) (Table 9.2) [32, 37–41]. In addition, results of randomized trials show that the Toupet hemifundoplication has less side effects in the follow-up period and shows less necessity for reoperations. This is confirmed in several meta-analyses, demonstrating an advantage of Toupet hemifundoplication over the Nissen fundoplication (Table 9.2). These results have been discussed controversially many times on surgical meetings and also within guideline committees because other evidence mainly from large centers with large series with Nissen fundoplication shows a lower rate of side effects and dysphagia [34, 37, 39]. This remains controversial.

An explanation for these controversial results can be explained by individual experience of surgeons with one or the other technique. It may be well true that even though these two techniques are not that much different, one surgeon can create a

Table 9.2 Overview on results of meta-analyses for laparoscopic Toupet hemifundoplication

Author/ year	Study comparison	*n*	Morbidity (%)	Dysphagia (%)	Reflux recurrence (%)	Redo (%)	Comment
Catarci [32] 2004	Total vs. partial wrap	388 405	9.4 13.1	16.8 10.1	16.5 14.9	9.6 1.6	Partial fundoplication better
Neufeld [37] 2007	Total vs. partial wrap	898	–	–	Four studies: No difference Four studies: Partial wrap better		
Davis [38] 2010	Total vs. partial wrap	1302	Major morbidity: Total: 0–7 Partial: 0–5	17 8	7 9		Toupet: Dysphagia better
Broeders [40] 2010	Total vs. partial	371 261	2.5 4.4	13.5 8.6	22.6 18.2	6.9 3.1	Toupet better
Fein [34] 2010	Total vs. partial	1061	0–8 1–10	2–19 0–8	0.4–19.1 0–15.3	–	Depends on surgeon
Tan [41] 2011	Total vs. partial	478 461	No major difference	16.4 6.9	13.1 13	–	Depends on surgeon

better experience and better results with the Nissen technique and another surgeon has a better result with the Toupet technique [34, 39]. This issue was discussed in several guideline committees, and it was suggested that it should be the surgeon's preference what technique she or he uses [35, 36]. Surgeons should use the one where the team has the most experience with. Sufficient information should be given to the patients to involve them in the decision process.

Conclusion

Laparoscopic posterior Toupet hemifundoplication is a very successful antireflux procedure with a rather low rate on side effects postoperatively. Based on current evidence-based criteria and meta-analyses, the Toupet hemifundoplication is superior to the Nissen fundoplication due to lower postoperative dysphagia rates and lower reoperation rate.

References

1. Allison PR. Reflux esophagitis, sliding hernia and the anatomy of repair. Surg Gynecol Obstet. 1951;92:419–31.
2. Nissen R. Eine einfache Operation zur Beeinflussung des Refluxösophagitis. Schweiz Med Wochenschr. 1956;86:590.
3. Skinner DB, Belsey RH. Surgical management of esophageal reflux and hiatus hernia. Long-term results with 1,030 patients. J Thorac Cardiovasc Surg. 1967;53(1):33–54.

4. Allison PR. Hiatus hernia; a 20 year retrospective survey. Ann Surg. 1973;178:273–6.
5. DeMeester TR, Johnson LF, Kent AH. Evaluation of current operations for the prevention of gastroesophageal reflux. Ann Surg. 1974;180:511–25.
6. Stylopoulos N, Rattner DW. The history of hiatal hernia surgery: from Bowditch to laparoscopy. Ann Surg. 2005;241(1):185–93.
7. Lerut T, Coosemans W, Christiaeus R, Gruwez JA. The Belsey Mark IV antireflux procedure. Indications and long-term results. In: Little AG, Ferguson MK, Skinner DP, editors. Diseases of the esophagus, Vol II: Benign diseases. Mount Kisco: Futura; 1990. p. S.181–8.
8. Thor KBA, Silander T. A long-term randomized prospective trial of the Nissen procedure versus a modified Toupet technique. Ann Surg. 1989;220:719–24.
9. Watson A, Jenkinson LR, Bell CS, Barlow AP, Norris TL. A more physiological alternative to total fundoplication for the surgical correction of resistant gastro-oesophageal reflux. Br J Surg. 1991;78:1088–94.
10. Walker SJ, Holt S, Sanderson CJ, Stoddard CJ. Comparison of Nissen total and Lind partial transabdominal fundoplication in the treatment of gastro-oesophageal reflux. Br J Surg. 1992;79:410.
11. Toupet A. Technique d'oesophago-gastroplastie avec phrenogastropexie appliqueè dans la cure radicale des hernies hiatales et comme complement de l'operation d'Heller dans les cardiospasmes. Mem Acad Chir. 1963;89:394–9.
12. Swanström LL, Hunter JG. Laparoscopic partial fundoplication. In: Peters JH, DeMeester TR, editors. Minimally invasive surgery of the foregut. St Louis: QMP; 1994. p. S.159–75.
13. Lundell L, Abrahamsson H, Ruth M, Sandberg L, Olbe L. Lower esophageal sphincter characteristics and esophageal acid exposure following partial or 360° fundoplication: results of a prospective, randomized, clinical study. World J Surg. 1991;15:115–21.
14. Cuschieri A, Hunter J, Wolfe B, Swanstrom LL, Hutson W. Multicenter prospective evaluation of laparoscopic antireflux surgery. Surg Endosc. 1993;7:505–10.
15. Lundell L, Abrahamsson H, Ruth M, Rydberg L, Lonroth H, Olbe L. Long-term results of a prospective randomized comparison of total fundic wrap (Nissen-Rossetti) or semifundoplication (Toupet) for gastro-oesophageal reflux. Br J Surg. 1996;83(6):830–5.
16. Wetscher GJ, Glaser K, Wieschemeyer T, Gadenstätter M. Tailored antireflux surgery for gastroesophageal reflux disease: effectiveness and risk of postoperative dysphagia. World J Surg. 1997;21:605–10.
17. McKernan JB, Champion JK. Minimal invasive antireflux surgery. Am J Surg. 1998;175:271–6.
18. Rydberg L, Ruth M, Abrahamsson H, Lundell L. Tailoring antireflux surgery: a randomized clinical trial. World J Surg. 1999;23:612–8.
19. Fibbe C, Layer P, Keller J, Strate U, Emmermann A, Zornig C. Esophageal motility in reflux disease before and after fundoplication: a prospective, randomized, clinical, and manometric study. Gastroenterology. 2001;121:5–14.
20. Zornig C, Strate U, Fibbe C, Emmermann A, Layer P. Nissen vs Toupet laparoscopic fundoplication. Surg Endosc. 2002;16(5):758–66.
21. Freys SM. Die laparoskopische partielle Fundoplikatio nach Toupet. In: Fuchs KH, Freys SM, Fein M, Thiede A, editors. Laparoskopische Antirefluxchirurgie. Heidelberg: Kaden Verlag; 2003. p. 57–68.
22. Watson DI, Jamieson GG, Ludemann R, Game PA, Devitt PG. Laparoscopic total versus anterior 180 degree fundoplication – Five year follow-up of a prospective randomised trial. Dis Esophagus. 2004;17(suppl 1):A 81,8.
23. Baigrie RJ, Cullis SNR, Ndhluni AJ, Cariem A. Randomized double-blind trial of laparoscopic Nissen fundoplication versus anterior partial fundoplication. Br J Surg. 2005;92:819–23.
24. Ludemann R, Watson DI, Jamieson GG, Game PA, Devitt PG. Five-year follow up of a randomized clinical trial of laparoscopic total versus anterior 180 degrees fundoplication. Br J Surg. 2005;92(2):240–3.
25. Spence GM, Watson DI, Jamieson GG, Lally CJ, Devitt PG. Single center prospective randomized trial of laparoscopic Nissen versus anterior 90 degrees fundoplication. J Gastrointest Surg. 2006;10:698–705.

26. Engström C, Lonroth H, Mardani J, Lundell L. An anterior or posterior approach to partial fundoplication? Long-term results of a randomized trial. World J Surg. 2007;3:1221–5.
27. Guerin E, Betroune K, Closset J, Mehdi A, Lefebre JC, Houben JJ, Gelin M, Vaneukem P, El Nakadi I. Nissen versus Toupet fundoplication: results of a randomized and multicenter trial. Surg Endosc. 2007;21:1985–90.
28. Fein M, Bueter M, Thalheimer A, Pachmayer V, Heimbucher J, Freys SM, Fuchs KH. Ten year outcome of laparoscopic antireflux procedures. J Gastrointest Surg. 2008;12:1893–9.
29. Strate U, Emmermann A, Fibbe C, Layer P, Zornig C. Laparoscopic fundoplication: Nissen versus Toupet two-year outcome of prospective randomized study of 200 patients regarding preoperative esophaegal motility. Surg Endosc. 2008;22:21–30.
30. Fuchs KH, Heimbucher J, Freys SM, Thiede A. Management of gastro-esophageal reflux disease 1995. Tailored concept of anti-reflux operations. Dis Esophagus. 1994;7:250–4.
31. Freys SM, Fuchs KH, Heimbucher J, Thiede A. Tailored augmentation of the lower esophageal sphincter in experimental antireflux operations. Surg Endosc. 1997;11(12):1183–8.
32. Catarci M, Gentileschi P, Papi C, Carrara A, Marrese R, Gaspari AL, Grassi GB. Evidenced based appraisal of antireflux fundoplication. Ann Surg. 2004;239:325–37.
33. Horvath KD, Jobe BA, Herron DM, Swanstrom LL. Laparoscopic Toupet fundoplication is an inadequate procedure for patients with severe reflux disease. J Gastrointest Surg. 1999;3:583–91.
34. Patti MG, Robinson T, Galvani C, Gorodner MV, Fisichella PM, Way LW. Total fundoplication is superior to partial fundoplication even when esophageal peristalsis is weak. J Am Coll Surg. 2004;198:863–9.
35. Stefanidis D, Hope WW, Kohn GP, Reardon PR, Richardson WS, Fanelli RD, SAGES Guideline Committee. SAGES Guidelines for surgical treatment of GERD. Surg Endosc. 2010;24:2647–69.
36. Fuchs KH, Babic B, Breithaupt W, Dallemagne B, Fingerhut A, Furnee E, Granderath F, Horvath OP, Kardos P, Pointner R, Savarino E, Van Herwarden-Lindeboom M, Zaninotto G. EAES recommendations for the management of gastroesophageal reflux disease. Surg Endosc. 2014;28:1753–73.
37. Neufeld M, Graham A. Levels of evidence available for techniques in antireflux surgery. Dis Esophagus. 2007;20:161–7.
38. Davis CS, Baldea A, Johns JR, Joehl RJ, Fisichella PM. The evolution and long-term results of laparoscopic antireflux surgery for the treatment of gastroesophageal reflux disease. JSLS. 2010;14(3):332–41.
39. Fein M, Seyfried F. Is there a role for anything other than a Nissen's operation? J Gastrointest Surg. 2010;14(suppl):S67–74.
40. Broeders JAJL, Mauritz FA, Ahmed Ali U, Draaisma WA, Ruurda JP, Gooszen HG, Smout AJPM, Broeders IAMJ, Hazebroek EJ. Systematic review and metaanalysis of laparoscopic Nissen versus Toupet fundoplication for gastro-esophageal reflux disease. Br J Surg. 2010;97:1318–30.
41. Tan G, Yang Z, Wang Z. Metaanalysis of laparoscopic total Nissen versus posterior Toupet fundoplication for GERD based on randomized clinical trials. ANZ J Surg. 2011;81:246–52.
42. Broeders JA, Sportel IG, Jamieson GG, Nijjar RS, Granchi N, Myers JC, Thompson SK. Impact of ineffective oesophageal motility and wrap type on dysphagia after laparoscopic fundoplication. Br J Surg. 2011;98:1414–21.
43. Fuchs HF, Gutschow CA, Brinkmann S, Herbold T, Bludau M, Schröder W, Bollschweiler E, Hölscher AH, Leers JM. Effect of laparoscopic antireflux surgery on esophageal motility. Dig Surg. 2014;31(4–5):354–8.
44. Watson DI, Jamieson GG, Bessell JR, Devitt PG. Laparoscopic fundoplication in patients with an aperistaltic esophagus and gastroesophageal reflux. Dis Esophagus. 2006;19:94–8.

Controversies Regarding Mesh Implantation for Hiatal Reinforcement in GERD and Hiatal Hernia Surgery

10

Ryan C. Broderick

Introduction

The failure of laparoscopic fundoplication and hiatal hernia repair has long been a vexing problem for surgeons and patients. Especially in large hiatal hernias, paraesophageal hernias, and upside-down stomachs, the recurrence rate is reported as high as 40% [1–7]. The underlying mechanism is a migration of the proximal stomach through the hiatal opening into the mediastinum. During primary antireflux procedures, the initial hiatal hernia is reduced by dissection and resection of the hernia sac and mobilization of the esophagus; therefore, an empty space remains in the lower mediastinum. Postoperatively, one can encourage patients to perform breathing exercises in order to allow for enlargement of the lower portions of the lungs to take over that space. However, usually the area around the distal esophagus in the lower mediastinum remains an empty space, which facilitates a migration of the proximal stomach upward if intra-abdominal pressure and esophageal tension remain high. The latter is supported heavily by intense physical body activity like hard work and straining, increased intra-abdominal fat, and increased esophageal tension by length shortening due to insufficient mobilization in the mediastinum during the first procedure.

Once the phreno-esophageal ligament is dissected and the lower mediastinum is opened, the risk for migration is there and can only be reduced by sufficient mobilization of the esophagus to avoid vertical tension [8–10]. This mechanism plays a major role in patients with migration after primary antireflux surgery. It must be emphasized that the weakened tissue at the hiatus, once a hernia has developed, remains a problem

R. C. Broderick (✉)
Division of Minimally Invasive Surgery, Department of Surgery,
University of California San Diego, La Jolla, CA, USA
e-mail: rbroderick@ucsd.edu

© Springer Nature Switzerland AG 2020

S. Horgan, K.-H. Fuchs (eds.), *Management of Gastroesophageal Reflux Disease*,
https://doi.org/10.1007/978-3-030-48009-7_10

chronically. During the initial experience of laparoscopic fundoplication, it became evident that the recurrence rate of hiatal hernia seemed to be somewhat higher than in open surgery [3]. Clinical evidence showed that in some patients, the hiatal structures such as the crura were quite weak with thin muscle, especially in older patients and in patients with large hiatal hernias. Another technical challenge that was encountered was the inability to fully approximate the crura with sutures, as the muscle had become so thin and fragile that some sutures would just cut through the muscle. As a consequence, several authors searched for solutions to solve this problem.

Basic Pathophysiology of Hiatal Hernias

The development of hiatal hernias is due to a persistent strain on the tissue at the hiatus, which separates chest from abdomen and therefore creates two different pressure environments [8, 9]. The elements of fixation of the distal esophagus to the hiatus are created by the diaphragm, the crura, the hiatal arch, and the phreno-esophageal ligament. Over time, these structures are exposed to daily stress and strain between the pressure gradient between the thorax and the often increased intra-abdominal pressure environment [9]. If a patient's tissue is weak, this will eventually lead to elongation and weakening of the structures at the esophagogastric junction and subsequently to a complete enlargement and destruction of the phreno-esophageal ligament transforming into the hernia sac. In addition, the hiatal crura may also weaken and stretch, especially in obese patients, with reduction of muscle substrate and an increase in fat.

A constant focus over the past decades has been to find an operative solution for hiatal hernia. The goals of surgery include not only strengthening the hiatal structures but also securing a stable position of the esophagus in the hiatus after a primary antireflux procedure. Current techniques usually accomplish these goals by mobilization of the esophagus and crural approximation, however, high rates of hiatal hernia recurrence after primary antireflux surgery demonstrate that current surgical techniques are not optimal [6, 8–10].

Initial Experience with Hiatal Enforcement

From general "hernia surgery," it is known that enforcing sutures and weak tissue with a nonabsorbable mesh would prevent hernia recurrence effectively, and therefore, some authors tested this concept at the hiatus [11–14]. During laparoscopic antireflux procedures, the mesh was introduced in the abdomen and usually fixed at the weak crura with either sutures or clips/screws to the hiatal muscle in order to compensate for the weak muscle substrate. The initial clinical experience was very promising, showing a significantly lower recurrence rate for hernias in patients when a nonabsorbable mesh was implanted at the hiatus [11–14]. Three early randomized trials pushed this development in practice, as all these trials showed favorable results for the implantation of nonabsorbable meshes (Table 10.1) [11, 14, 15]. A significant increase in rate of mesh implantation in laparoscopic antireflux

Table 10.1 Literature review of mesh implantation in hiatal hernia surgery and GERD

Author	year	study	patients(n)	Indication	Mesh material	Mesh shape	Hernia sac excision	Primary hiatal suture	Mesh placement	Antireflux procedure	Follow-upmonths	Recurrencerate(%)
Hawlasi + Zonca	1998	–	27	PEH	PP	Oval	+	+	Circular/anterior	Gastropexy	1–56	0
Basso et al.	2000	–	70	GERD/HH	PP	Rectangle	+/–	–	Posterior	Fundoplication	12	1,8
Kamolz et al.	2000	Prosp	100	–	PP	Rectangle	Not given	+	Posterior	Fundoplication	12	1
Granderath et al.	2000	–	170	GERD/HH	PP	Rectangle	K. A.	+	Posterior	Fundoplication	12–30	0,6
Frantzides et al.	2002	Prosp	36	HH > 8 cm	ePTFE	Oval	–	+	Circular	Fundoplication	–	0
Champion u. Rock	2003	Retros	52	GERD/HH > 5 cm	PP	Rectangle	–	+	Posterior	Fundoplication	12	1,9
Casaccia et al.	2005	Retros	27	PEH	PP/PTFE	A-shape	–	+/–	Posterior	Fundoplication	6–46	3,7
Granderath et al.	2005	Prosp	50	GERD	PP	Rectangle	+	+	Posterior	Fundoplication	12	8
Gryska + Vernon	2005	–	135	GERD/PEH/RH	PTFE/ePTFE	V-shape	+	–	Posterior	Fundoplication	>6	0,8
Oelschlager et al.	2006	Prosp	51	PEH	SIS	Rectangle	+	+	Posterior	Fundoplication	6	9
Ringley et al.	2006	Prosp	22	HH > 5 cm	HADM	U-shape	K. A.	+	Posterior	Fundoplication	12	0
Granderath et al.	2007	Prosp	23	GERD	PP/PPCC/PTFE	Rectangle/U-shape	K. A.	+/–	Posterior	Fundoplication	3–12	0
Turkcapar et al.	2007	Prosp	164	GERD	PP	U-shape	K. A.	+	Posterior	Fundoplicatio	>24	1,8
Jacobs et al.	2007	Retros	92	–	SIS	–	–	+	Posterior	Fundoplication/Gastropexy	38	3,3
Lubezky et al.	2007	Retros	59	PEH/RPEH	PTFE/ePTFE/PECC	–	+	+	–	Fundoplication	6–92	35,6

(continued)

Table 10.1 (continued)

Author	year	study	patients(n)	Indication	Mesh material	Mesh shape	Hernia sac excision	Primary hiatal suture	Mesh placement	Antireflux procedure	Follow-upmonths	Recurrencerate(%)
Zaninotto et al.	2007	Retros	35	PEH Typ III	ePTFE	Rectangle	+	+	Circular	Fundoplication	>12	5,7
Granderath et al.	2008	Prosp	33	RH	PP	Oval	+	+	Circular	Fundoplication	60	6,1
Hazebroek et al.	2008	Prosp	40	Large HH	PPTC	-	−	+	Posterior	Fundoplication	12	5,6
Lee et al.	2008	Retros	52	HH > 5 cm	HADM	U-shape	+	+	Posterior	Fundoplication	12–24	3,8
Müller-Stich et al.	2008	Prosp	22	GERD	PP	Circular	−	+	Circular	Gastropexy	12	22,7
Soricelli et al.	2009	Retros	138	HH	PP	Rectangle	+	+/−	Posterior	Fundoplication	95	2,4
Zehetner et al.	2010	Retros	21	PEH	Polyglactin	–	−	+	Posterior	Fundoplication	12	9,5
Antonakis et al.	2016	Prosp	13	PEH	Bio-Mesh	Circular	+	+	Circular	Fundoplication	26	10
Koetje et al.	2017	Retros	189	Large HH PEH	Timesh	U-shape	+	+	Posterior	Fundoplication	39	26

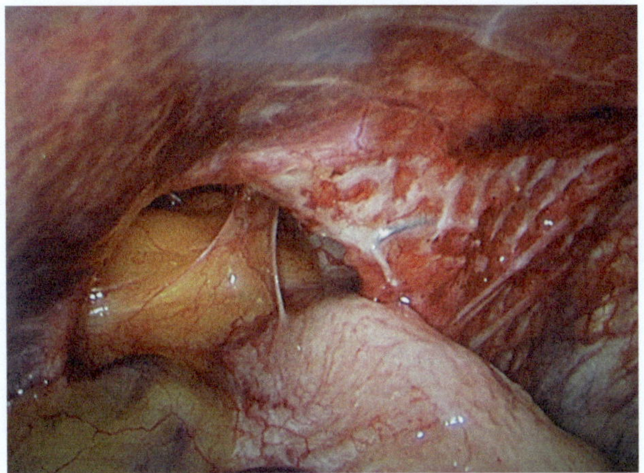

Fig. 10.1 Circular-shaped mesh for hiatal enforcement placed at primary laparoscopic antireflux procedure during redo-surgery for mediastinal migration of the stomach

surgery was seen in the past 15 years [16–36]. However, with the increasing spread of this technique, reports emerged detailing severe complications due to the use of a mesh at the hiatus including erosion, dysphagia, and severe hiatal scarring [37–45]. Each of these is discussed in greater detail below. Furthermore, recurrence of hiatal hernia also could occur despite a hiatal enforcement with mesh (Fig. 10.1).

Side Effects and Complications from Mesh Implantation at the Hiatus

Reports have been published about severe side effects/complications from mesh implantation [37–45]. It also must be emphasized that likely the number of publications underscores the true incidence of these complications, as many discussions at conferences and meetings have indicated a higher risk for severe mesh complications. The different types of problems are discussed below.

Mesh Erosion

The presence of foreign bodies in the mediastinum or at the hiatus always carries a certain risk for erosion into the GI tract [38, 42–44]. The reason for this is a constant movement at the cardia due to swallowing and breathing. The structures at the hiatal opening experience the movement of the heartbeat, the thoracic respiratory mechanism, the vertical mobility of the esophagus during swallowing, and the changing diameter of the esophagus during the passage of food. These movements may facilitate the stepwise penetration of such a foreign body through the esophageal or gastric wall. In retrospect, the erosion phenomenon should have been expected with the implantation of non-resorbable mesh at the hiatus. However, it was still surprising to surgeons and gastroenterologists when the first cases of mesh erosion occurred from their original position at the crura (usually fixed by sutures or clips) and then after 1 or 2 years dislocated into the esophageal lumen [42–45] (Fig. 10.2). Once the mesh was eroded, revisional surgery was indicated. Often these revisional procedures were high risk for complications and required performing an esophageal and/or gastric resection [43–45].

Frozen Cardia and Hiatus

Another frequent problem after mesh implantation, often observed in revisional procedures for dysphagia or recurrence, is the development of severe scarring within the hiatus [42–45]. Sometimes all structures of the cardia and the hiatus are stuck together in one big tissue block as if it was frozen or glued together (Fig. 10.3). This phenomenon, termed "frozen cardia," is dramatic, because no surgical dissection is really in a traditional way possible due to obliteration of tissue planes. Patients with

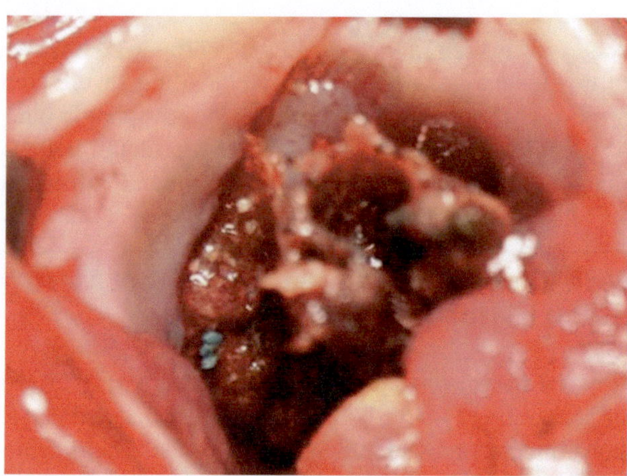

Fig. 10.2 Penetration of a U-shaped nonabsorbable mesh into the esophageal lumen after 1–2 years, causing therapy-refractory pain and dysphagia

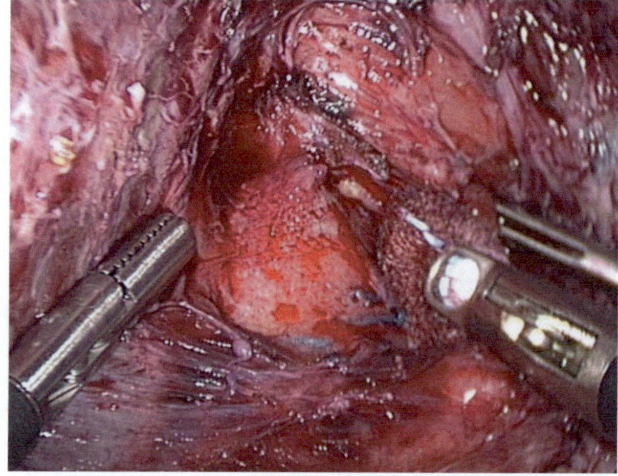

Fig. 10.3 After implantation of a mesh, sometimes the tissues around the cardia and hiatus develop a severe rigid "scaring tissue block," which can hardly be dissected without destroying the structures. We call this phenomenon "frozen cardia," which usually will lead to a resection of the stomach and/or esophagus

frozen cardia usually present with increasing pain and dysphagia. Even after several episodes of dilatation or bouginage, the symptoms do not disappear, and the situation usually ends in an inability to keep up a normal nutrition.

One can and should try to dissect these adhesions; however, the tissues give the impression of being welded together. Often during dissection and attempting to separate the target organs, destruction of the hiatal structures occurs requiring more extensive resection and reconstruction. It is well known that in some patients, scarring is more expressed than in others, but this phenomenon as described above is seen very frequently in revisional surgery after the implantation of mesh. Unfortunately in many cases, this devastating situation can only be resolved by resection of the esophagus and/or stomach.

Gastroparesis

Clinical evidence has shown that secondary gastroparesis can develop after implantation of a mesh at the hiatus [59, 60]. These patients may develop vagal lesions after primary antireflux procedure and may have only limited symptoms in the first year postoperatively. While normal postoperative scarring may remodel and become softer in most patients over time, scarring around an implanted mesh may develop more severe and rigid scars later with foreign body reaction. When the posterior vagal trunk is exposed directly to the mesh at the hiatus, the nerve can become involved in the scaring process. When the vagus nerve becomes embedded in scar, it may lose function after an initial symptom-free interval.

Fatal Complications (Rare)

Fatal complications have been reported after implantation of a mesh at the hiatus when special screwlike clips were used to fix the mesh at the diaphragm [37]. These screwlike clips, when applied laparoscopically, may penetrate the diaphragm and reach the pericardium and the heart. Several cases have been discussed at meetings with such complications, which may even cause the death of a patient [37–44].

Current Mesh Implantation Types and Techniques

The use of mesh for mechanical enforcement at the hiatus is currently characterized by few standards, as many authors apply this technique at their own preference and decision. There is no clear evidence when to use a mesh and what material, what size, and what shape of mesh should be applied in laparoscopic antireflux surgery. There are suggestions from centers and reviews available [46–52]. Validated guidelines are lacking, and the current use reflects the diversity of opinions and also the diversity of the different materials.

Table 10.2 Overview on results of randomized controlled trials regarding mesh implantation for hiatal enforcement during primary antireflux procedures

Author/ year	n	Mesh material	Follow-up months	Recurrence with sutures %	Recurrence with mesh %	p
Frantzides 2002	72	PTFE	6	22	0	0.017
Granderath 2005	100	PP	12	26	8	0.023
Oelschlager 2006	108	SIS	6	24	9	0.058
2011			58	59	54	1.0
Watson 2015	126	Titan SIS	6	23.1	21.8	1.0
Oor 2018	68	TiMesh	12	19.4	25.0	0.581

Some authors use mesh only in patients with large hiatal hernias (e.g., larger than 5 cm) [46]. There are other authors who use mesh enforcement only very selectively in cases. In these cases, it is determined intraoperatively that a severe anatomical weakness of the crura exists, or the approximation by suturing is insufficient, and mesh is placed in attempt to compensate for these deficiencies [46]. Alternatively, there are surgeons that use mesh implantation in every single case of antireflux surgery or hiatal hernia repair.

Granderath et al. have developed an indication for mesh by objectively measuring intraoperatively the area of hiatal opening [19, 24]. They calculate the hiatal surface area (HSA) and have started a concept of tailoring the use of a mesh according to the HSA [24, 53]. Others have followed and report on rates of hiatal hernia recurrence (Table 10.2) [53, 54].

Other factors may play a role such as the material, the size, and the shape of the size of mesh. Several materials are currently in use: polypropylene (PP), polytetrafluorethylene (PTFE), small intestine submucosa (SIS), human acellular dermal matrix (HADM), collage-coated polypropylene (PPCC), collagen-coated polyester (PECC), polyglycolic acid (PGA), and titanium-coated polypropylene (PPTC) [55]. These materials were also experimentally tested [55]. Experimental tests show differences in effect of shrinking and foreign body reactions, and the optimal materials regarding shrinking are probably polypropylene and polyester, while regarding scaring, probably the best materials are nonabsorbable mesh [55].

The configuration and shaping of the mesh may be important for its function (Fig. 10.4). The configuration of the mesh may be a small band or rectangle that connects the crura posteriorly [12]. Alternatively, the mesh may be U-shaped, or it can be implanted in a circular fashion on the crura around the esophagus (Fig. 10.1). The mesh configuration and shape may also play a major role in some complications, because a circular mesh around the hiatus may influence the esophageal wall and may cause erosion of the esophageal wall as published in several reports [37–45]. Some authors like to routinely use a circular mesh with the justification that this

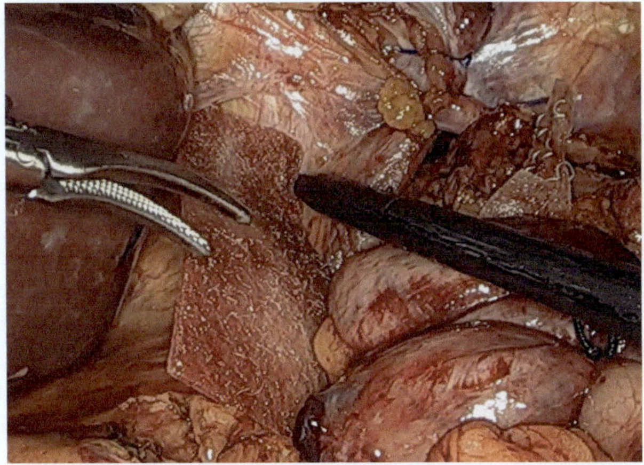

Fig. 10.4 U-shaped mesh for hiatal enforcement positioned around the esophagus at the hiatus

circular mesh best stabilizes the hiatal opening. However, clinical evidence shows that this stabilization of the hiatal opening may lead to severe scaring of the hiatal border resulting in a quite rigid crural edge of the hiatus. The latter can cause a technical problem during revisional surgery, as the crura may become so rigid to not allow any manipulation or further approximation. Effects of shrinking and foreign body reactions cannot be foreseen and may result in strange postoperative configurations, as seen in cases of revisional surgery.

Another controversial issue is the fixation of the mesh on the muscle or ligamentous structure of the diaphragm. The mesh can be sutured at the border of the underlying diaphragm. It can be fixed with screwlike-structured staples to the muscle or other clips. All these different options are often discussed during meetings quite controversially between protagonists and critics of mesh use. Given there is not enough good data to inform specific recommendations, it can be expected that this will continue to raise debate for some time.

Current Data and Recommendations on Mesh Implantation

Table 10.1 demonstrates the available and representative data of mesh application during antireflux and hiatal hernia surgery from the past 15 years, which was recently summarized by Granderath [11, 14–36]. The data shows from retrospective and prospective series that most authors use a posterior implantation of the mesh for augmentation of the hiatus. The material used varies widely among the authors (Table 10.1). Follow-up time is reported between 1 and 92 months with an overall recurrence rate between 0% and 36% with a median of 3.5%. In most of these publications, the authors use a fundoplication as antireflux procedure [14–36].

A few randomized trials are available and show favorable results for the mesh application in early follow-up (Table 10.2) [11, 14, 15, 56–58]. However, the power of these early studies is limited due to low case numbers [11, 14]. Regarding mesh implantation in patients with small- and moderate-size hiatal hernias, one randomized trial shows that there is an advantage for patients with mesh augmentation in decreased hernia recurrence rate (2% versus 26%) [14]. However, in the follow-up of this study, it could be shown that after 3 months, the dysphagia rate was increased in the patient group with mesh augmentation (16% versus 4%) [14]. After 1 year, the reflux-related symptoms did not show any difference between the groups which demonstrated that the effect of mesh implantation would have only limited influence on the overall result.

More long-term randomized studies with follow-up time of around 5 years show that the recurrence rate of hiatal hernias is similar between cases in which the hiatal approximation was performed by suture versus those performed by a mesh implantation (20–50%) [15, 56]. In the study from Oelschlager et al., the 5-year results were identical with 50% recurrence rate between sutured crura hiatus and mesh implantation [56]. In a randomized trial by Watson et al., three different groups of patients (suture hiatoplasty versus mesh implantation with titanium mesh versus mesh implantation with biologic mesh) were compared [57]. The results do not show any differences in follow-up, since the recurrence rates were 23% versus 22% with mesh implantation [58]. These results are confirmed by the latest study in showing no substantial advantage regarding symptom control, necessity for reoperations, and hernia recurrence [58].

Other studies show positive results with biologic meshes, in which the long-term complication rate may be lower [47, 56]. However, further follow-up is needed to monitor for evolving complications in the absorbable mesh groups. Clinical evidence shows that there can be also troublesome side effects developing with absorbable/biologic meshes, since either these substances can cause also severe scarring or the material can dissolve leaving some viscous fluid at the mesh implantation site with a possible recurrence of the hernia (Fig. 10.5).

Several meta-analyses have been published regarding mesh use (Table 10.3) [47–52]. The protagonists of mesh implantation rely often on the early comparative studies regarding mesh implantation, showing a lower early recurrence rate of hiatal

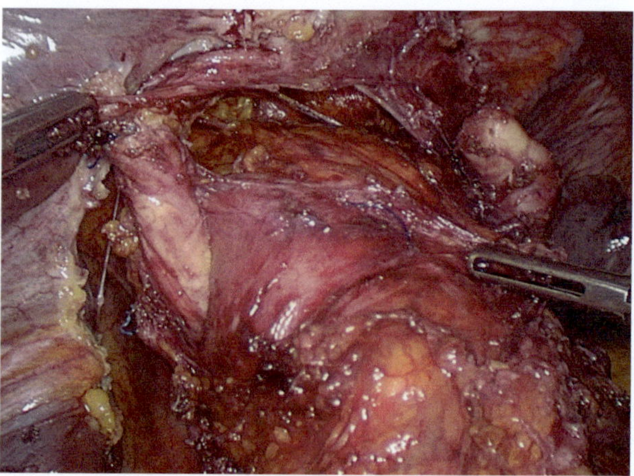

Fig. 10.5 The posterior positioned absorbable mesh for hiatal enforcement has shrunk to a strand-like structure, causing dysphagia after a 1-year symptom-free interval

Table 10.3 Overview on meta-analyses regarding mesh implantation at the hiatus

Author/year	n	Studies	Summarized results	Conclusions
Müller-Stich 2015	915	3 RCT 9 CS	Recurrence: 12.1 versus 20.5% Mortality: 1.6 versus 1.8%	Clear advantage for mesh
Tam 2016	1194	13 Studies	Recurrence: 0.42; $p = 0.014$	Minor advantage for mesh
Memon 2016	406	4 RCT	Recurrence: OR 2.01; $P < 0.07$	Similar results
Zhang 2017	1474	4 RCT 9 Case control	Recurrence: 2.4 versus 9.4% Quality of life: SF36: BioMesh better GIQLI: similar Suture: less dysphagia	Similar results

hernias [11, 14]. These authors emphasize one of the main arguments for mesh implantation is the reduction in additional surgery after the primary antireflux procedure with mesh. One meta-analysis showed that using mesh augmentation in patients with large hiatal hernias led to a significant decrease of revisional surgery after primary surgery with mesh implantation (Odds ratio 3.73) [50]. There was no difference in short-term complications. This was a very important result for the protagonists of mesh, as it promised a significant reduction for revisional surgery [50]. The critics of mesh implantation emphasize the severe complications of mesh implantation [42–45].

These findings were used by Müller-Stich et al. in a subsequent analysis, using a Markov model for calculation to evaluate the cost-benefit ratio for the use of mesh in 915 large hiatal hernia patients [48]. The rate of recurrent hiatal hernias could be reduced by mesh implantation, from 20.5% to 12.1%, after close to 3-year follow-up [48]. The study showed an overall higher benefit for patients with mesh implantation, because the complication rate was similar between mesh implantation and without mesh implantation (14.2% versus 15.3%). This was based on the prerequisite that the rate of necessary revisional surgery was lower with the use of the mesh. The authors concluded mesh implantation may reduce redo-surgery and reduce the overall risk of antireflux surgery [48, 50].

However, the findings from Müller-Stich et al. are not supported by recent meta-analysis and another randomized trial [52, 57, 58]. This meta-analysis shows an improved rate of early hernia recurrence with the use of mesh but equal results in recurrent reflux symptoms and possibly more dysphagia associated with mesh implantation [52].

Furthermore, in the recent randomized Dutch trials, it was shown that there is a comparable rate of radiolographic and symptomatic recurrence rate between patients with and without mesh augmentation [36, 58]. Interestingly, there was no decrease in the necessity of revisional surgery with mesh augmentation [36, 58]. The authors conclude and recommend that mesh implantation should be considered, but no clear advantage could be demonstrated [58].

Table 10.4 Overview on necessity for major esophageal and/or gastric resections during revisional surgery after mesh implantation at the hiatus during primary antireflux surgery

Author/year	Patients n	Type of primary procedure n	Necessity for major resection during redo-surgery %
Parker 2010	69	69 redo-surgery: 10 with mesh implantation 59 without mesh implantation	40% after mesh implantation 6% after suture hiatoplasty
Nandipati 2013	26	26 redo-surgery after mesh implantation	41% resection: 22% gastric resections 19% esophageal resections
Fuchs 2017	322	322 redo-surgery: 42 with mesh implantation 280 with suture hiatoplasty	43% after mesh implantation 8% after suture hiatoplasty

Mesh implantation should be considered in large hiatal hernias; however, severe complications may occur, and therefore, patients must have an accurate informed consent about these possibilities. Based on currently available data, it is difficult to give a precise recommendation for the use of mesh at the hiatus. It remains an individual decision of the surgeon. Even though mesh implantation has been shown to be of advantage in general hernia surgery, it seems to be a different situation at the hiatus. The enlarged opening at the hiatus cannot be closed completely like in other hernias (ventral hernia and inguinal hernia), since at the hiatus there is the necessity to leave sufficient space for the passage of the esophagus, which may be technically difficult to solve by a mesh. Furthermore, experience in literature shows that the risk of mesh problems in redo-antireflux surgery may lead to the necessity of major gastric or esophageal resections, as shown in Table 10.4 [43–45].

It must be also emphasized that an insufficient mobilization of the esophagus in the mediastinum cannot be compensated by enforcing the hiatus with mesh, as remaining tension will cause the migration upward.

Conclusions

Many laparoscopic surgeons use mesh augmentation at the hiatus with non-resorbable or absorbable mesh currently. Substantial controversies are present, and surgical meetings often feature controversial discussions. Based on the available evidence, it can be summarized that the implantation of mesh in a regular GERD patient with a small- to midsize hiatal hernia cannot be recommended as a routine procedure, since the advantages seem to be quite limited with recurrence and risk of long-term complication. In large hiatal hernias (>5 cm), current evidence and meta-analysis suggest that the use of a mesh can be considered, but the risk for complications is substantial, and therefore, the patient should be informed about these risks. Early results on bioabsorbable mesh are promising for reduction in early recurrence, but longer-term data is needed to determine durability of the repair. In centers of antireflux surgery with a large experience in upper GI surgery, the use of a mesh may not reduce the necessity of revisional surgery even in large hiatal hernias. Therefore, the indication for mesh implantation should be tailored and focused to each individual patient. It is the opinion of the authors that permanent mesh should not be placed for hiatal reinforcement under any circumstance due to the potentially devastating consequences of erosion or frozen hiatus. Early reports of bioabsorbable mesh placement are promising but require longer-term follow-up.

References

1. Altorki NK, Yankelevitz D, Skinner DB. Massive hiatal hernias: the anatomic basis of repair. J Thorac Cardiovasc Surg. 1998;115(4):828–35.
2. Maziak DE, Todd TR, Pearson FG. Massive hiatus hernia: evaluation and surgical management. J Thorac Cardiovasc Surg. 1998;115(1):53–60; discussion 61-2.
3. Hashemi M, Peters JH, DeMeester TR, Huprich JE, Quek M, Hagen JA, Crookes PF, Theisen J, DeMeester SR, Sillin LF, Bremner CG. Laparoscopic repair of large type III hernia: objective followup reveals high recurrence rate. J Am Coll Surg. 2000;190:553–60.
4. Stylopoulos N, Gazelle GS, Rattner DW. Paraesophageal hernias: operation or observation? Ann Surg. 2002;236(4):492–500; discussion 500-501.
5. Draaisma WA, Gooszen HG, Tournoij E, Broeders IA. Controversies in paraesophageal hernia repair: a review of literature. Surg Endosc. 2005;19(10):1300–8.
6. Stylopoulos N, Rattner DW. The history of hiatal hernia surgery: from Bowditch to laparoscopy. Ann Surg. 2005;241:185–93.
7. Furnée EJ, Draaisma WA, Broeders IA, Gooszen HG. Surgical reintervention after failed antireflux surgery; a systematic review of the literature. J Gastrointest Surg. 2009;13:1539–49.
8. Allison PR. Peptic ulcer of the oesophagus. Thorax. 1948;3(1):20–42.
9. DeMeester TR. Etiology and natural history of gastroesophageal reflux disease and predictors of progressive disease. In: Yeo CJ, DeMeester SR, Mc Fadden DW, editors. Shackelford's surgery of the alimentary tract. 8th ed. Philadelphia: Elsevier; 2019. p. 204–20.
10. DeMeester SR. Laparoscopic paraesophageal hernia repair: critical steps and adjunct techniques to minimize recurrence. Surg Laparosc Endosc Percutan Tech. 2013;23(5):429–35. https://doi.org/10.1097/SLE.0b013e3182a12716.
11. Frantzides CT, Madan AK, Carlson MA, Stavropoulos GP. A prospective, randomized trial of laparoscopic polytetrafluoroethylene (PTFE) patch repair vs simple cruroplasty for large hiatal hernia. Arch Surg. 2002;137(6):649–52.
12. Granderath FA, Schweiger UM, Kamolz T, Pasiut M, Haas CF, Pointner R. Laparoscopic antireflux surgery with routine mesh-hiatoplasty in the treatment of gastroesophageal reflux disease. J Gastrointest Surg. 2002;6(3):347–53.
13. Zilberstein B, Eshkenazy R, Pajecki D. Laparoscopic mesh repair antireflux surgery for treatment of large hiatal hernia. Dis Esophagus. 2005;18:166–9.
14. Granderath FA, Schweiger UM, Kamolz T, Asche KU, Pointner R. Laparoscopic Nissen fundoplication with prosthetic hiatal closure reduces postoperative intrathoracic wrap herniation: preliminary results of a prospective randomized functional and clinical study. Arch Surg. 2005;140:40–8.
15. Oelschlager BK, Pellegrini CA, Hunter JG, Soper N, Brunt M, Sheppard B, Jobe B, Polissar N, Mitsumori L, Nelson J, Swanstrom LL. Biologic prosthesis reduces recurrence after laparoscopic paraesophageal hernia repair: a multicenter, prospective, randomized trial. Ann Surg. 2006;244:481–90.
16. Hawlasi A, Zonca S. Laparoscopic repair of paraesophageal hernia repair. JSLS. 1998;2:269–72.
17. Basso N, De Leo A, Genco A. 360° laparoscopic fundoplication with tension-free hiatoplasty in the treatment of symptomatic gastroesophageal reflux disease. Surg Endosc. 2000;14:164–9.

18. Kamolz T, Bammer T, Wykypiel HJ, Pasuit M, Pointner R. Quality of life and surgical outcome after laparoscopic Nissen and Toupet fundoplication: one year follow up. Endoscopy. 2000;32:363–8.
19. Granderath FA. Operative Therapie bei Hiatushernie. Der Chirurg: Evidenz zur Netzeinlage; 2017. https://doi.org/10.1007/s00104-016-0338-3.
20. Champion JK, Rock D. Laparoscopic mesh cruroplasty for large paraesophageal hernias. Surg Endosc. 2003;17:551–3.
21. Cassacia M, Torelli P, Panaro F. Laparoscopic tension-free repair of large paraesophageal hiatal hernias with a composite shaped mesh: two year follow-up. J Laparoendosc Adv Surg Tech. 2005;15:279–84.
22. Gryska PV, Vernon JK. Tension-free repair of hiatal hernia during laparoscopic fundoplication: a ten-year experience. Hernia. 2005;9:150–5.
23. Ringley CD, Bochkarev V, Ahmed SI. Laparoscopic hiatal hernia repair with human acellular dermal matrix patch: our initial experience. Am J Surg. 2006;192:767–72.
24. Granderath FA, Schweiger UM, Pointner R. Laparoscopic antireflux surgery: tailoring the hiatal closure to the size of hiatal surface area. Surg Endosc. 2007;21:542–8.
25. Turkcapar A, Kepenekci I. Laparoscopic fundoplication with prosthetic hiatal closure. World J Surg. 2007;31:2169–76.
26. Jacobs M, Gomez E, Plasencia G. Use of Surgisis mesh in laparoscopic repair of hiatal hernias. Surg Laparosc Endosc Percutan Tech. 2007;17:365–8.
27. Lubezky N, Sagie B, Keidar A. Prosthetic mesh repair of large and recurrent diaphragmatic hernias. Surg Endosc. 2007;21:737–41.
28. Zaninotto G, Portale G, Constantini M. Objective follow-up after laparoscopic repair of large type III hiatal hernia. Assessment of safety and durability. World J Surg. 2007;31:2177–83.
29. Granderath FA, Granderath UM, Pointner R. Laparoscopic revisional fundoplication with circular hiatal mesh prosthesis: the long-term results. World J Surg. 2008;32:999–1007.
30. Hazebroek EJ, Ng A, Yong DHK. Clinical evaluation of laparoscopic repair of large hiatal hernias with TiMesh. ANZ J Surg. 2008;78:914–7.
31. Lee YK, James E, Bochkarev V. Long-term outcome of cruroplasty reinforcement with human acellular dermal matrix in large paraesophageal hiatal hernia. J Gastrointest Surg. 2008;12:811–5.
32. Müller-Stich BP, Linke GR, Borovicka J. Laparoscopic mesh-augmented hiatoplasty as a treatment of gastroesophageal reflux disease and hiatal hernias – preliminary clinical and functional results of a prospective case series. Am J Surg. 2008;195:749–56.
33. Soricelli E, Basso N, Genco A. Long-term results of hiatal hernia mesh repair and antireflux laparoscopic surgery. Surg Endosc. 2009;23:2499–504.
34. Zehetner J, Lipham JC, Ayazi S. A simplified technique for intrathoracic stomach laparoscopic fundoplication with Vicryl mesh and reinforcement. Surg Endosc. 2010;24:675–9.
35. Antonakis F, Köckerling F, Kalinowski F. Functional results after repair of large hiatal hernia by use of a biologic mesh. Front Surg. 2016;3:16.
36. Koetje JH, Oor JE, Roks DJ, Van Westreenen HL, Hazebroek EJ, Nieuwenhuijs VB. Equal patient satisfaction, quality of life and objective recurrence rate after laparoscopic hiatal hernia repair with and without mesh. Surg Endosc. 2017; https://doi.org/10.1007/s00464-016-5405-9.
37. Kemppainen E, Kiviluoto T. Fatal cardiac tamponade after emergency tension-free repair of a large paraesophageal hernia. Surg Endosc. 2000;14:593.
38. Coluccio G, Ponzio S, Ambu V. Dislocation into the cardial lumen of a PTFE prosthesis used in the treatment of voluminous hiatal sliding hernia, a case report. Minerva Chir. 2000;55:341–5.
39. Arendt T, Stuber E, Monig H, Folsch UR, Katsoulis S. Dysphagia due to transmural migration of surgical material into the esophagus nine years after Nissen fundoplication. Gastrointest Endosc. 2000;51:607–10.
40. Targarona EM, Bendahan G, Balague C, Garriga J, Trias M. Mesh in the Hiatus A controversial issue. Arch Surg. 2004;139:1286–96.

41. Rathore MA, Andrabi SIH, Bhatti MI, Najfi SMH, McMurray A. Meta analysis of recurrence after laparoscopic repair of paraesophageal Hernia. JSLS. 2007;11(4):456–60.
42. Stadlhuber RJ, Sherif AE, Mittal SK, Fitzgibbons RJ, Brunt LM, Hunter JG, DeMeester TR, Swanstrom LL, Smith CD, Filipi CJ. Mesh complications after prosthetic reinforcement of hiatal closure: a 28-case series. Surg Endosc. 2009;23:1219–26.
43. Parker M, Bowers SP, Bray JM, Harris AS, Belli EV, Pfluke JM, Preissler S, Asbun HJ, Smith CD. Hiatal mesh is associated with major resection at revisional operation. Surg Endosc. 2010;24(12):3095–10.
44. Nandipati K, Bye M, Yamamoto SR, Pallati P, Lee T, Mittal SK. Reoperative intervention in patients with mesh at the hiatus is associated with high incidence of esophageal resection--a single-center experience. J Gastrointest Surg. 2013;17(12):2039–44. https://doi.org/10.1007/s11605-013-2361-8.
45. Fuchs KH. Revisionseingriffe nach Antirefluxchirurgie. In: Fuchs KH, editor. Management der Gastroösophagealen Refluxkrankheit. Berlin: De Gruyter Verlag; 2018. p. 183–208.
46. Fuchs KH, Babic B, Breithaupt W, Dallemagne B, Fingerhut A, Furnee E, Granderath F, Horvath P, Kardos P, Pointner R, Savarino E, Van Herwaarden-Lindeboom M, Zaninotto G. EAES recommendations for the management of gastroesophageal reflux disease. Surg Endosc. 2014;28(6):1753–73.
47. Antoniou SA, Müller-Stich BP, Antoniou GA, Köhler G, Kuketina RR, Koch OO, Pointner R, Granderath FA. Laparoscopic augmentation of the diaphragmatic hiatus with biologic mesh versus suture repair: a systematic review and meta analysis. Langenbeck's Arch Surg. 2015;400:577–83.
48. Müller-Stich BP, Kenngott HG, Gondan M, Stock C, Linke GR, Fritz GR, Nickel F, Diener MK, Gutt CN, Wente M, Büchler MW, Fischer L. Use of Mesh in laparoscopic paraesophageal hernia repair: a meta-analysis and risk-benefit analysis. PLoS One. 2015;10(10):e0139547.
49. Tam V, Winger DG, Nason KS. A systematic review and metaanalysis of mesh vs suture cruroplasty in laparoscopic large hiatal hernia repair. Am J Surg. 2016;211:226–38.
50. Memon MA, Memon B, Yunus RM, Khan S. Suture Cruroplasty versus prosthetic hiatal herniorrhaphy for large hiatal hernia: a metaanalysis and systematic review of randomized controlled trials. Ann Surg. 2016;263:258–66.
51. Huddy JR, Markar SR, Ni MZ, Morino M, Targarona EM, Zaninotto G, Hanna GB. Laparoscopic repair of hiatus hernia: does mesh type influence outcome? A meta-analysis and European survey study. Surg Endosc. 2016;30(12):5209–21.
52. Zhang C, Liu D, Li F, Watson DI, Gao X, Koetje JH, Luo T, Yan C, Du X, Wang Z. Systematic review and metaanalysis of laparoscopic mesh versus suture repair of hiatus hernia: objective and subjective outcomes. Surg Endosc. 2017; https://doi.org/10.1007/s00464-017-5586-x.
53. Grubnik VV, Malynovskyy AV. Laparoscopic repair of hiatal hernias: new classification supported by long-term results. Surg Endosc. 2013;27(11):4337–46. https://doi.org/10.1007/s00464-013-3069-2.
54. Antoniou SA, Pointner R, Granderath FA. Hiatal surface area as a basis for a new classification of hiatal hernia. Surg Endosc. 2014;28(4):1384–5. https://doi.org/10.1007/s00464-013-3292-x.
55. Müller-Stich BP, Senft JD, Lasitschka F, Shevchenko M, Billeter AT, Bruckner T, Kenngott HG, Fischer L, Gehring T. Polypropylene, polyester or polytetrafluoroethylene - is there an ideal material for mesh augmentation at the esophageal hiatus ? Results from an experimental study in a porcine model. Hernia. 2014;18:873–81.
56. Oelschlager BK, Pellegrini CA, Hunter JG. Biologic prosthesis to prevent recurrence after laparoscopic paraesophageal hernia repair: long- term follow-up from a multicenter, prospective, randomized trial. J Am Coll Surg. 2011;213:461–8.
57. Watson DI, Thompson SK, Devitt PG, Smith L, Woods SD, Aly A, Gan S, Game PA, Jamieson GG. Laparoscopic repair of very large Hiatus hernia with sutures versus absorbable mesh versus nonabsorbable mesh: a randomized controlled trial. Ann Surg. 2015;261:282–9.

58. Oor JE, Roks DJ, Koetje JH, Broeders JA, van Westreenen HL, Nieuwenhuijs VB, Hazebroek EJ. Randomized clinical trial comparing laparoscopic hiatal hernia repair using sutures versus sutures reinforced with non-absorbable mesh. Surg Endosc. 2018;32(11):4579–89. https://doi.org/10.1007/s00464-018.
59. Van Rijn S, Roebroek YGM, Conchillo JM, Bouvy ND, Masclee AAM. Effect of Vagus nerve injury on the outcome of antireflux surgery: an extensive literature review. Dig Surg. 2016;33:230–9.
60. Bhayani NH, Sharata AM, Dunst CM, Kurian AA, Reavis KM, Swanstrom LL. End of the road for dysfunctional end organ: laparoscopic gastrectomy for refractory gastroparesis. J Gastrointest Surg. 2015;19:411–7.

Robotic Hiatal Hernia Repair

11

Joslin N. Cheverie, Ryan C. Broderick, Robert F. Cubas, and Santiago Horgan

Introduction

Paraesophageal hernias present a clinical and anatomical entity that must be fully appreciated for safe and effective management. They are an uncommon form of hiatal hernia that tend to present clinically in the population of patients over 65 years of age. The most common symptomatic presentations of a paraesophageal hernia (PEH) include dysphagia, regurgitation, gastroesophageal reflux, dyspnea, chest or epigastric pain or pressure, and anemia. Weight loss in this patient population may be common and dramatic. Acute presentations may demonstrate signs and symptoms of bleeding (due to friction ulcer) or obstruction (due to gastric volvulus). The risk of hemorrhage and ischemia in the acute setting is a particular subset of PEH presentation.

There are four types of hiatal hernias as depicted below (Fig. 11.1). Type 1 hernias account for 90% of all hiatal hernias and are often asymptomatic or present with predominantly reflux symptoms. Type 2, type 3, and type 4 reflect the paraesophageal component and involve movement of the gastric fundus through the hiatus into the thorax. Type 3 or "mixed" hernias are the most common representing

J. N. Cheverie (✉) · R. F. Cubas
Division of Minimally Invasive Surgery, Department of Surgery, University of California San Diego Medical Center, La Jolla, CA, USA
e-mail: jcheverie@ucsd.edu

R. C. Broderick
Division of Minimally Invasive Surgery, Department of Surgery, University of California San Diego, La Jolla, CA, USA

University of California San Diego, Department of Surgery, Center for the Future of Surgery, La Jolla, CA, USA

S. Horgan
Division of Minimally Invasive Surgery, Department of Surgery, University of California San Diego, La Jolla, CA, USA

© Springer Nature Switzerland AG 2020
S. Horgan, K.-H. Fuchs (eds.), *Management of Gastroesophageal Reflux Disease*,
https://doi.org/10.1007/978-3-030-48009-7_11

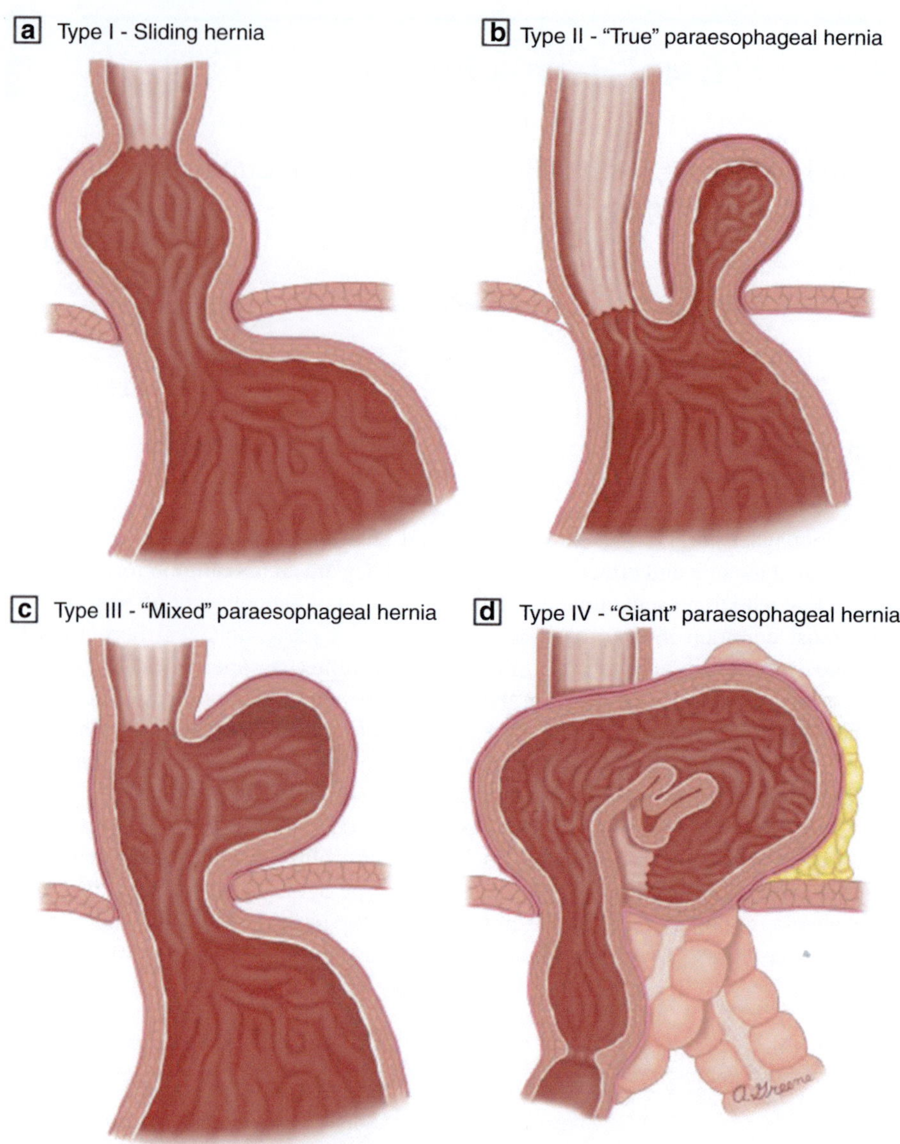

Fig. 11.1 Types of hiatal hernias

90% of all PEH. Giant PEH are defined as types 2, 3, or 4 but with over 50% of the stomach in an intrathoracic position [1, 2].

Symptomatic hernias should be repaired unless there are clinical parameters precluding safe and effective surgical intervention. The timing and preoperative evaluation vary depending on the patient and disease factors and will be discussed below. Elective repair in the symptomatic patient has been associated with an increase in patient quality of life with satisfaction rates in the literature ranging between 85 and 96%. Revisional surgery is known for its technical difficulty, higher complication rate, and decreased patient satisfaction. Clinical assessment and perioperative considerations are imperative in this group in order to properly stratify surgical candidates and optimize outcomes [3, 4].

Robotic repair of a paraesophageal hernia is an efficient and ergonomic approach to this challenging anatomical problem. Added precision and extended accessibility and visualization of the thorax from an abdominal approach make the robotic repair a preferred surgical method. In addition to the mentioned clinical manifestations, this chapter will review the preoperative workup required. Surgical technique will then focus on the robotic approach in a stepwise fashion. Evidentiary review of outcomes will highlight this approach as a feasible if not superior approach [5, 6].

Special considerations for emergent and prophylactic repair, esophageal lengthening, crural closure with regard to mesh, and relaxing incisions will be addressed. In addition, a brief comparative cost analysis with robotic and laparoscopic approach will be highlighted.

Preoperative Evaluation

As with all foregut surgery, preoperative preparation is critical. A carefully documented history of current symptoms, previous treatment modalities and outcomes, and comorbid cardiac and pulmonary processes must be completed. This may alter the pathway to surgery with involvement of other respective specialists to investigate further any underlying cardiac, pulmonary, or systemic disease processes. In addition to symptomatology, patient characteristics and comorbidities may help alter or adjust operative approach.

The proposed workup in our institution consists of esophagogastroduodenoscopy, pH testing (only performed if patients had disabling reflux symptoms), upper GI series, and high-resolution manometry. Variations to this may be reasonable depending on the patient symptoms, the surgical approach, and the acute presentations. In the case of acute volvulus, CT scan of the chest and abdomen may suffice but would lack more specific functional information which may preclude knowledge of underlying motility disorders.

Upper Endoscopy

Endoscopy is performed for every patient to assess the anatomy with regard to esophageal length, size of hernia, esophagitis, presence of Cameron's erosions at the level of the diaphragm, and assessment of gastric volvulus. Retroflexion views as well as assessment of the GEJ are crucial.

Barium Swallow

This contrast study demonstrates size, location, orientation, and reducibility of the paraesophageal component. It also gives functional information with regard to dysphagia and regurgitation. Esophageal length is also assessed.

High-Resolution Esophageal Manometry

Esophageal manometry is indicated in the assessment of dysphagia or noncardiac chest pain in patients without evidence of mechanical obstruction, ulceration, or inflammation. It is imperative for surgical planning when an anti-reflux procedure is indicated.

The fundamental difference between conventional manometry and high-resolution manometry (HRM) is the number of pressure sensors used and the spacing between them. In contrast to conventional manometry where sensors are spaced at 3–5 cm intervals, in HRM, sensors are typically spaced 1 cm apart along the length of the manometric assembly. Catheters with up to 36 sensors distributed longitudinally and radially in the esophagus allow for simultaneous pressure readings spanning both sphincters and the interposed esophagus [7].

pH Monitoring

Ambulatory pH monitoring is performed by placing a wireless pH capsule (Bravo system) 6 cm above the upper border of the LES. At the time of endoscopy completion, the Bravo delivery catheter is introduced through the mouth, and the capsule is attached to the esophageal mucosa. The patient wears a Bravo pH receiver around the waist. Data is transmitted to a receiver worn by the patient, and data recording is carried out for 48 hours. A standard DeMeester scoring is compiled for objective assessment [8].

Operative Technique

Paraesophageal hernia repair may be performed via a transthoracic or transabdominal approach. Open, laparoscopic, and robotic technique may be applied.

We prefer the robotic system for transabdominal paraesophageal hernia repair in our institution for both elective and emergency settings provided a suitable clinical scheme. The operation is performed using the da Vinci Surgical System (Intuitive Surgical, Sunnyvale, CA), which combines robotics and computer imaging to enable microsurgery in a laparoscopic environment. The most notable benefit of the robot with this approach is the 7 degrees of freedom provided by the instrument arms. Tip articulation mimics the up/down and side-to-side flexibility of the human wrist. These articulations extend the surgeon's minimally invasive abilities within the confines of the intracorporeal space [9].

OR Setup

OR size must accommodate the robotic system consisting of three to four integrated components. The patient cart is draped with sterility and is advanced toward the patient over the head (Si system) or from the side (Xi system). This cart is physically docked with the patient through robotic arms and adapting robotic trocars. A variety of robotic instruments exist which are manually connected and inserted at the patient cart. A vision cart, which includes the system processors, sits at side of the patient and allows for a camera and energy interface between patient cart and the surgical console.

The endoscope is calibrated through the vision cart accordingly. The surgical console may be single or dual depending on the requirements of the institution. The integration of visual cues allows for precise activation and control of the robotic arms with the surgical field. All of the unit components must be appropriately positioned with spatial allowance to accommodate regular intraoperative conduct. Before the patient is brought into the room, it should be confirmed that all appropriate equipment is present, turned on, and functioning properly including all three components of the da Vinci® Robotic System; for this matter, an experienced OR and robotic support staff is crucial [10].

Patient Positioning

The patient is initially placed in the supine position over a beanbag. Pneumatic compression stockings are routinely placed on the lower extremities. All pressure points are comfortably padded. After satisfactory induction of general endotracheal anesthesia, the legs are placed in split leg attachments and the arms out to the side on padded arm boards (Fig. 11.2). Preoperative antibiotics are given, and the abdomen is prepped from the nipples down to the pubic symphysis and as far lateral as possibly, especially on the left side.

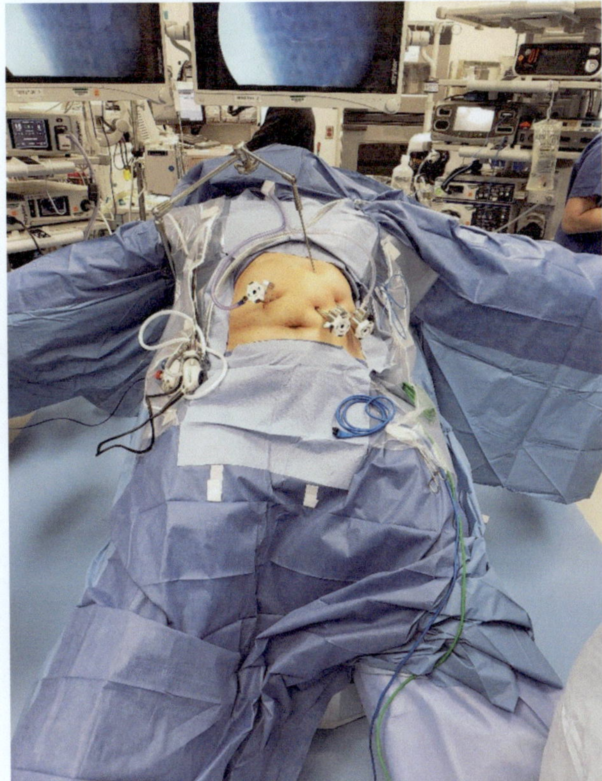

Fig. 11.2 Patient in supine position with outstretched arms to 80° and split legs in steep reverse Trendelenburg

Trocar Placement

A 12 mm, 8.5 mm, or 8 mm trocar (depending on the system being used; Si vs. Xi) is initially placed, under direct vision using an optical trocar system, in the left mid abdomen two fingerbreadths lateral to the umbilicus and one palm width inferior to the left costal margin. This port is used for the robotic camera. Two additional robotic 8 mm trocars are then placed: one on the left subcostal midclavicular line and one on the right subcostal midclavicular line. A 5 mm assistant trocar is positioned in the left flank and is used during the case for retraction. It may be upsized to a 12 mm trocar to accommodate sutures or mesh as desired. The patient is positioned in steep reverse Trendelenburg. A small subxiphoid incision is used for the placement of the Nathanson liver retractor (Fig. 11.3).

Docking

At this point, the robotic surgical cart is approximated into position, and the arms are attached to the three specific trocars (Fig. 11.4). The position of the patient cart will depend on the system used; the Si will have to come in from the patient's left

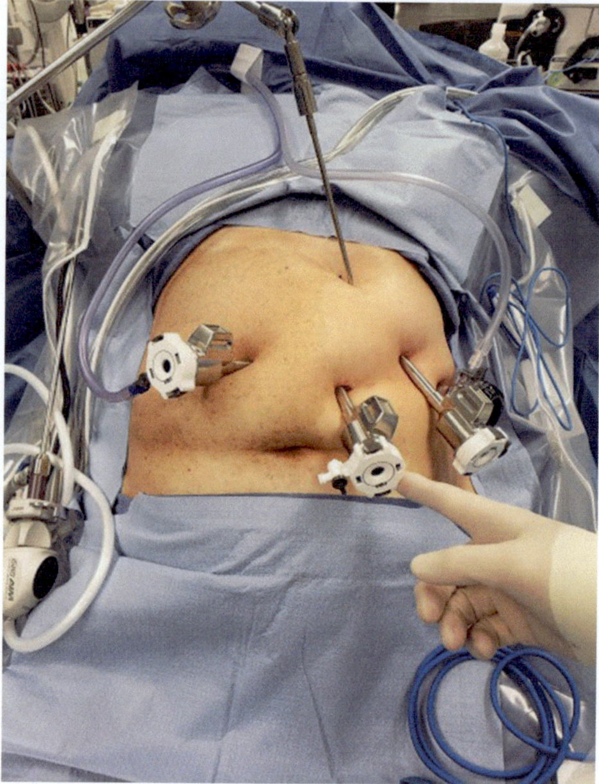

Fig. 11.3 Assistant's finger pointing at the camera port. Insufflation cannula connected to the 12 mm assistant port and smoke evacuator cannula connected to the right 8 mm port

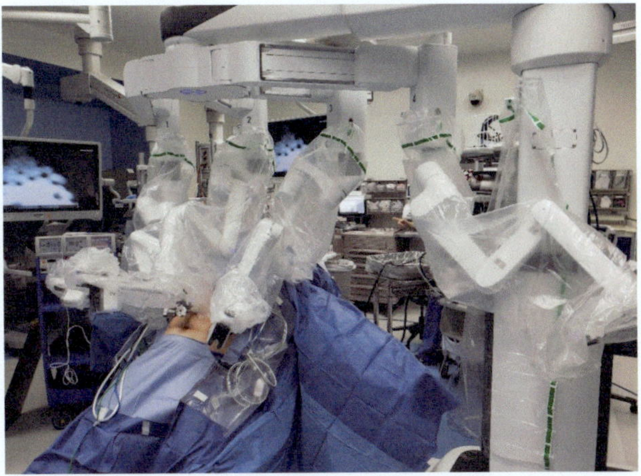

Fig. 11.4 da Vinci Xi; patient cart approaching perpendicularly from the left side, with the boom rotated 90° counterclockwise

shoulder or head, whereas the Xi can approach the patient perpendicularly from the left or right side, and the boom will have to rotate 90 degrees counterclockwise or clockwise, respectively. A Cadiere Forceps or Forced Bipolar instrumentation is placed in the surgeon's left hand, and in the right hand, the articulated robotic vessel sealer device is introduced. The assistant at the bedside usually performs the setup of the robot. The assistant surgeon is positioned on the patients' left side. During the case, the assistant is in charge of switching the robotic instruments and introducing and extracting the sutures, Penrose, or mesh (if used) for the operating surgeon. For this reason, basic training in laparoscopic surgery and robotics is essential for the assistant surgeon.

Visualization

The left mid-abdominal port is used for the 30 degree robotic camera selecting the downward view. After the left lobe of the liver is retracted anteriorly using the Nathanson retractor, the hiatus is exposed. At this point, the hernia is visualized (Fig. 11.5). Often, with positioning, herniated contents will reduce spontaneously at this point.

Reduction of Hernia

The herniated contents are reduced manually, as required, and the robotic vessel sealer may be used (along with the Force Bipolar) in a hand-over-hand manner. An additional formal grasper, such as the Cadiere, may be required. The left crus approach is preferred (Fig. 11.6) beginning with division of the short gastric vessels using the robotic vessel sealer from the level of the inferior pole of the spleen allowing for left crural exposure. In the event of massive herniation, the surgical approach

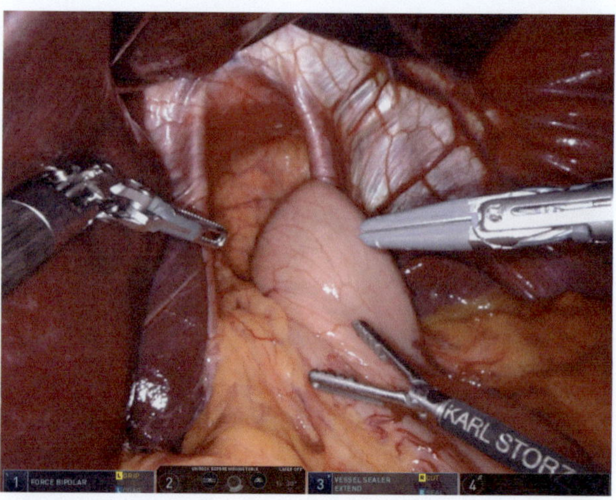

Fig. 11.5 Exposure of the hiatus with a large paraesophageal hernia

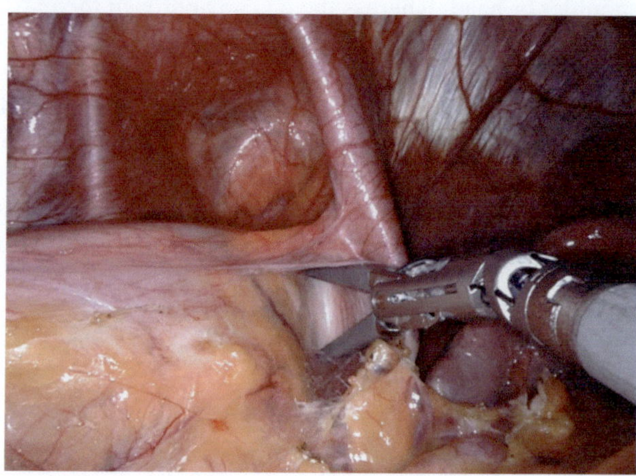

Fig. 11.6 Left crus approach

may have to be modified with initial dissection commencing at the interface of the hernia sac and the left crura avoiding excessive short gastric vessel division. Incision of the hernia sac is started at its junction with the left crus and continued around the rim of the hiatus in a circumferential fashion. Entry into the correct plane will ease the dissection and minimize bleeding and disorientation. Reduction of the sac is performed as much as possible from this position while avoiding injury to the anterior vagus nerve. Once the left crus is exposed, the dissection is then focused on the right side of the esophagus. The pars flaccida is opened, and the right crus is mobilized with a combination of blunt dissection, hook dissection, and robotic vessel sealer, reducing further the intrathoracic component of the hernia and sac. A retro-esophageal window is created and a Penrose drain passed and secured with an 0-PDS Endoloop which is used for further manipulation and retraction by the assistant as the dissection continues into the mediastinum.

Fig. 11.7 Hernia sac dissected off the mediastinum

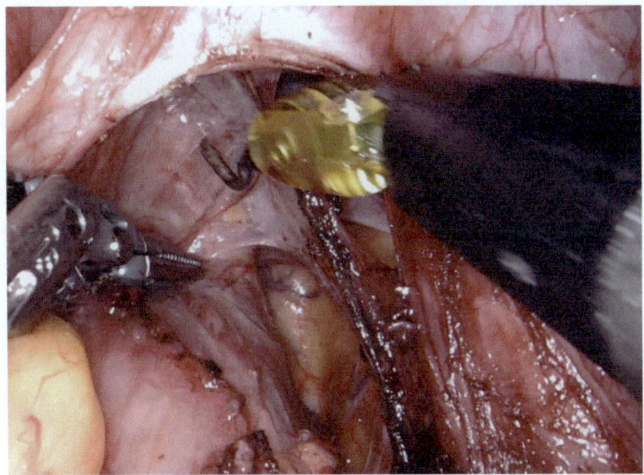

Next, the hernia sac is dissected off its mediastinal attachments (Fig. 11.7). This can be a tedious process requiring technical precision and circumferential approach. Care must be taken to identify the pleural attachments that are often intimate with the hernia sac. Any violation of the pleura should be addressed by means of immediate closure with suture or clip placement. Subsequent desufflation of the abdomen and 1 minute of bag ventilation per anesthesia will obviate any clinical implication.

The aorta is identified posteriorly and the esophageal attachments divided allowing for circumferential mobilization. The anterior and posterior vagus nerves are identified and are kept with the esophagus. Once tension-free intra-abdominal esophagus has been achieved, the hernia dissection is complete [11].

Esophageal Lengthening

If a 3 cm intra-abdominal esophageal length cannot be obtained with esophageal mobilization alone, a Collis gastroplasty may be performed to obtain additional esophageal length. Failure to lengthen a shortened esophagus can lead to recurrence as it produces strain on the repair. The Collis procedure entails the creation of a gastric tube by vertically stapling the proximal stomach from the angle of His, parallel to a large bougie placed alongside the gastric lesser curvature. This neoesophagus permits that the new esophagogastric junction be located intra-abdominally. Collis gastroplasty is not without its complications. The neoesophagus created by the gastroplasty does not display the normal peristaltic activity of the esophagus and can lead to dysphagia. Persistent parietal cells can also lead to recurrent heartburn and esophagitis. In addition, the presence of a staple line can lead to leak rates of 1–3% even in high-volume, experienced centers [12]. We prefer a modality of lengthening that involves pulling down the fundus so that level of the angle of His is pulled into the jaws of the blue load stapling device in a parallel fashion necessitating a single staple line.

Crural Closure

The esophagus is retracted anteriorly and to the left. Closure of the diaphragmatic defect is started at the junction of the right and left crus to decrease tension on every stitch and is carried out cephalad. The closure is performed using a running 0 non-absorbable barbed suture (Fig. 11.8). A 52 Fr bougie is passed down the esophagus during the repair to tailor the closure and to avoid undue angulation as the esophagus passes through the hiatus. We also ensure visualization of the aorta and keep this structure away from the approximating suture. Furthermore, a C-shaped GORE® Bio-A is used routinely to reinforce the closure of the diaphragmatic defect. The mesh is secured in place to the antero- and retro-esophageal diaphragm using fibrin sealant. Additional anchoring sutures may be required. In the event that the diaphragmatic crura cannot be approximated primarily without tension, a relaxing incision may be necessary [13].

Relaxing Incisions

Relaxing incisions are typically performed on the right side unless excessive scarring or close proximity to the inferior vena cava (IVC) is prohibitive in which case a left-sided incision is performed. A right-sided relaxing incision is made by incising the diaphragm 2 cm lateral to the crus, between the right crus and IVC, and carrying this full thickness without violating the pleural space. Caution must be taken to avoid the anterior crural vein and the thoracic duct near the aortic hiatus. A left-sided incision is performed in a similar fashion between the left crus and the left seventh rib taking care not to injure the left-sided phrenic nerve. In cases where a unilateral relaxing incision is not sufficient, bilateral relaxing incisions can be performed. The crural closure and relaxing incisions should be reinforced and covered with a mesh [14].

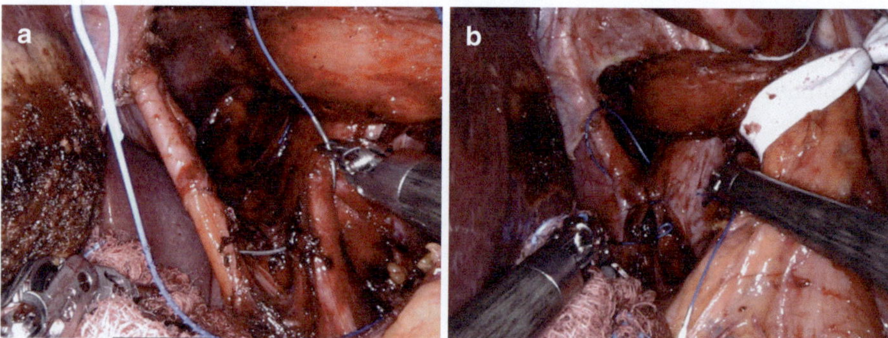

Fig. 11.8 (**a, b**) Posterior crural closure using a running nonabsorbable barbed suture

Fundoplication

The creation of a floppy tension-free 360 degree fundoplication is gauged over a 52F bougie. If the fundus is not completely free of hiatal or posterior attachments, then additional dissection is performed. The fundus is then placed up on the left crura and is grasped from the posterior retroesophageal window. The shoeshine maneuver is fundamental to ensure the proper orientation of the wrap demonstrating a "short gastric to short gastric" association (Fig. 11.9). This confirms proper fundal placement of the wrap preventing wrap herniation. It also avoids undue twisting of the fundus as it comes around the esophagus. Once this maneuver is satisfied, an initial 2-0 silk suture attaches stomach to the stomach using the divided short gastric vessels as landmarks for approximation (Fig. 11.10). The Penrose drain is removed at this point. A second 2-0 silk suture then encompasses the stomach, esophagus, and stomach to truly anchor the wrap

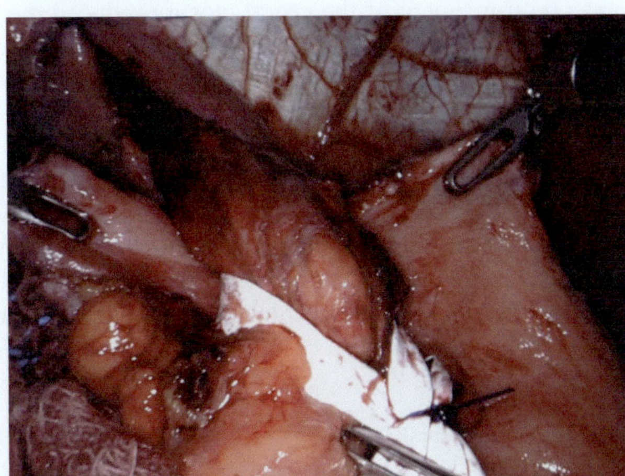

Fig. 11.9 Shoeshine maneuver

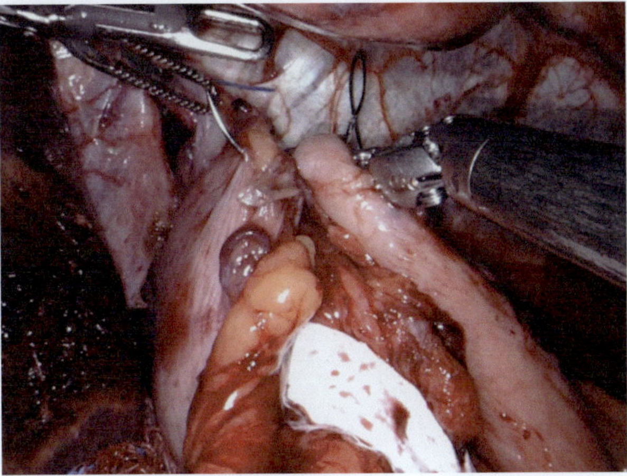

Fig. 11.10 Floppy Nissen fundoplication

in a proper location. A final suture incorporating only the stomach may be placed. We prefer to anchor the wrap posteriorly to the midline crura. Other techniques of fixation such as lateral crural suture fixation may be used with caution not to alter the orientation of the wrap. Upper endoscopy is performed at the completion of the case to check the indemnity of the mucosa of the esophagus and stomach and to verify the adequacy, orientation, and patency of the fundoplication. In the presence of impaired or unknown esophageal motility, a partial (270 degree) Toupet fundoplication is preferred.

Mesh Reinforcement

Both permanent and biologic meshes have been shown to be effective in reducing early recurrences in separate randomized trials. In a 2016 meta-analysis of four randomized trials including 406 patients, compared with suture closure alone, mesh reinforcement of the crural closure reduced the rate of reoperation but not recurrence or complication rates. On the other hand, no comparative large studies have been performed on the use of bioabsorbable mesh (Fig. 11.11); however, these short studies demonstrated its safety and effectiveness [15, 16].

The ideal hernia repair should result in a permanent retention of the stomach in the abdominal cavity. However, the recurrence rate following PEH repair is high because of a pressure gradient resulting from the positive intra-abdominal pressure and negative intrathoracic pressure. While not routinely applied at our institution, such fixation techniques are described below and may be useful in acute presentations or in giant hernias for which the boggy reduced and enlarged stomach seems functionally impaired [11].

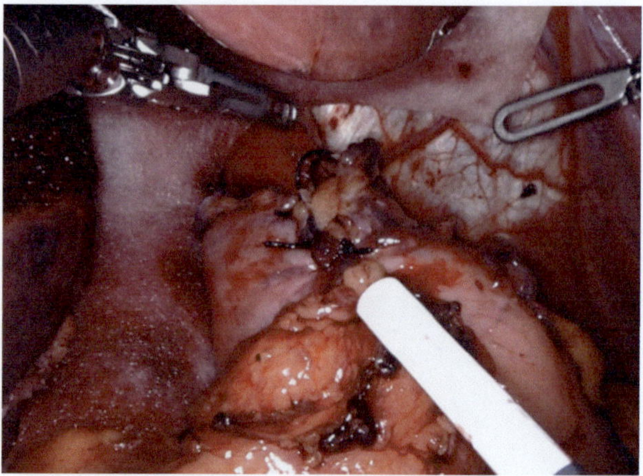

Fig. 11.11 Bio-A mesh (GORE®) placed in a C-shape to reinforce the anterior and posterior hiatus

Anterior Gastropexy with Sutures

Gastropexy with sutures to the anterior abdominal wall may be performed at the end of a PEH repair.

Posterior Gastropexy with Sutures (Hill Repair)

Sutures placed from the lower esophageal sphincter to the arcuate ligament are performed less often due to its technical difficultness and poor results. An anterior gastropexy is preferred [17].

Anterior Gastropexy with PEG Tubes

An endoscopic hernia reduction with or without laparoscopic assistance, followed by anterior gastropexy with two PEG tubes, may be performed for patients who are too frail to undertake a formal PEH repair or for patients in an emergency setting. The placement of two PEG tubes reduces the potential risk of stomach volvulus around a single PEG tube. This procedure relieves symptoms from a paraesophageal hernia, prevents the occurrence of gastric volvulus, and does not preclude a formal hernia repair at a later time [18].

Perioperative Complications

Pneumothorax

Violation of the pleura is a common complication of the challenging dissection of the hernia sac in the mediastinum. This usually has minimal clinical consequences, but immediate communication with anesthesia is imperative. Primary closure with suture or clips is appropriate. This sometimes requires further dissection to remove tension of the scarred sac off of the pleura. Abdominal desufflation and handbag mask ventilation can alleviate any notable capnothorax. Of course, one must be prepared for more aggressive intervention such as thoracostomy tube if clinically warranted. However, it is important in the perioperative setting to remember the mechanism of pneumothoraces in this surgical patient population.

Vagal Injury

Inadvertent injury to the anterior and posterior vagus nerves is possible at multiple points of the procedure. Both traction and sharp/thermal are possible. Rates range from 10–42%. Injury may cause clinically relevant gastroparesis presenting with nausea and vomiting as well as diarrhea. Careful dissection and early as well as continued identification are key to avoid inadvertent injury [19].

While there is a concern for gastroparesis and gastric outlet obstruction after vagal injury, Oelschlager et al. performed a review of 30 patients who underwent a vagotomy during the course of an esophageal lengthening procedure, 20 anterior, six posterior, and four bilateral, and compared the results with 72 patients that did not have a vagotomy. The primary presenting symptoms were improved in both groups. Similarly, there was no difference in the severity of abdominal pain, bloating, diarrhea, or early satiety between the vagotomy and no vagotomy groups at follow-up (median of 19 months). No patient required a subsequent operation for gastric outlet obstruction [20].

Esophageal Perforation

Although rare, esophageal perforation can be a catastrophic complication leading to mediastinitis and death if not recognized and managed appropriately. They are frequently associated to Collis gastroplasty (88%), and its overall occurrence and presentation as a postoperative leak is 2.5% [4]. Our preference would be complete exposure including endoscopic evaluation followed by primary full-thickness repair.

Gastric Perforation

Inadvertant gastric injury with perforation is rare (0.3%) and should be managed as above with full exposure and primary repair. The location will often be optimally incorporated in the fundoplication [4]. Endoscopic evaluation may be beneficial for complete evaluation.

Bleeding

A most common source of bleeding may be from the short gastric vessels following transection with thermal energy. It is often due to blighting at the angle of division and subsequent temporary retraction.

A more concerning intrathoracic bleeding event may occur from small arterial vessels branching from the aorta during the posterior dissection. Larger vessel bleeding may occur. Inflammation of the sac can lead to diffuse oozing during the mediastinal dissection. Regardless of location, general principles of surgery including pressure, communication, exposure, and control are necessary. The robotic forum adds 3-D visualization and ergonomic ease of access in confined spaces. We prefer initial control with pressure by insertion of Raytec® gauze. Adjuncts such as 10 mm suction devices may be useful. Assessment and definitive control through application of thermal energy device or clips may then ensue. Communication with anesthesia is crucial.

Dysphagia

As with many hiatal surgery, dysphagia may ensue and has multiple possible etiologies. Thorough evaluation by means of UGIS, EGD, and manometry is often required. Common causes can be undue angulation of the esophagus as it enters the abdomen due to the crural closure. A wrap may be functionally too tight. Both of these may be alleviated by serial endoscopic dilatation. Wrap slippage may necessitate revisional surgery.

Reflux

According to a prospective study of 111 patients performed at Johns Hopkins University where a validated gastroesophageal reflux disease-specific quality of life (QOL) tool was administered to patients before and at 2, 12, and 36 months after the procedure (higher QOL scores represented greater severity of symptoms). Overall, patients experienced significant symptom improvement at postoperative months 2 (mean QOL score, 10.18 [7.39]), 12 (mean QOL score, 9.74 [8.69]), and 36 (mean QOL score, 10.58 [9.14]) compared with baseline (mean QOL score, 28.50 [11.13]) *(P < 0.001)* [21].

Outcomes

PEH is a potentially devastating condition frequently manifesting in patients of advanced age with other substantial medical problems.

The pressure gradient across the abdominal and thoracic cavities predisposes the patient to a recurrence after a PEH repair. A meta-analysis of 13 studies, including 965 patients, reported an overall recurrence of 10.2% and a "true" recurrence rate of 25.5% when a follow-up barium esophagogram was used [22].

Most patients with a radiographic recurrence after PEH repair are asymptomatic, and patients with a clinical recurrence often have reflux symptoms that can be controlled with proton pump inhibitors. Only a small fraction of patients will require a reoperation for complications or intractable symptoms.

Robotic-assisted paraesophageal hernia repair is a safe procedure that has a learning curve of about 36 cases. Upon review of the literature, this approach seems to have the same benefits as those of the laparoscopic approach in terms of total surgical time, complication rate, length of hospital stay, and quality of life; in addition, the robotic platform may be associated with a lower recurrence rate than the laparoscopic approach according to small retrospective series [23].

Reoperative Considerations

Reoperation for a symptomatic paraesophageal hernia should be performed by highly experienced surgeons, as these procedures present a significant technical challenge, especially if permanent mesh has been placed at the time of the index operation. In this setting, the robotic platform presents an invaluable approach, as it contributes to decrease the rate of conversion to an open procedure, especially in the presence of perforation, ischemia, or significant blood loss, and intraoperative complications that can still be fixed while sitting in the console.

In more complex reoperative cases (patients who failed numerous transabdominal repairs), a transthoracic approach can offer a virgin territory for repair.

Emergent Repair: Timing and Indication

Over 40 years ago, life-threatening complications such as gastric ischemia, perforation, or severe hemorrhage were thought to occur in up to 30% of patients diagnosed with PEH. As a result, operative repair of any PEH was sought, irrespective of symptoms. Recent literature and modern operative techniques challenge these historical estimates. Stylopoulos used a Markov Monte Carlo model to predict clinical outcomes related to elective laparoscopic hernia repair and watchful waiting. He found an annual probability of developing acute complications requiring emergent surgery of 1.1% in the watchful waiting group and a mortality rate of 1.4 and 5.4% for laparoscopic elective surgery and emergency surgery, respectively.

Giant paraesophageal hernias may present acutely with Borchardt's triad: severe epigastric pain, retching, and inability to pass a nasogastric tube. The best timing for an operative repair after an acute presentation is a subject of ongoing debate. Although any clinical or radiological suspicion of acute ischemia or perforation requires immediate surgical management, most acute presentations can be initially managed conservatively providing the opportunity for semi-elective repair [24].

Cost Analysis of Laparoscopic Versus Robotic Fundoplication

Robotic compared to laparoscopic Nissen fundoplication and hiatal hernia repair have been demonstrated to be associated with increased costs in previously published studies. Müller-Stich et al. conducted a randomized controlled trial comparing laparoscopic to robotic fundoplication. They identified a shorter operative time for robotic fundoplication at 88 min, compared to 102 min for laparoscopic ($p = 0.033$). Costs were higher for robotic compared to laparoscopic procedures (€3244 vs. €2743, respectively; $p = 0.003$). A study on robotic fundoplication costs using the United Health System Consortium database included 12,079 patients who underwent robotic, laparoscopic, or open fundoplication. When laparoscopic was compared to robotic fundoplication, there was no significant difference in morbidity, mortality, or length of stay. Robotic fundoplication was associated with an increased 30-day readmission rate compared to a laparoscopic approach (3.6 vs. 1.8%; $p < 0.05$). Costs were also higher in robotic procedures in this study ($10,644 robotic vs. $7968 laparoscopic; $p < 0.05$). Another large database study, this time using the Nationwide Inpatient Sample, evaluated 297,335 patients undergoing robotic compared to laparoscopic gastrointestinal surgery, including both fundoplication and gastroenterostomy without gastrectomy. In the fundoplication cohort, there was no difference in the length of stay or complications. Costs were significantly higher with robotic fundoplication ($37,638 vs. $32,947; $p < 0.0001$).

According to Higgins RM et al., after retrospectively evaluating 22 robotic and 115 laparoscopic fundoplication procedures, robotic cases were associated with a statistically significant increase in operative time and overall supply cost. The mean and median number of robotic instruments used for fundoplication was 4.9 and 4.0, respectively. The mean total cost of robotic instruments, excluding outliers, was $1320.7 and $2925.2 including outliers. Among the 22 robotic fundoplications performed, 13 outlier instruments were used (individual case cost of >$1000). These instruments included primarily bowel graspers and cautery spatulas. To account for the amortized upfront cost of the robotic instruments, an additional analysis of standardizing the cost of each robotic instrument as $200 per case was performed. From this, it was determined that there was no difference in total supply cost between robotic and laparoscopic fundoplications [25].

Conclusion

Robot-assisted laparoscopic hiatal hernia repair has demonstrated low short-term clinical recurrence rates with morbidity and quality of life comparable to the literature for laparoscopic repair, even in older patients and those with high operative risks. With increasing numbers of robotic-trained general surgeons in the community, a wider application of the robotic platform for the repair of paraesophageal hernia, even in complex cases, is expected which will bring shorter operative times. It will also allow wider application of minimally invasive technique although surgeon experience and knowledge of anatomy may not be substituted. The ergonomic and visual advantages of the robotic platform add surgical precision and potentially lower recurrence rates.

References

1. Geha AS, Massad MG, Snow NJ, Baue AE. A 32-year experience in 100 patients with giant paraesophageal hernia: the case for abdominal approach and selective antireflux repair. Surgery. 2000;128(4):623–30. https://doi.org/10.1067/msy.2000.108425. PubMed PMID: 11015096.
2. Seetharamaiah R, Romero RJ, Kosanovic R, Gallas M, Verdeja JC, Rabaza J, Gonzalez AM. Robotic repair of giant paraesophageal hernias. JSLS. 2013;17(4):570–7. https://doi.org/10.4293/108680813X13654754534594. PubMed PMID: 24398199; PMCID: PMC3866061.
3. Hall T, Warnes N, Kuchta K, Novak S, Hedberg H, Linn JG, Haggerty S, Denham W, Joehl RJ, Ujiki M. Patient-centered outcomes after laparoscopic paraesophageal hernia repair. J Am Coll Surg. 2018;227(1):106–14. https://doi.org/10.1016/j.jamcollsurg.2017.12.054. PubMed PMID: 29454100.
4. Luketich JD, Nason KS, Christie NA, Pennathur A, Jobe BA, Landreneau RJ, Schuchert MJ. Outcomes after a decade of laparoscopic giant paraesophageal hernia repair. J Thorac Cardiovasc Surg. 2010;139(2):395–404, e1. https://doi.org/10.1016/j.jtcvs.2009.10.005. PubMed PMID: 20004917; PMCID: PMC2813424.
5. Vasudevan V, Reusche R, Nelson E, Kaza S. Robotic paraesophageal hernia repair: a single-center experience and systematic review. J Robot Surg. 2018;12(1):81–6. https://doi.org/10.1007/s11701-017-0697-x. PubMed PMID: 28374223.

6. Dunnican WJ, Singh TP, Guptill GG, Doorly MG, Ata A. Early robotic experience with para-esophageal hernia repair and Nissen fundoplication: short-term outcomes. J Robot Surg. 2008;2(1):41–4. https://doi.org/10.1007/s11701-008-0079-5. PubMed PMID: 27637217.

7. Wirsching A, Zhang Q, McCormick SE, Hubka M, Low DE. Abnormal high-resolution manometry findings and outcomes after paraesophageal hernia repair. J Am Coll Surg. 2018;227(2):181–8 e2. https://doi.org/10.1016/j.jamcollsurg.2018.03.033. PubMed PMID: 29605727.

8. Pohl D, Tutuian R. Reflux monitoring: pH-metry, Bilitec and oesophageal impedance measurements. Best Pract Res Clin Gastroenterol. 2009;23(3):299–311. https://doi.org/10.1016/j.bpg.2009.04.003. PubMed PMID: 19505660.

9. Diez Del Val I, Martinez Blazquez C, Loureiro Gonzalez C, Vitores Lopez JM, Sierra Esteban V, Barrenetxea Asua J, Del Hoyo Aretxabala I, Perez de Villarreal P, Bilbao Axpe JE, Mendez Martin JJ. Robot-assisted gastroesophageal surgery: usefulness and limitations. J Robot Surg. 2014;8(2):111–8. https://doi.org/10.1007/s11701-013-0435-y. PubMed PMID: 27637520.

10. DeUgarte DA, Hirschl RB, Geiger JD. Robotic repair of congenital paraesophageal hiatal hernia. J Laparoendosc Adv Surg Tech A. 2009;19(Suppl 1):S187–9. https://doi.org/10.1089/lap.2008.0185.supp. PubMed PMID: 19331624.

11. Galvani CA, Loebl H, Osuchukwu O, Samame J, Apel ME, Ghaderi I. Robotic-assisted para-esophageal hernia repair: initial experience at a single institution. J Laparoendosc Adv Surg Tech A. 2016;26(4):290–5. https://doi.org/10.1089/lap.2016.0096. PubMed PMID: 27035739.

12. Zaman JA, Lidor AO. The optimal approach to symptomatic paraesophageal hernia repair: important technical considerations. Curr Gastroenterol Rep. 2016;18(10):53. https://doi.org/10.1007/s11894-016-0529-6. PubMed PMID: 27595155.

13. Asti E, Sironi A, Bonitta G, Lovece A, Milito P, Bonavina L. Crura augmentation with Bio-A((R)) mesh for laparoscopic repair of hiatal hernia: single-institution experience with 100 consecutive patients. Hernia : the journal of hernias and abdominal wall surgery. 2017;21(4):623–8. Epub 2017/04/12. https://doi.org/10.1007/s10029-017-1603-1. PubMed PMID: 28396955.

14. Crespin OM, Yates RB, Martin AV, Pellegrini CA, Oelschlager BK. The use of crural relaxing incisions with biologic mesh reinforcement during laparoscopic repair of complex hiatal hernias. Surg Endosc. 2016;30(6):2179–85. https://doi.org/10.1007/s00464-015-4522-1. PubMed PMID: 26335079.

15. Memon MA, Memon B, Yunus RM, Khan S. Suture Cruroplasty versus prosthetic hiatal hernior-rhaphy for large hiatal hernia: a meta-analysis and systematic review of randomized controlled trials. Ann Surg. 2016;263(2):258–66. https://doi.org/10.1097/SLA.0000000000001267. PubMed PMID: 26445468.

16. Tam V, Winger DG, Nason KS. A systematic review and meta-analysis of mesh vs suture cruroplasty in laparoscopic large hiatal hernia repair. Am J Surg. 2016;211(1):226–38. https://doi.org/10.1016/j.amjsurg.2015.07.007. PubMed PMID: 26520872; PMCID: PMC5153660.

17. Park Y, Aye RW, Watkins JR, Farivar AS, Louie BE. Laparoscopic Hill repair: 25-year follow-up. Surg Endosc. 2018;32(10):4111–5. https://doi.org/10.1007/s00464-018-6150-z. PubMed PMID: 29602997.

18. Kercher KWMB, Ponsky JL, Goldstein SL, Yavorski RT, Sing RF, Heniford BT. Minimally invasive management of paraesophageal herniation in the high-risk surgical patient. Am J Surg. 2001;182(5):510–4.

19. Van Rijn S et al., Effect of vagus nerve injury on the outcome of antireflux surgery: an extensive literature review. dig surg. 2016;33:230–9.

20. Oelschlager BK, Yamamoto K, Woltman T, Pellegrini C. Vagotomy during hiatal hernia repair: a benign esophageal lengthening procedure. J Gastrointest Surg. 2008;12(7):1155. https://doi.org/10.1007/s11605-008-0520-0.

21. Lidor AO, Steele KE, Stem M, Fleming RM, Schweitzer MA, Marohn MR. Long-term quality of life and risk factors for recurrence after laparoscopic repair of paraesophageal hernia. JAMA Surg. 2015;150(5):424–31. https://doi.org/10.1001/jamasurg.2015.25.

22. Rathore MA, Andrabi SI, Bhatti MI, Najfi SM, McMurray A. Metaanalysis of recurrence after laparoscopic repair of paraesophageal hernia. JSLS. 2007;11(4):456–60. Epub 2008/02/02. PubMed PMID: 18237510; PMCID: PMC3015848.
23. Brenkman HJ, Parry K, van Hillegersberg R, Ruurda JP. Robot-assisted laparoscopic hiatal hernia repair: promising anatomical and functional results. J Laparoendosc Adv Surg Tech A. 2016;26(6):465–9. https://doi.org/10.1089/lap.2016.0065. PubMed PMID: 27078499.
24. Wirsching A, El Lakis MA, Mohiuddin K, Pozzi A, Hubka M, Low DE. Acute vs. elective paraesophageal hernia repair: endoscopic gastric decompression allows semi-elective surgery in a majority of acute patients. J Gastrointest Surg. 2018;22(2):194–202. https://doi.org/10.1007/s11605-017-3495-x. PubMed PMID: 28770418.
25. Higgins RM, Frelich MJ, Bosler ME, Gould JC. Cost analysis of robotic versus laparoscopic general surgery procedures. Surg Endosc. 2017;31(1):185–92. https://doi.org/10.1007/s00464-016-4954-2. PubMed PMID: 27139704.

Management of the Short Esophagus in GERD

12

Steven R. DeMeester

Introduction

In the normal anatomic arrangement, several centimeters of the distal esophagus and the gastroesophageal junction (GEJ) lie below the esophageal hiatus within the abdomen. This allows the lower esophageal sphincter to be within the hiatus, such that crural contraction with inspiration augments sphincter resistance to the flow of gastric contents into the thoracic esophagus during times of increased abdominal pressure. When the GEJ, the fundus of the stomach, or both migrate into the chest above the hiatus, a hiatal hernia is present. Sliding hiatal hernias are characterized by the GEJ remaining above the fundus of the stomach, while with paraesophageal hernias (PEH), the fundus of the stomach is above the GEJ and located next to the esophagus. In most patients with a PEH, the GEJ has also migrated above the diaphragm into the chest.

Intrinsic to the repair of a hiatal hernia is the need to bring the GEJ, stomach, and distal esophagus back into the abdomen. However, since 1950, it has been known that in some patients, this can be challenging, particularly those with severe gastroesophageal reflux disease (GERD) or a large hiatal hernia. In these patients, esophageal shortening can lead to loss of intra-abdominal esophageal length and put the repair of the hernia under tension. Tension during repair of any hernia is known to increase the risk for hernia recurrence. Consequently, in 1957, Dr. J. Leigh Collis described a technique to address acquired esophageal shortening and reduce tension during hiatal hernia repair [1]. His technique, now referred to as a Collis gastroplasty, creates an extension to the esophagus by creating a tube of neoesophagus from the upper stomach. His gastroplasty was done as a transthoracic procedure, but subsequently, several techniques have been developed to create the gastroplasty using a laparoscopic approach. The laparoscopic management of a short esophagus

S. R. DeMeester (✉)
Thoracic and Foregut Surgery, The Oregon Clinic, Portland, OR, USA
e-mail: sdemeester@orclinic.com

© Springer Nature Switzerland AG 2020
S. Horgan, K.-H. Fuchs (eds.), *Management of Gastroesophageal Reflux Disease*,
https://doi.org/10.1007/978-3-030-48009-7_12

is challenging, and as a result, there is a tendency by many surgeons to ignore esophageal length and proceed with a standard repair. However, tension is the enemy of any hernia repair, and long-term successful outcomes with hiatal hernia repairs, as for all other abdominal hernias, require addressing tension when encountered.

Identifying the Short Esophagus

Patients at risk for acquired esophageal shortening include those with advanced GERD with esophagitis, stricture, long-segment Barrett's esophagus, a history of sarcoidosis, caustic ingestion, scleroderma, and a large sliding or paraesophageal hernia [2, 3]. In some reports, patients with a PEH have the highest frequency of a short esophagus [4].

The presence of a foreshortened esophagus in patients with severe GERD is understandable since exposure to refluxed gastric juice causes mucosal injury and can lead to transmural inflammation, fibrosis, and collagen contraction. An esophageal stricture is strongly associated with a shortened esophagus and the need for a gastroplasty. The presence of both a large hiatal hernia (>5 cm) and an esophageal stricture further increases the risk of a shortened esophagus [2]. In addition, a history of a previous failed antireflux procedure with recurrent hiatal hernia should raise suspicion that the length of the esophagus is short. The etiology of esophageal shortening in patients with a PEH is unclear but may be related to loss of elasticity in the longitudinal esophageal muscle related to chronic loss of intra-abdominal fixation of the gastroesophageal junction. While any of these histories should increase the suspicion that a patient may have a short esophagus, none are definitive.

The preoperative workup for any patient presenting with a hiatal hernia or GERD symptoms should include a thorough history and objective studies to understand the relevant pathophysiology. Potentially important objective studies include upper endoscopy, esophageal manometry, 24 or 48 hour pH monitoring, and a video-esophagram. The indication for repair of a sliding hiatal hernia is the presence of documented GERD, while for a PEH, it is the presence of symptoms, age 65 or under, or a type IV hernia with the stomach and another organ in the chest [5]. Symptoms in patients with a PEH may be GERD related but often consist of shortness of breath or chest discomfort after meals, dysphagia, or the presence of anemia. The objective studies will define the size, type, and reducibility of any hiatal hernia, presence of a stricture or erosive esophagitis, esophageal function, and the presence and severity of increased esophageal exposure to refluxed gastric juice. A foreshortened esophagus can effectively be ruled out when a hiatal hernia fully reduces on barium esophagram, but in any nonreducing hiatal hernia, a short esophagus may be present. Therefore, while objective studies can rule out a short esophagus, none can accurately identify its presence. Instead, a foreshortened esophagus can only be confirmed by the intraoperative inability to reduce the gastroesophageal junction below the hiatus by 2–3 cm after mediastinal esophageal mobilization and posterior crural closure.

Management of the Short Esophagus

Although the existence and frequency of a foreshortened esophagus remains debated, failure to obtain an adequate length of intra-abdominal esophagus during hiatal hernia repair has been proposed as a leading cause for reherniation, slippage, or breakdown of the repair [6]. It has been reported that 20–33% of patients with an inadequate intra-abdominal length will fail after a fundoplication [3]. The primary method of esophageal lengthening during repair of a hiatal hernia is mediastinal esophageal mobilization. In addition, patients with a large hiatal hernia, particularly a PEH, are often kyphotic, and closing the hiatus posteriorly brings the esophagus anterior and adds intra-abdominal length. In order to accomplish a fundoplication without tension, there should be 2–3 cm of intra-abdominal esophagus below the hiatal closure (Fig. 12.1).

The amount of intra-abdominal esophagus during laparoscopic surgery is deceptive since the pneumoperitoneum artificially elevates the diaphragm and gives the appearance of more esophageal length than what is actually present. With deflation of the pneumoperitoneum, the diaphragm descends, and some of the apparent esophageal length is lost. Thus, if posterior crural closure and mediastinal esophageal mobilization are insufficient to provide 2–3 cm of abdominal esophagus, esophageal lengthening is recommended. In addition, creation of a capnothorax during laparoscopic surgery is well tolerated, particularly if done bilaterally, and will put the diaphragm in neutral position. This reduces crural closure tension and also permits a more realistic assessment of intra-abdominal esophageal length [7].

My preferred approach for a Collis gastroplasty has been previously published and is based on the wedge fundectomy Collis gastroplasty (WFCG) technique described by Terry and colleagues [8]. After determining that intra-abdominal length is less than 3 cm, a 52 French bougie is passed and kept along the lesser

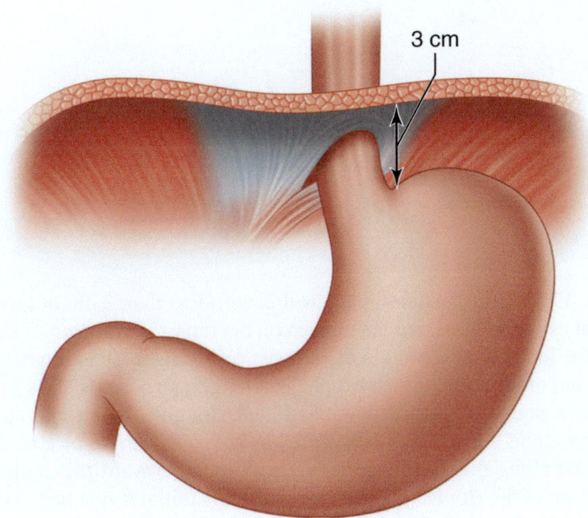

Fig. 12.1 An important concern for reducing hiatal hernia recurrence is obtaining adequate esophageal length. Most surgeons consider 3 cm of intra-abdominal length, the requisite length when measured from the left crus to the angle of His and gastroesophageal junction

curvature of the stomach. The aim is to establish 3 cm of intra-abdominal esophagus or neoesophagus, so if the GEJ was 1 cm below the hiatus, a 2 cm Collis is created, and if the GEJ was at the hiatus, a 3 cm gastroplasty is created. The planned length of the Collis gastroplasty is marked on the lesser curve by measuring down from the angle of His 1, 2, or 3 cm as needed to obtain 3 cm of intra-abdominal esophagus.

The gastroplasty is started with a staple line from the greater curve headed toward the angle of His in order to minimize the amount of fundus that is ultimately resected (Fig. 12.2a–c). Subsequent staple lines sequentially cut through the inferior staple line, gradually working down toward the mark initially made along the lesser curvature (Fig. 12.3a, b). My preference is a 45 mm purple load with a powered stapler that allows precise adjustment of the angle of the stapler. The last staple line toward the bougie should have the bougie on each side of the jaws of the stapler such that

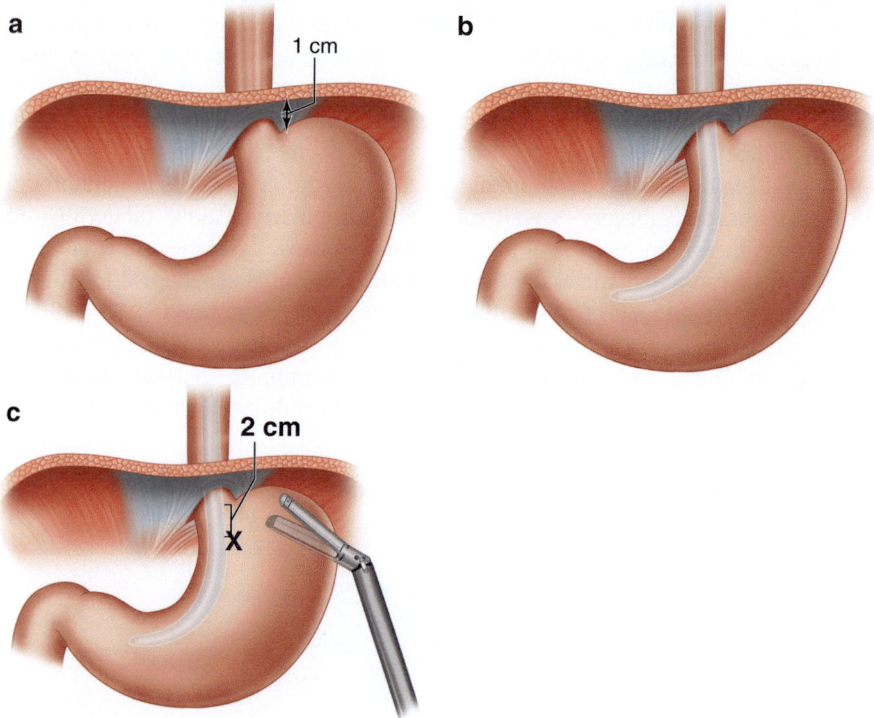

Fig. 12.2 (**a**) In patients such as this with less than 3 cm of intra-abdominal length, a Collis gastroplasty is added to reduce tension on the repair. The length of the Collis gastroplasty is dependent on the location of the angle of His/gastroesophageal junction below the left crus. In this case, there is 1 cm of intra-abdominal esophageal length, so a 2 cm Collis gastroplasty will be added. (**b**) A 52 French bougie is passed down and kept along the lesser curvature of the stomach. (**c**) A mark is made along the lesser curvature 2 cm below the angle of His. The 45 mm articulating stapler is placed along the greater curvature and aimed toward the angle of His to minimize the ultimate amount of the stomach that is resected. This initial staple line is not directed at the "X" making the spot 2 cm below the angle of His

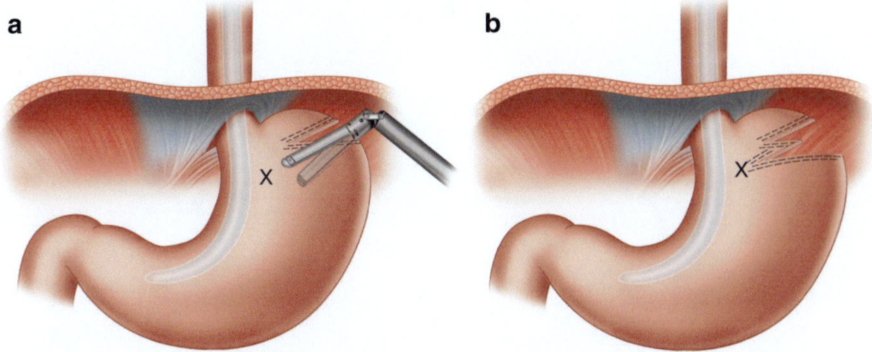

Fig. 12.3 (**a**) The subsequent stapler application is placed across the inferior staple line from the initial staple cut, gradually working down toward the mark created on the lesser curve 2 cm below the angle of His. Depending on how far down the mark is, it may take several staple lines, each through the inferior staple line of the prior stapler application, to reach the mark. (**b**) In this way, a "starfish"-shaped piece of fundus is gradually created

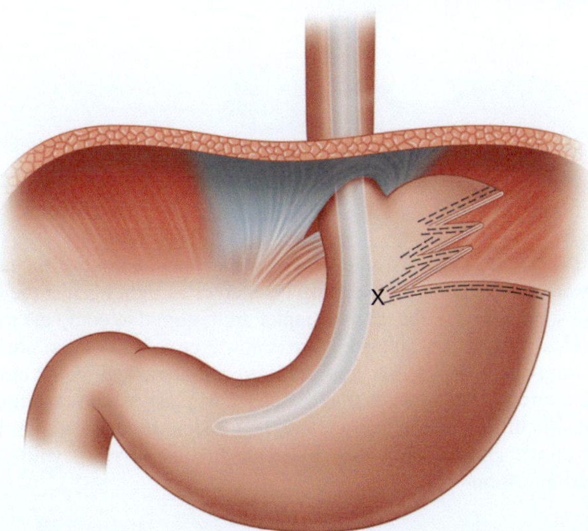

Fig. 12.4 Once the mark is reached, the stapler is aimed directly across the mark with one blade above and one below the bougie. When the stapler is closed, it will bounce off the bougie. This will ensure that the final staple line is as close as possible to the bougie

when it is closed, the jaws bounce off the bougie. This allows the staple line to get as close to the bougie as possible (Fig. 12.4). Once the staple line is as close as possible to the bougie, the stapler is aimed upward toward the angle of His parallel to the bougie (Fig. 12.5a–c). It is important to keep the stapler as tight onto the bougie as possible since the gastroplasty tube is aperistaltic. The objective is to have the lumen of the gastroplasty smaller than the native esophagus, so the funnel effect moves food from the distal esophagus through the gastroplasty to the stomach. The final resected piece of fundus has a starfish-shaped appearance. This is removed in a specimen-retrieval bag. The staple line should be inspected to ensure hemostasis and integrity. I do not use any staple line reinforcement material.

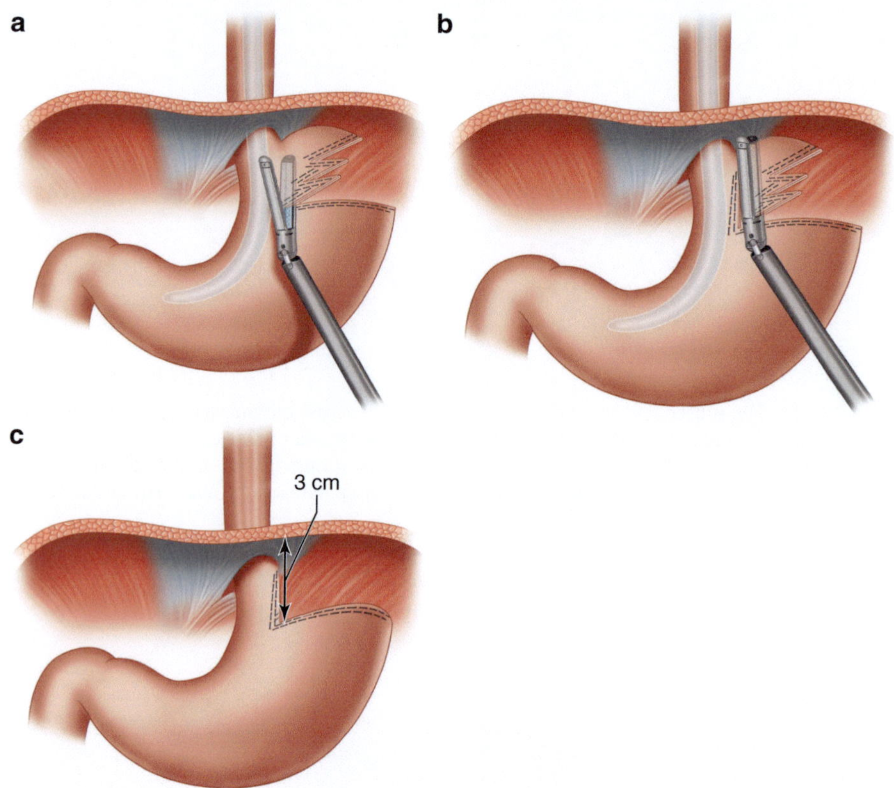

Fig. 12.5 (**a**) Once the staple line has reached the bougie, the next staple load is directed upward toward the angle of His, keeping the stapler as tight against the bougie as possible. (**b**) Typically, 2–3 staple loads of the 45 mm stapler are required to complete the resection of the small wedge of fundus. (**c**) Once completed, there is now 3 cm of intra-abdominal "esophagus." The original 1 cm of intra-abdominal esophagus had been supplemented with 2 cm of neoesophagus from the lesser curvature of the stomach (the Collis gastroplasty). The resulting staple line will be buried with creation of the fundoplication, and the residual fundus left after the wedge fundectomy technique as shown gives a very nice piece of fundus to work with for either a Toupet or a Nissen fundoplication

If a Toupet fundoplication is planned, the bougie can be removed and the crural closure completed prior to performing the Toupet. For a Nissen fundoplication, I leave the 52 bougie in place and do the Nissen fundoplication first and then remove the bougie and complete the crural closure. In both cases, with a Toupet or Nissen, the staple lines should be buried by the anterior fundus and the esophagus. This step minimizes the risk of any leak. Another important principle is that the fundoplication should be kept as high on the gastroplasty as possible, preferably at the top near the gastroesophageal junction. This will depend on how short the esophagus was initially. In most patients, the native GEJ lies below the hiatus after good esophageal mobilization and reduction of the hernia, and in these patients, the fundoplication can be placed around the Collis gastroplasty with the top at the native GEJ. In this situation, the fundoplication will lie nicely below the hiatus without tension, and all of the gastric-acid-secreting mucosa of the gastroplasty is within or below the fundoplication. In some patients, the esophagus is so short that the native GEJ is at or above the hiatus, which means the Collis gastroplasty extends into or above the hiatus. In these patients, since the fundoplication should remain in the abdomen, there will be a short length of Collis gastroplasty above the fundoplication. The importance of this is the fact that the gastroplasty is made from the stomach, and acid production by the gastric mucosa of the Collis gastroplasty above the fundoplication can lead to erosive esophagitis in the distal esophageal squamous mucosa in some patients [3, 9]. For this reason, I perform upper endoscopy on all patients 3 months after Collis gastroplasty, and if esophagitis is present, the patients are placed back on some form of acid suppression medication.

In our center, the type of fundoplication, partial or complete, is based on the patient's preoperative symptoms and objective test results. In elderly patients, or those with dysphagia, poor motility on high-resolution manometry, or impaired bolus clearance on videoesophagram, a partial (Toupet) fundoplication is preferred. Others are given a complete (Nissen) fundoplication. Since the gastroplasty tube is aperistaltic, bolus transport through the gastroplasty relies on the motility of the distal esophagus above the gastroplasty. Consequently, we are more liberal with the use of a partial fundoplication in patients that have a Collis gastroplasty.

Outcome with a Collis Gastroplasty

Before the introduction of laparoscopic surgery, most antireflux procedures were performed in patients with severe GERD, often with impaired esophageal body function. A Collis gastroplasty in these patients frequently led to protracted postoperative dysphagia. In a series reported in 1998, a transthoracic Collis gastroplasty in the presence of preoperative dysphagia was significantly associated with a poor postoperative outcome. Many of these patients had strictures and severe reflux disease [10]. The availability of potent acid-suppressing medications has led to a reduction in the acid-related complications of reflux disease including strictures. Furthermore, the number of patients presenting for elective repair of a paraesophageal hernia in the era of laparoscopic surgery is increasing. In these patients, a Collis gastroplasty seems to be better tolerated. In contrast to our earlier series, a recent evaluation of our laparoscopic Collis gastroplasties showed that severe reflux disease was less common [9]. The Collis gastroplasty was done in 72% of patients either for a PEH or during reoperation for a failed fundoplication. Dysphagia was a common preoperative symptom; however, it resolved in the majority of patients (71%) postoperatively. Importantly, new-onset dysphagia occurred in only two patients (5.5%) and resolved after one endoscopic dilatation in both patients. Dysphagia that was present preoperatively and persisted was typically mild and did not significantly impact the patient's diet or lifestyle. The relief of dysphagia in most patients was likely related to repair of the large hiatal hernia and healing of esophagitis. However, we also attributed the low rate of new-onset dysphagia to our "tailored approach" for a fundoplication, using a Toupet rather than a Nissen in patients with manometric evidence of ineffective esophageal motility [9].

A second potential issue with a Collis gastroplasty is acid production by the neoesophagus above the fundoplication. In our recent series, we found that the prevalence of esophagitis after laparoscopic Collis gastroplasty was much lower (11%) than reported by others. It is not clear why our prevalence was much less than the 36% rate reported by Jobe et al., but it may in part be related to our efforts to keep the fundoplication as high on the neoesophagus as possible without inducing excessive tension on the repair [9, 11]. It is also possible that the degree of shortening in our patients was less than that in the series by Jobe et al., because in patients with a very short esophagus the Collis gastroplasty can extend above the hiatus. In that circumstance, it is not possible to position the fundoplication at the top of the gastroplasty. Importantly, esophagitis in these patients is often asymptomatic. Consequently, I recommend that an early postoperative endoscopy be done after a Collis gastroplasty to evaluate for esophagitis. If esophagitis is found in the setting of an intact fundoplication treatment with acid suppression, medication is recommended to prevent stricture formation or other complications related to ongoing mucosal injury.

A transthoracic Collis gastroplasty has been associated with complications not typically seen with standard antireflux surgery, including staple line leaks, abscesses, and fistulas [12]. We are always careful to ensure adequate perfusion of the Collis segment and would avoid a Collis gastroplasty if there was any compromise of the lesser curve blood supply due to interruption of the left gastric artery. In our series of laparoscopic wedge fundectomy Collis gastroplasties, we did not have any of these complications. We routinely cover the Collis staple line with the fundoplication to minimize the risk of a leak or fistula. Further, the wedge fundectomy technique may lead to a wider and more robust portion of fundus that lessens the tension that was sometimes present with a fundoplication after a traditional transthoracic Collis gastroplasty.

The key issue of course with a Collis gastroplasty is whether it reduces hernia recurrence rates. In a recent publication on 50 elective laparoscopic PEH repairs, a Collis gastroplasty was used in 42%, and on 1-year objective follow-up, the hernia recurrence rate overall was 8%, but no patient with a Collis gastroplasty had a recurrent hernia [13]. It would seem logical that if the esophagus was deemed short in patients that had a Collis gastroplasty and a short esophagus should induce tension on the repair and increase the risk for hernia recurrence, then, if the Collis was not helping to reduce tension, these patients should have the highest rate of recurrent hernia on follow-up. Instead, none of these patients had a recurrent hernia, suggesting that the Collis gastroplasty is a useful adjunct to reduce tension and hernia recurrence in patients judged to have a short esophagus intraoperatively.

Conclusion

Patients found to have a short esophagus during laparoscopic hiatal hernia repair are likely at increased risk for breakdown of the repair and a recurrent hiatal hernia. The first steps to gain esophageal length are mediastinal esophageal mobilization and posterior crural closure. If these steps are inadequate, a Collis gastroplasty should be added. The wedge fundectomy technique allows esophageal lengthening laparoscopically and is associated with a low rate of complications. Clear-cut evidence that a laparoscopic Collis gastroplasty reduces hernia recurrence rates is lacking; however, tension on the repair of any hernia is associated with an increased failure rate. Consequently, a Collis gastroplasty in the setting of a foreshortened esophagus is likely to prove beneficial in the long term and should be part of the armamentarium of modern laparoscopic esophageal surgeons.

References

1. Collis JL. An operation for hiatus hernia with short esophagus. J Thorac Surg. 1957;34:768–78.
2. Gastal OL, et al. Short esophagus: analysis of predictors and clinical implications. Arch Surg. 1999;134(6):633–6; discussion 637-8.
3. Horvath KD, Swanstrom LL, Jobe BA. The short esophagus: pathophysiology, incidence, presentation, and treatment in the era of laparoscopic antireflux surgery. Ann Surg. 2000;232(5):630–40.
4. Herbella FAM, Del Grande JC, Colleoni R. Short esophagus: literature incidence. Dis Esophagus. 2002;15(2):125–31.
5. Stylopoulos N, Gazelle GS, Rattner DW. Paraesophageal hernias: operation or observation? Ann Surg. 2002;236(4):492–500; discussion 500-1.
6. Hashemi M, et al. Laparoscopic repair of large type III hiatal hernia: objective followup reveals high recurrence rate. J Am Coll Surg. 2000;190(5):553–60; discussion 560-1.
7. Davila Bradly D, et al. Assessment and reduction of diaphragmatic tension during hiatal hernia repair. Surg Endosc. 2015;29:796–804.
8. Terry ML, Vernon A, Hunter JG. Stapled-wedge Collis gastroplasty for the shortened esophagus. Am J Surg. 2004;188(2):195–9.
9. Zehetner J, et al. Laparoscopic wedge fundectomy for collis gastroplasty creation in patients with a foreshortened esophagus. Ann Surg. 2014;260(6):1030–3.
10. Ritter MP, et al. Treatment of advanced gastroesophageal reflux disease with Collis gastroplasty and Belsey partial fundoplication. Arch Surg. 1998;133(5):523–8; discussion 528-9.
11. Jobe BA, Horvath KD, Swanstrom LL. Postoperative function following laparoscopic collis gastroplasty for shortened esophagus. Arch Surg. 1998;133(8):867–74.
12. Patel HJ, et al. A 25-year experience with open primary transthoracic repair of paraesophageal hiatal hernia. J Thoracic Cardiovasc Surg. 2004;127(3):843–9.
13. Abdelmoaty W, et al. Combination of surgical technique and bioresorbable mesh reinforcement of the crural repair leads to low early hernia recurrence rate with laparoscopic paraesophageal hernia repair. J Gastrointest Surg. 2019: p. in press.

Overview and Management of Paraesophageal Hernias

13

Arielle Lee, Kai Neki, José Bezerra Câmara Neto, and Karl-Hermann Fuchs

Introduction and Classifications

At present, controversy exists regarding the management of hiatal hernia and its associated conditions, such as gastroesophageal reflux disease (GERD) and chronic anemia [1–6]. The majority of the controversy stems from the variable definitions of hernia types based on anatomical changes at the hiatus and the accuracy of diagnostic tests in differentiating these anatomical abnormalities [1, 2, 5]. In general, hiatal hernia can be defined as migration of either the stomach or esophagogastric junction and occasionally other visceral organs into the mediastinum, in the setting of deterioration of the phreno-esophageal ligament and widening of the hiatus.

The history of hiatal hernia surgery was best summarized by Stylopoulos and Rattner in 2005 [7]. The original definition and classification of hiatal hernias, in association with the most frequently associated disease, GERD, can be traced to 1948, when Allison published his fundamental paper on *Peptic Ulcers of the Esophagus* [8]. The first descriptions of post-traumatic and congenital diaphragmatic hernias date back to the sixteenth century [7]. In the first half of the twentieth century, several authors published their clinical experiences with hiatal hernias [7].

In 1948, Philip Allison described his clinical experience with several types of hiatal hernia, supported by radiographic studies [8]. He classified his experience into four different morphologic types (Fig. 13.1). In the first figure, he shows a true paraesophageal hernia, which he names as such (Fig. 13.1a). In the second figure, he demonstrates a sliding hiatal hernia with esophageal shortening (Fig. 13.1b). In the third figure, a sliding hiatal hernia is described, complicated by a paraesophageal pouch (Fig. 13.1c). The fourth figure demonstrates a "bulging hernia"

A. Lee · K. Neki · J. B. C. Neto · K.-H. Fuchs (✉)
University of California San Diego, Center for the Future of Surgery, La Jolla, CA, USA

© Springer Nature Switzerland AG 2020
S. Horgan, K.-H. Fuchs (eds.), *Management of Gastroesophageal Reflux Disease*,
https://doi.org/10.1007/978-3-030-48009-7_13

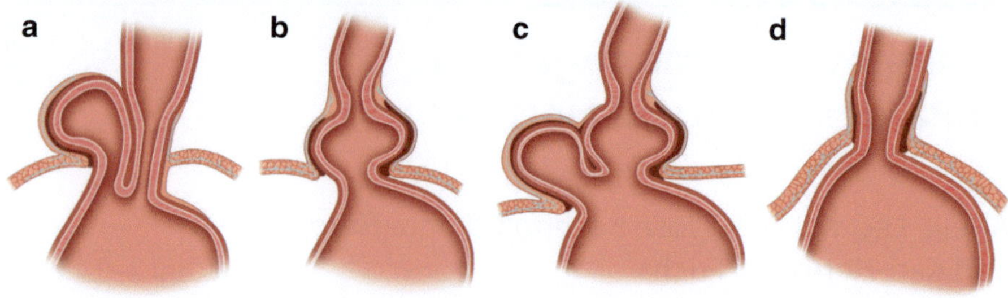

Fig. 13.1 The types of hiatal hernias as described by Allison 1948. His first drawing showed a true paraesophageal hernia (**a**), followed by a sliding hernia (**b**). The third was a mixed hernia (**c**) with both cardia and fundus migrated. The forth type (**d**) was a bulging of the diaphragm without migration of the stomach

(Fig. 13.1d). Of note, this image demonstrates a "bulging diaphragm" with an intact cardia at the hiatal opening. The topographic migration of the cardia and proximal stomach does not cause a true hernia, nor does the cardia protrude through the hiatus. Weakening of the diaphragm around the hiatus allows for cephalad movement of the center portion of the diaphragm along with the cardia, with preservation of the adhesive structures at the cardia.

Allison's early classification system, together with his pexy operation, was popularized in the 1950s by many surgeons. The subsequent experience with GERD patients with hiatal hernia led to a more thorough understanding of these two entities and their association [8–12]. Allison's fundophrenicopexy and Nissen's early experience with fundoplication stimulated a more scientific focus on these conditions [11, 12].

After another decade of clinical experience, Skinner and Belsey, who published a number of papers in the 1950s and 1960s, summarized their comprehensive experience in 1967 with a report encompassing over 1000 patients with hiatal hernia [9, 10, 13, 14]. In this publication, they documented the hiatal hernia classification that remains in use internationally [15]. Figure 13.2 demonstrates this classification with four types of hiatal hernia (Fig. 13.2a). Type I, a sliding hernia, accounts for approximately 85 to 90% of all hiatal hernias in the vast majority of subsequent publications [13–15]. Type II is a true paraesophageal hernia with intact position of the cardia at the hiatal level (Fig. 13.2b). Type II is further characterized by a small defect or weakening in the phreno-esophageal ligament, causing herniation of the fundic flap into the paraesophageal mediastinal area through the hiatus. Type III is a complete dislocation of the proximal stomach, with movement of both the cardia and fundus into the lower mediastinum (Fig. 13.2c). Type IV is defined as a large Type III hernia combined with cranial migration of other organs such as the colon, small bowel, or even the spleen into the mediastinum (Fig. 13.2d). Types II, III, and IV combined occur only in 5–15% of patients with hiatal hernia. Skinner and his group have propagated this classification, which many surgeons now follow [1–3, 5, 6].

In a subsequent publication on massive hiatal hernia, Skinner again reiterated that he reserves the term "paraesophageal hernia" to apply strictly to a true Type

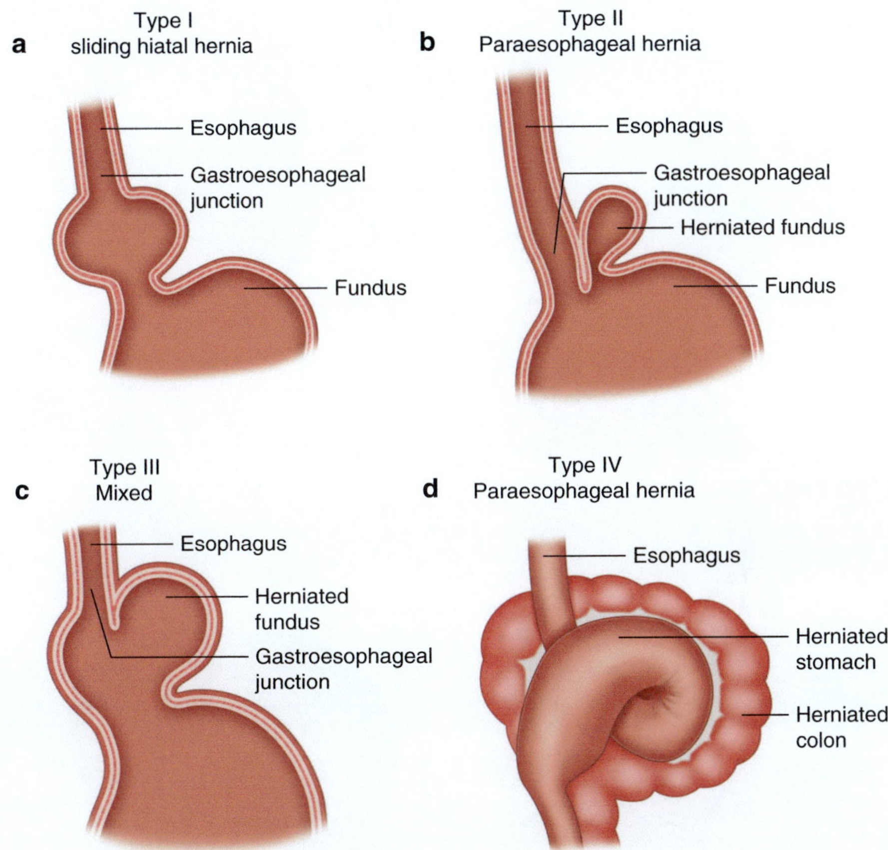

Fig. 13.2 Skinner's and Belsey's classification of hiatal hernias, as it is used still today by many physicians: Type I, sliding hernia (**a**); Type II, true paraesophageal hernia (**b**); Type III, mixed hernia with both cardia and fundus migrated (**c**); Type IV, upside-down stomach with accompanying viscera (**d**)

II paraesophageal hernia. Despite this, many surgeons broadly apply the term "paraesophageal hernia" to Types II, III, and IV [13, 15]. Skinner believed Type II hernia to be "an uncommon situation with the esophagogastric junction remaining securely anchored in the abdomen" [13, 15]. In contrast, the term paraesophageal hernia is currently used for all hernias with the exception of small- to midsize sliding Type I hernias. Particularly in the United States, all large hiatal hernias are described as paraesophageal hernias, if the fundus has migrated into the chest [1–3, 5, 6].

At some institutions in Europe, Skinner's classification was modified in daily practice based on anatomical and clinical observations [16, 17]. Some European gastroenterologists and surgeons differentiated between (Fig. 13.3a–d) first, a sliding hernia hiatal hernia; second, a mixed hiatal hernia with migration of both the

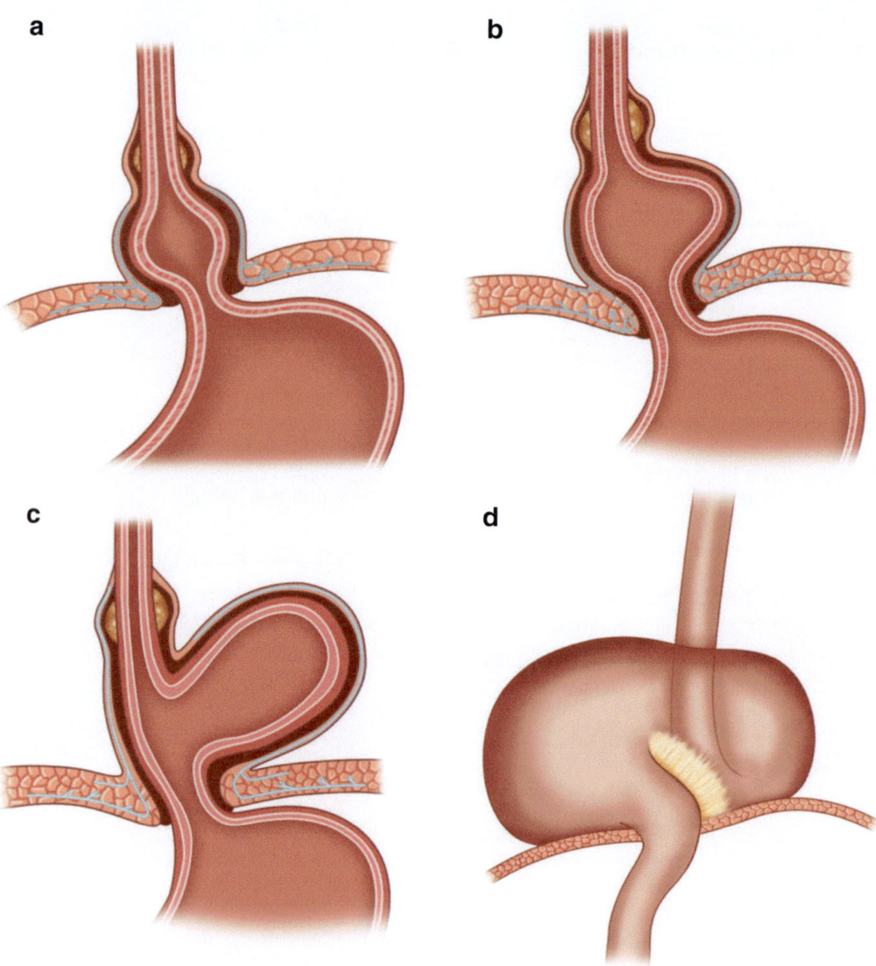

Fig. 13.3 Endoscopic classification mainly used in Europe: First, axial sliding hernia (**a**); second, mixed hernia with both cardia and fundus migrated (**b**); third, true paraesophageal hernia (**c**); forth, upside-down stomach with or without other viscera (**d**)

cardia and fundus; third, a true paraesophageal hernia with stable cardia and migration of a paraesophageal fundic flap alone (true paraesophageal hernia); and fourth, an upside-down stomach with possible migration of other viscera. This classification represented more the development of a hiatal hernia associated with GERD in Type 1 and Type 2, separated from rarely occurring true paraesophageal hernias and upside-down stomach (Type 3 and Type 4).

Another classification, based on endoscopic findings, was created and published by Lucius Hill in 1995, describing the findings of the hiatus and cardia in endoscopic retroflexion (Fig. 13.4) [18, 19]. Hill differentiated the following:

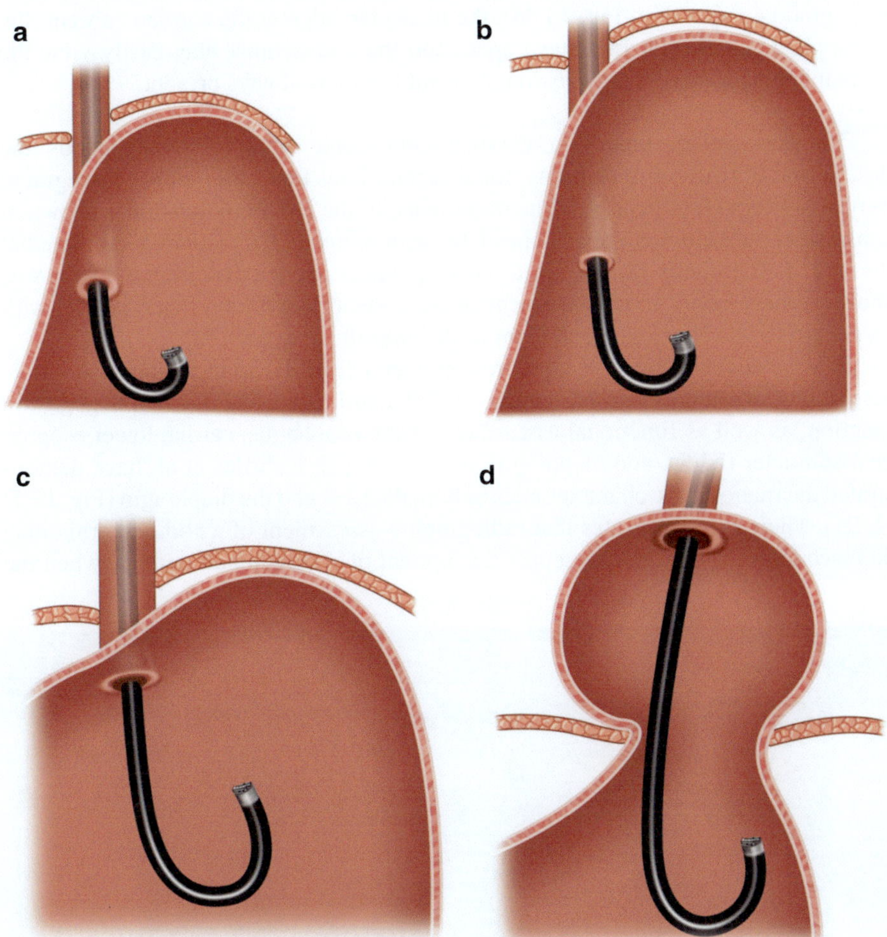

Fig. 13.4 The endoscopic Hill classification for describing the flap valve in endoscopic retroflexion: grade 1, muscular tissue of the cardia is tight around the endoscope (**a**); grade 2, ridge of muscular tissue at the cardia is less well defined, and there is some oral displacement of the cardia as well as a certain opening of the angle of His (**b**); grade 3, the ridge of the muscular structure at the gastric entrance is barely present anymore, and the cardia is widened, allowing a view into the esophageal lumen next to the scope (**c**); grade 4, the normal muscular ridge is completely gone, and the entrance of the stomach stays always open (**d**). The endoscopist can look into the esophagus, and there is always a hiatal hernia present

- A grade 1 flap valve (Fig. 13.4a): the ridge of the tissue at the cardia is preserved and closely approximated to the shaft of the retroflexed scope, extending 3–4 cm along the lesser curvature.
- A grade 2 flap valve (Fig. 13.4b): the ridge at the cardia is less pronounced and may open with respiration.
- A grade 3 flap valve (Fig. 13.4c): a diminished ridge of the cardia is noted, along with failure to close around the endoscope, often accompanied by a hiatal hernia.

- A grade 4 flap valve (Fig. 13.4d): the muscular ridge at the cardia is absent; the esophagogastric junction stays open, and the endoscopist may easily view the esophageal lumen in retroflexion. A hiatal hernia is always present.

This description, based on detailed endoscopic observations, expands the description of features of a sliding hiatal hernia. Thus far, it has not been integrated into the current classifications. The importance of the Hill classification is shown in subsequent publications, since it correlates with reflux activity and may even predict the size of the hiatus [2, 20]. In a recent publication, the Hill classification was shown to be superior to measurement of the vertical length of a hiatal hernia, with respect to the mechanical assessment of the antireflux barrier [20].

With the advent of high-resolution manometry (HRM), an increasingly accurate assessment of the mechanical features and dynamic status of the esophagogastric junction, as well as functional assessment of the esophagus, cardia, lower esophageal sphincter (LES), and diaphragm, is possible [2]. Kahrilas et al. have demonstrated the manometric characteristics of both the LES and the diaphragm (Fig. 13.5) [2, 21]. Their study indicates that radiographic assessment of a sliding hernia may be inaccurate, similar to endoscopic assessment of sliding hiatal hernias, when the

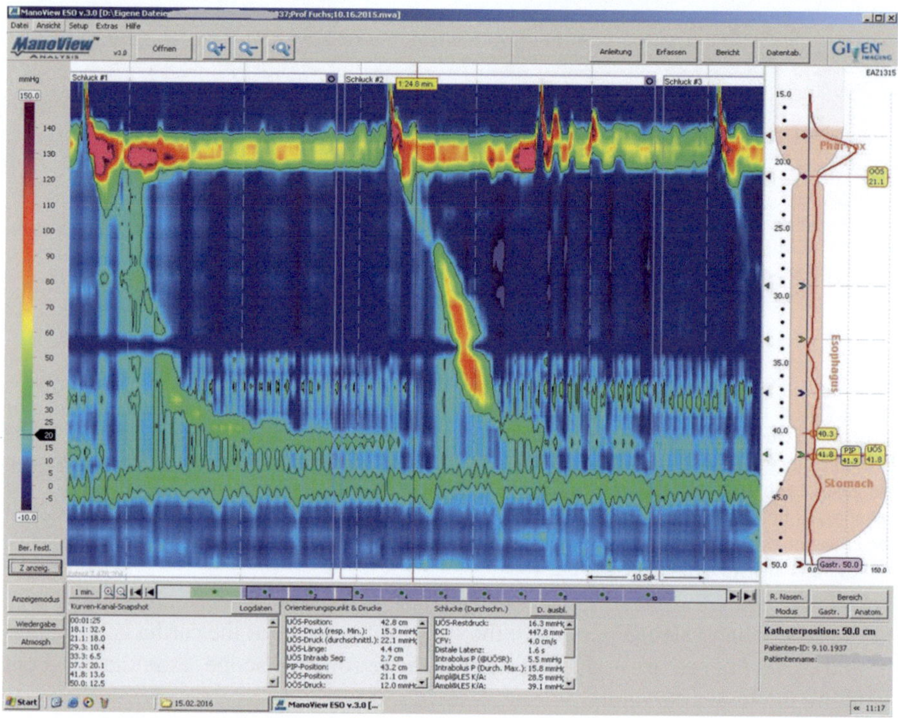

Fig. 13.5 Demonstration of the high-resolution manometry profile of a patient with a hiatal hernia as measured with multiple pressure sensors, which allows for a precise assessment. Note the separated pressure level of the LES and the diaphragm due to the hernia

endoscopic protocol does not account for physiologic movement of the esophagus due to longitudinal tension, and vertical movements of the LES during swallowing [2, 21]. Furthermore, he emphasizes that "unless a strict protocol for endoscopic measurement of the esophagogastric junction is tightly adhered to, the identification of Type I hernias less than 3 cm in size with endoscopy is unreliable."

It can be challenging to identify the exact position of the esophagogastric junction, as the beginning of the gastric mucosal folds is used as a visual landmark during endoscopy. This identification may be particularly difficult in the cardia of a patient with long-term GERD and Barrett's esophagus. In these patients, the distal esophageal segment within the deteriorated sphincter may carry columnar lined epithelium and folds due to effacement of the LES. As a result, the distal esophageal segment with the LES may be widened and appear to be part of the gastric wall. The improved accuracy of HRM in assessing hiatal hernia size has been confirmed by other authors [2, 21–23].

Granderath and Pointner introduced the term hiatal surface area (HSA) as another classification of hiatal size measurement and assessment of the severity of hiatal deterioration during GERD [24]. Based on the clinical dilemma of hiatal closure in larger hernias, the authors began calculating HSA as a criterion for decision-making regarding mesh use. HSA is an intraoperative measurement, quantifying the crural length (in cm), as well as the semicircle between both ventral crural edges representing the hiatal arch. With these values, the crural angle can be calculated and subsequently the HSA between the crurae. The authors use the HSA to differentiate between hiatal closure with versus without mesh [24]. Others have used this method to stratify their patients with different sizes of hiatal hernia [24–26]. Smaller hernias are classified as <10 cm^2; large hiatal hernias 10–20 cm^2, and a third group, patients with >20 cm^2 as giant hernias.

Special Issues Regarding Paraesophageal Hernias

In this manuscript, we will use the term "paraesophageal hernia" for all larger hiatal hernias including true paraesophageal hernias, mixed hernias, and upside-down stomach, as most authors especially in North America do [2, 6, 15, 22, 23]. It must be emphasized that in patients with a true paraesophageal hernia and concomitant upside-down stomach, the cardia and LES remain at the level of the hiatus, permitting reasonable function of the antireflux barrier. These patients usually do not have associated GERD symptoms [4–6].

Patients with large mixed hiatal hernias, with migration of the fundus and the cardia into the chest, usually have severe GERD [4, 5]. Additionally, these patients may develop short esophagus over time due to inflammation and scarring of the esophagus, which may lead to further surgical challenges [5] (see Chap. 12).

Patients with massive hernias may develop severe respiratory sequelae over time, as pulmonary capacity may be reduced due to the size and mass effect of the hernia. These patients are frequently elderly, increasing their risk for pulmonary complications at baseline [27]. Thus, the assessment, diagnosis, and surgical decision-making process should be managed expeditiously in these particular patients, prior to loss of pulmonary reserve.

The diagnostic management of these patients entails assessment of anatomical changes, as well as an extensive functional workup via GI function studies to evaluate all possible pathophysiologic causes. This includes a precise diagnosis according to the previously described classifications [4, 5, 23]. Patients must also be evaluated for presence of insufficient esophageal motility and involvement of delayed gastric emptying, which may initially be confounding factors in the diagnosis. Precise endoscopic evaluation of the esophagus and stomach is imperative. The presence of Barrett's esophagus must be verified or excluded. In the stomach, the presence of gastric ulcers and/or Cameron lesions must be verified [6]. Other causes of chronic anemia must be worked up and excluded as well.

As mentioned above, paraesophageal hernias occur infrequently and represent approximately 5–15% of all hiatal hernias [13, 23]. Since the hernia sac can be large, with significant intramediastinal involvement, the operative management of these patients should be undertaken by skilled surgeons, experienced in both abdominal and thoracic surgery. These patients should be treated in centers with a comprehensive knowledge of esophageal disorders and sufficiently high surgical volume. The management of an error in diagnostic workup, or technical problems during surgery, is best managed at a facility with appropriate resources and experienced staff. It is not surprising that some of the best results regarding surgical treatment of paraesophageal hernias were published via open transthoracic approach within an experienced group [28].

Two decades ago, the surgical management of patients with giant hernias remained associated with a certain level of mortality, which had to be taken into consideration when establishing indications for hiatal hernia surgery in elderly patients [7, 13, 15, 29]. Watchful waiting was considered an acceptable option, particularly in high-risk patients, as the mortality rate with surgery for paraesophageal hernia repair could be substantial [29].

With the advent and advancement of minimally invasive surgical techniques, impact of operative intervention on these patients has changed, access trauma has been reduced, and overall likelihood of mortality has been reduced [29–35]. Several publications show favorable outcomes with laparoscopic reduction of hernia and fundoplication for treatment of paraesophageal hernias [35].

Emergency Procedures for Paraesophageal Hernias

With respect to large hiatal hernias, both upward migration of the hernia and the paraesophageal extent of intramediastinal dislocation are based on the degree of stomach mobility. With sufficient mobility, patients are at increased risk for development of gastric volvulus within the mediastinum, resulting in strangulation of the stomach and potentially other organs following the stomach into the chest. Since paraesophageal hernias are a rare phenomena, such surgical emergencies are also rather infrequent [29, 35]. However, in certain centers, they may represent a substantial percentage of cases due to referral patterns [36, 37]. It must be emphasized that the relationship between the percentage of emergency cases and elective operations is variably reported in the literature, raising the question of whether cases are accurately reported as emergent, since the percentage of patients ranges from 3% to 15% [35–37].

In practice, these emergent cases are frequently managed by the on-call general or thoracic surgeons. Indications for emergency surgery include ischemia, gastrointestinal bleeding from a Cameron ulcer, gastric outlet obstruction, cardiopulmonary decompensation due to intrathoracic pressure increase, and aspiration events [36].

The literature shows that these patients have an elevated risk of both postoperative complications and mortality, as they are often decompensated from baseline due to the acute pathophysiologic process occurring [35–37]. The technical principles of the paraesophageal hernia repair remain the same during emergent surgery. Due to strangulation and occasional perforation, the need for gastric resection and more complex procedures is elevated in comparison to elective cases [36].

The morbidity rate in the setting of emergent paraesophageal hernia repair is reported to be between 20% and 45% [35–37]. The mortality rate may be as high as 5–16.4% [34–36]. In emergent cases, the necessity of open operation is increased, and longer hospital stays are documented as well [35, 36].

The Technique of Surgical Treatment of Paraesophageal Hernias

True Paraesophageal Hernias

The majority of patients with true paraesophageal hernia suffer from postprandial pain. It is uncommon for these patients to have massive gastroesophageal reflux. The diagnosis of a true paraesophageal hernia is generally established by radiography and/or upper GI endoscopy. Attention to detail is mandatory during endoscopic retroflexion to accurately observe fundic movements during respiration. A less experienced endoscopist is liable to miss the endoscopic subtleties of a paraesophageal herniation. Therefore, it is critical to spend time in retroflexion, observing the respiratory movements of the gastric wall and diaphragm. One may be able to observe migration of a small portion of fundic flap above the diaphragm through a small defect in the phreno-esophageal ligament.

After a few steps of laparoscopic exploration and dissection of the hiatus, the migration of the fundus will be readily apparent. It is infrequent that the localized defect in the phreno-esophageal ligament is appropriately managed without further dissection of the hiatus. Once the hiatal region is dissected and the hernia visualized, weakening of the hiatal structure, particularly the phreno-esophageal ligament, can be noted. A formal hiatal dissection is necessary to delineate the anatomical landmarks of both the crurae and the hiatal arch.

In general, a full hiatal dissection is completed in these cases. With the esophagus is mobilized from all attachments at the hiatus, there is concern for elevated risk of secondary reflux postoperatively; thus, fundoplication after formal hiatal approximation via posterior cruroplasty should be performed, in our opinion.

Upside-down Stomach

Patients with upside-down stomach with or without additional migration of other viscera often present with a chief complaint of retrosternal and thoracic pain. Prior to referral to an esophageal center, they have, for the most part, undergone either upper GI swallow study or cross-sectional imaging, and the diagnosis is established beforehand. Functional assessment of esophageal and gastric function should be performed to assess for the presence of motility disorders.

Laparoscopic exploration frequently demonstrates complete rotation of the stomach into the chest, with or without other viscera. If the colon has migrated into the thorax, it can be easily reduced into the abdominal cavity by gently pulling it caudad. The stomach should then be pulled down into the abdomen, and a thorough inspection should be performed of the hiatus and the hernia sac, with evaluation of the position and length of intra-abdominal esophagus. In each case, one can confirm an adhesive strand from the left crus to the fundus, which represents the axis of rotation of the stomach into the chest.

The dissection of the hiatus is started at the left crus after division of the short gastric vessels (Fig. 13.6). Full mobilization of the hernia out of the mediastinum is critical, since it needs to be reduced completely. The hernia sac can be grasped at the left crus, proceeding with full mediastinal mobilization of the hernia sac via gentle blunt dissection, resulting in minimal to no blood loss. The sac is then pulled down in the abdominal cavity to be resected. With reduction of the hernia, the esophagus along with the vagal trunks can be fully appreciated in the mediastinum. These structures must be preserved, and lesions to the esophagus must be avoided. We advocate against leaving any hernia sac in the mediastinum, since it may hinder the

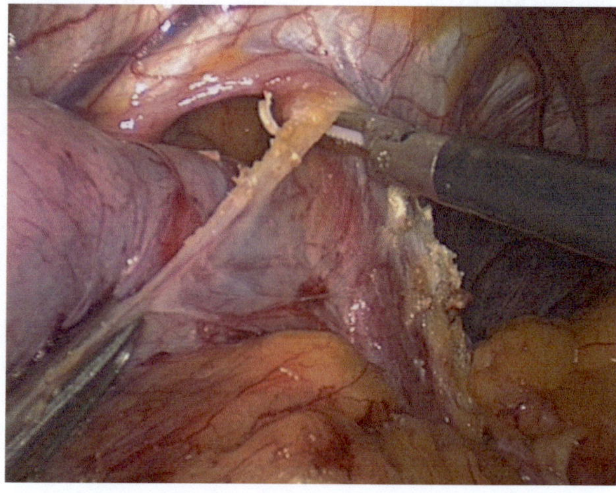

Fig. 13.6 The start of the dissection of a massive hiatal hernia at the left crus to divide the hernia sac for further mobilization in the mediastinum and complete hernia sac resection

full anatomical assessment of the intramediastinal structures. Furthermore, it may disturb mobilization of the esophagus and distort the shaping of the fundoplication. Additionally, residual hernia sac left within the mediastinum may make a future dissection even more challenging should a revision surgery be necessary.

In patients with upside-down stomach, there is usually no risk for a shortened esophagus, since the cardia is at the level of the hiatus. It is often difficult to handle the weakened hiatal diaphragm, which may be widened and attenuated over the years. Hiatal approximation is important, and we usually perform this with two figure-of-8-stitches posteriorly and an additional one to two stitches anteriorly. This combined anterior and posterior hiatoplasty provides a sufficient hiatal approximation; in the majority of cases, mesh reinforcement is not needed. However, in some cases, a crural gap remains and tension is high. In these cases, we use mesh to bridge the hiatal gap.

We are aware of the current controversial discussion about the arguments both in favor of and against the use of mesh reinforcement at the hiatus. As a center for referrals of redo surgery, we have seen many complications after mesh implantation and therefore use mesh reinforcement at the hiatus only selectively (see Chap. 10).

Management of (Paraesophageal) Mixed Hernias

These types of hernias are likely the most frequent paraesophageal hernias [4, 5, 35]. Involved patients usually suffer from prolonged symptoms of GERD and require a full gastrointestinal functional assessment regarding their reflux disease and possible Barrett's esophagus. In paraesophageal mixed hernias, the hernia develops due to a circular defect of the phreno-esophageal ligament. With the ongoing process of strain in this region, in conjunction with increasing weakening of the supportive connective tissue structures of the cardia, the LES moves higher up into the mediastinum (Fig. 13.7). These patients have a large vertical extension of their

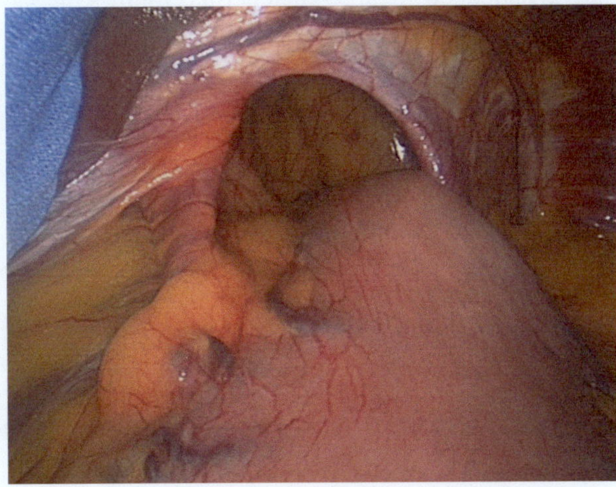

Fig. 13.7 Laparoscopic view in a large mixed hiatal hernia with possible shortening of the esophagus

Table 13.1 Overview on the application of technical details among specialized surgeons to treat paraesophageal hernias

Technical details	Arafat FO, 2012	DeMeester SR, 2013	Cohn TD, Soper NJ, 2017	Dallemagne B, 2018	Sorial RK, 2019
Dissection + identification vagus	+	+	+	+	+
Hernia sac excision	+	+	+	+	+
High esophageal mobilization	+	+	+	+	+
Crural approximation suture	+	+	+	+	+
Crural absorbable mesh enforcement always Selective	– –	+	+	+	+
Right-side release selective	–	+	+	–	–
Esophageal lengthening Collis	+	+	+	+	+
Fundoplication always	+	+	+	+	+
Partial fundoplication in esophageal motility disorders	+	+	+	+	

hernia, along with a particularly elevated risk of developing short esophagus (see Chap. 12).

Prior to hernia surgery, patients deemed to potentially require intraoperative esophageal lengthening should be evaluated by surgeons in esophageal centers, as such complex anatomical situations are managed most efficaciously during primary surgery. The technique of laparoscopic hiatal hernia reduction, closure of the hiatus, and laparoscopic fundoplication is described in detail in other chapters. The procedure in patients with large/giant hernias follows the same technical principles.

There are a few particular issues that are important for the success of these techniques in patients with large paraesophageal mixed hernias. Table 13.1 demonstrates some important surgical concepts that most experts follow to manage patients with paraesophageal hernias based on both clinical experience and evidence from the literature [32–37]. The following list of technical steps describes these details:

1. The surgeon should be experienced in a variety of esophageal procedures, which may range from simple, straightforward, laparoscopic fundoplication to the necessity for a Collis gastroplasty or resection.
2. It is important to have sufficient liver retraction to gain an optimal view of the hiatus and subsequently the mediastinum.
3. The first step is the dissection of the hiatal sac and its resection as mentioned above. This can be best done via constant downward tension applied to the cardia

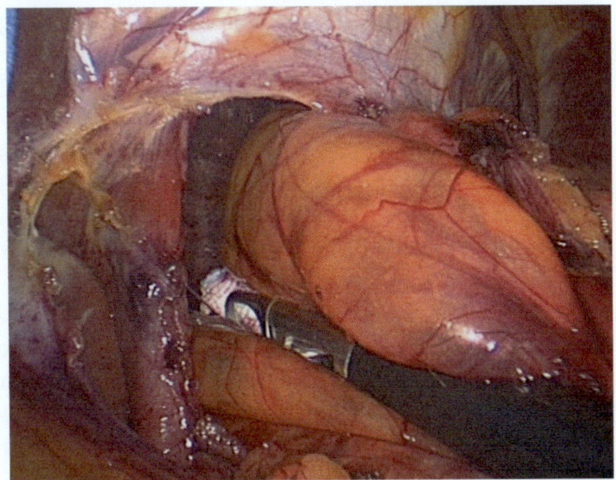

Fig. 13.8 Blunt mobilization of the hernia sac of a large mixed hernia in the mediastinum, which will allow for an optimal view on the esophagus and the vagal trunks

in order to achieve adequate exposure of the esophagus and mediastinum (Fig. 13.8).

4. Careful dissection of the cardia with resection of all fatty tissue and elements of the hernia sac is important for the definition of all anatomical structures, especially the anterior and posterior vagus.

5. The identification and preservation of the vagal trunks are critical in preventing postoperative gastroparesis.

6. A loop around the LES facilitates the atraumatic pull-down of the esophagus while exerting adequate strength. This will facilitate esophageal mobilization to the level of the pulmonary vessels in the mediastinum. Tension-free positioning of the LES in the abdominal cavity is a key element contributing to the future function of the fundoplication as an antireflux barrier. This step is of utmost importance, because mesh reinforcement of the hiatus will never compensate for insufficient mobilization of the esophagus to create a tension-free position of the LES.

7. The narrowing of the hiatus can be performed with figure-of-8-stitches of braided suture material. Usually two to three stitches posteriorly are enough to create sufficient reapproximation. It is important to avoid any tenting of the esophagus by the posterior cruroplasty, since this can lead to postoperative "hiatal dysphagia." An anterior hiatoplasty should be added to complete the narrowing of the hiatus in these cases. The use of mesh reinforcement should be used selectively in those cases in which it is deemed necessary (see Chap. 10).

In cases of short esophagus, one should not hesitate to perform an esophageal lengthening procedure (see Chap. 12). A gastropexy may be added to the fundoplication, if there is a slight tension that does not appear significant enough to warrant performance of a Collis gastroplasty [38, 39].

Results of Surgical Therapy for Paraesophageal Hernia

Table 13.2 demonstrates an overview on the outcomes following surgical intervention for paraesophageal mixed hernias in the literature [31, 36, 40–45]. Early data from the laparoscopic era show the overall promise of this technique, given that length of hospital stay, postoperative complication rates, and mortality (0.3 versus 1.7%) were improved [30]. However, the debate regarding the role of minimally invasive techniques for this difficult surgical entity continued for several years. No randomized trials are currently available.

Reflecting on the available literature regarding these patients, it is critical to clearly delineate the difference between a good outcome and a bad outcome. Radiologic hernia recurrence, frequently used as a marker for assessment of outcomes, is easily measured. However, symptomatic and functional outcomes are likely to be more relevant. Quality of life is influenced by symptom patterns, i.e., reflux or dysphagia, while simple migration of the wrap into the chest may not alter quality of life for the patient [35]. Dallemagne et al. performed a review demonstrating that the average radiologic recurrence rate of hiatal hernia is between 16 and 66%, while the rate of redo operations was lower, ranging from 2% to 9% [35]. Table 13.2 shows a similar analysis based on Dallemagne's review [35]. The data show that the selected reports have a radiologic recurrence rate with a median of 32%, persistent and/or new onset of symptoms at 18%, and necessity for redo operation reported as 4% (2–9%) [31, 36, 40–45]. This is interesting, since the need for redo surgery is 4%, which is lower than the frequency of redo operations in regular antireflux procedures [46, 47]. In conjunction with evidence suggestive of reduced

Table 13.2 Overview on results after paraesophageal hernia surgery (based on Dallemagne [35])

Authors Year	n	Follow-up symptoms/ radiography months	Persist./ new-onset symptoms %	Radiolog. recurrence %	Redo surgery done %
Jobe 2002	52	39/37	19	32	4
Aly 2005	100	47	–	23	4
Zaninotto 2007	54	71/32	22	20	9
Luketich 2010	662	30/25	11	16	3
Dallemagne 2011	85	118/99	16	66	2
Oelschlager 2012	78	58	29	57	3
Targarona 2013	77	108	22	46	4
Shea 2019	199	–	11	32	7

mortality associated with the laparoscopic approach, one can conclude that this approach is likely advantageous.

Some surgical groups were initially critical about shifting approaches but with increasing experience reported favorable results with minimally invasive techniques [48]. The report of Dallemagne et al. was noteworthy, with a reoperation rate of only 2%, despite an objective hernia radiologic recurrence rate of 66% [35]. Luketich et al. reported a reoperation rate of 3.2% in 662 patients, with a reported radiologic recurrence rate of 16% [43].

In summary, patients with large or massive hiatal hernias do carry the infrequent but increased risk of presenting as a surgical emergency. Additionally, these patients may suffer long term from sequelae of aspiration and other respiratory problems. Thus, a critical assessment and diagnostic workup should be performed and elective laparoscopic repair undertaken when appropriate, following the aforementioned technical details.

References

1. Vakil N, van Zanten SV, Kahrilas PJ, Dent J, Jones R, the global consensus Group. The Montreal definition and classification of GERD: a global evidence-based consensus. Am J Gastroenterol. 2006;101:1900–20.
2. Kahrilas PJ, Kim HC, Pandolfino JE. Approaches to the diagnosis and grading of hiatal hernia. Best Pract Res Clin Gastroenterol. 2008;22(4):601–16. https://doi.org/10.1016/j.bpg.2007.12.007.
3. Stefanidis D, Hope WW, Kohn GP, Reardon PR, Richardson WS, Fanelli RD, SAGES Guideline committee. SAGES guidelines for surgical treatment of GERD. Surg Endosc. 2010;24(11):2647–69.
4. Fuchs KH, Babic B, Breithaupt W, Dallemagne B, Fingerhut A, Furnee E, Granderath F, Horvath OP, Kardos P, Pointner R, Savarino E, Van Herwarden-Lindeboom M, Zaninotto G. EAES recommendations for the management of gastroesophageal reflux disease. Surg Endosc. 2014;28:1753–73.
5. DeMeester TR. Etiology and natural history of gastroesophageal reflux disease and predictors of progressive disease. In: Yeo CJ, DeMeester SR, Mc Fadden DW, editors. Shackelford's surgery of the alimentary tract. 8th ed. Philadelphia: Elsevier; 2019. p. 204–20.
6. Cheverie JN, Lam J, Neki K, Broderick RC, Lee AM, Matsuzaki T, Cubas R, Sandler BJ, Jacobsen GR, Fuchs KH, Horgan S. Paraesophageal hernia repair: a curative consideration for chronic anemia? Surg Endosc. 2019; https://doi.org/10.1007/s00464-019-07014-3.
7. Stylopoulos N, Rattner DW. The history of hiatal hernia surgery: from Bowditch to laparoscopy. Ann Surg. 2005;241(1):185–93.
8. Allison PR. Peptic ulcer of the oesophagus. Thorax. 1948;3(1):20–42.
9. Belsey R. The symptoms and clinical diagnosis of hiatus hernia. Bristol Med Chir J. 1952;69(250):39–44.
10. Belsey R. Peptic ulcer of the oesophagus. Ann R Coll Surg Engl. 1954;14(5):303–22.
11. Nissen R. Eine einfache Operation zur Beeinflussung des Refluxösophagitis. Schweiz Med Wschr. 1956;86:590.
12. Allison PR. Hiatus hernia; a 20 year retrospective survey. Ann Surg. 1973;178:273–6.
13. Skinner DB, Belsey RH. Surgical management of esophageal reflux and hiatus hernia. Long-term results with 1,030 patients. J Thorac Cardiovasc Surg. 1967;53(1):33–54.
14. Skinner DB, Booth DJ. Assessment of distal esophageal function in patients with hiatal hernia and-or gastroesophageal reflux. Ann Surg. 1970;172(4):627–37.

15. Altorki NK, Yankelevitz D, Skinner DB. Massive hiatal hernias: the anatomic basis of repair. J Thorac Cardiovasc Surg. 1998;115(4):828–35.
16. Fuchs KH. Pathophysiologie. In: Fuchs KH, Stein HJ, Thiede A, editors. Gastrointestinale Funktionsstörungen. Berlin/Heidelberg: Springer; 1997. p. 495–513.
17. Zwerchfellhernien HA. In: H Becker und BM Ghadimi, Allgemein- und Viszeralchirurgie. Urban-Fischer-Elsevier 2012, pp. 168–173.
18. Hill LD, Kozarek RA, Kraemer SJ, Aye RW, Mercer CD, Low DE, Pope CE 2nd. The gastro-esophageal flap valve: in vitro and in vivo observations. Gastrointest Endosc. 1996;44(5):541–7.
19. Hill LD, Kozarek RA. The gastroesophageal flap valve. J Clin Gastroenterol. 1999;28(3):194–7.
20. Jobe BA, Kahrilas PJ, Vernon AH, Sandone C, Gopal DV, Swanstrom LL, Aye RW, Hill LD, Hunter JG. Endoscopic appraisal of the gastroesophageal valve after antireflux surgery. Am J Gastroenterol. 2004;99(2):233–43.
21. Kahrilas PJ, Bredenoord AJ, Fox M, Gyawali CP, Roman S, Smout AJPM, Pandolfino JE, International HRM Working group. Neurogastroenterol Motil. 2015;27:160–74.
22. Tolone S, Savarino E, Zaninotto G, Gyawali CP, Frazzoni M, de Bortoli N, Frazzoni L, Del Genio G, Bodini G, Furnari M, Savarino V, Docimo L. High-resolution manometry is superior to endoscopy and radiology in assessing and grading sliding hiatal hernia: a comparison with surgical in vivo evaluation. United European Gastroenterol J. 2018;6(7):981–9. https://doi.org/10.1177/2050640618769160.
23. Jobe BA, Richter JE, Hoppo T, Peters JH, Bell R, Dengler WC, DeVault K, Fass R, Gyawali CP, Kahrilas PJ, Lacy BE, Pandolfino JE, Patti MG, Swanstrom LL, Kurian AA, Vela MF, Vaezi M, DeMeester TR. Preoperative diagnostic workup before antireflux surgery: an evidence and experience-based consensus of the Esophageal Diagnostic Advisory Panel. J Am Coll Surg. 2013;217(4):586–97. https://doi.org/10.1016/j.jamcollsurg.2013.05.023.
24. Granderath FA, Schweiger UM, Pointner R. Laparoscopic antireflux surgery: tailoring the hiatal closure to the size of hiatal surface area. Surg Endosc. 2007;21(4):542–8.
25. Grubnik VV, Malynovskyy AV. Laparoscopic repair of hiatal hernias: new classification supported by long-term results. Surg Endosc. 2013;27(11):4337–46. https://doi.org/10.1007/s00464-013-3069-2.
26. Antoniou SA, Pointner R, Granderath FA. Hiatal surface area as a basis for a new classification of hiatal hernia. Surg Endosc. 2014 Apr;28(4):1384–5. https://doi.org/10.1007/s00464-013-3292-x.
27. Rantanen TK. Salo JA; GERD as a cause of death: analysis of fatal cases under conservative therapy. Scand J Gastroenterol. 1999;34(3):229–33.
28. Maziak DE, Todd TR, Pearson FG. Massive hiatus hernia: evaluation and surgical management. J Thorac Cardiovasc Surg. 1998;115(1):53–60; discussion 61-2.
29. Stylopoulos N, Gazelle GS, Rattner DW. Paraesophageal hernias: operation or observation? Ann Surg. 2002 Oct;236(4):492–500; discussion 500-501.
30. Draaisma WA, Gooszen HG, Tournoij E, Broeders IA. Controversies in paraesophageal hernia repair: a review of literature. Surg Endosc. 2005;19(10):1300–8.
31. Oelschlager BK, Petersen RP, Brunt LM, Soper NJ, Sheppard BC, Mitsumori L, Rohrmann C, Swanstrom LL, Pellegrini CA. Laparoscopic paraesophageal hernia repair: defining long-term clinical and anatomic outcomes. J Gastrointest Surg. 2012;16(3):453–9. https://doi.org/10.1007/s11605-011-1743-z.
32. Arafat FO, Teitelbaum EN, Hungness ES. Modern treatment of paraesophageal hernia: preoperative evaluation and technique for laparoscopic repair. Surg Laparosc Endosc Percutan Tech. 2012;22(4):297–303. https://doi.org/10.1097/SLE.0b013e31825831af.
33. DeMeester SR. Laparoscopic paraesophageal hernia repair: critical steps and adjunct techniques to minimize recurrence. Surg Laparosc Endosc Percutan Tech. 2013;23(5):429–35. https://doi.org/10.1097/SLE.0b013e3182a12716.
34. Cohn TD, Soper NJ. Paraesophageal hernia repair: techniques for success. J Laparoendosc Adv Surg Tech A. 2017;27(1):19–23. https://doi.org/10.1089/lap.2016.0496.

35. Dallemagne B, Quero G, Lapergola A, Guerriero L, Fiorillo C, Perretta S. Treatment of giant paraesophageal hernia: pro laparoscopic approach. Hernia. 2018;22(6):909–19. https://doi.org/10.1007/s10029-017-1706-8.
36. Shea B, Boyan W, Decker J, Almagno V, Binenbaum S, Matharoo G, Squillaro A, Borao F. Emergent repair of paraesophageal hernias and the argument for elective repair. JSLS. 2019;23(2). pii: e2019.00015 https://doi.org/10.4293/JSLS.2019.00015.
37. Sorial RK, Ali M, Kaneva P, Fiore JF Jr, Vassiliou M, Fried GM, Feldman LS, Ferri LE, Lee L, Mueller CL. Modern era surgical outcomes of elective and emergency giant paraesophageal hernia repair at a high-volume referral center. Surg Endosc. 2019; https://doi.org/10.1007/s00464-019-06764-4.
38. Ponsky J, Rosen M, Fanning A, Malm J. Anterior gastropexy may reduce the recurrence rate after laparoscopic paraesophageal hernia repair. Surg Endosc. 2003;17(7):1036–41.
39. Tsimogiannis KE, Pappas-Gogos GK, Benetatos N, Tsironis D, Farantos C, Tsimoyiannis EC. Laparoscopic Nissen fundoplication combined with posterior gastropexy in surgical treatment of GERD. Surg Endosc. 2010;24(6):1303–9. https://doi.org/10.1007/s00464-009-0764-0.
40. Jobe BA, Aye RW, Deveney CW, Domreis JS, Hill LD. Laparoscopic management of giant type III hiatal hernia and short esophagus. objective follow-up at three years. J Gastrointest Surg. 2002;6(2):181–8; discussion 188.
41. Aly A, Munt J, Jamieson GG, Ludemann R, Devitt PG, Watson DI. Laparoscopic repair of large hiatal hernias. Br J Surg. 2005;92(5):648–53.
42. Zaninotto G, Portale G, Costantini M, Fiamingo P, Rampado S, Guirroli E, Nicoletti L, Ancona E. Objective follow-up after laparoscopic repair of large type III hiatal hernia. Assessment of safety and durability. World J Surg. 2007;31(11):2177–83.
43. Luketich JD, Nason KS, Christie NA, Pennathur A, Jobe BA, Landreneau RJ, Schuchert MJ. Outcomes after a decade of laparoscopic giant paraesophageal hernia repair. J Thorac Cardiovasc Surg. 2010;139(2):395–404, 404.e1. https://doi.org/10.1016/j.jtcvs.2009.10.005.
44. Dallemagne B, Kohnen L, Perretta S, Weerts J, Markiewicz S, Jehaes C. Laparoscopic repair of paraesophageal hernia. Long-term follow-up reveals good clinical outcome despite high radiological recurrence rate. Ann Surg. 2011;253(2):291–6. https://doi.org/10.1097/SLA.0b013e3181ff44c0.
45. Targarona EM, Grisales S, Uyanik O, Balague C, Pernas JC, Trias M. Long-term outcome and quality of life after laparoscopic treatment of large paraesophageal hernia. World J Surg. 2013;37(8):1878–82. https://doi.org/10.1007/s00268-013-2047-0.
46. Furnée EJ, Draaisma WA, Broeders IA, Gooszen HG. Surgical reintervention after failed anti-reflux surgery; a systematic review of the literature. J Gastrointest Surg. 2009;13:1539–49.
47. Zhou T, Harnsberger C, Broderick R, Fuchs HF, Talamini M, Jacobsen G, Horgan S, Chang D, Sandler B. Reoperation rates after laparoscopic fundoplication. Surg Endosc. 2015;29:510–4.
48. Zehetner J, Demeester SR, Ayazi S, Kilday P, Augustin F, Hagen JA, Lipham JC, Sohn HJ, Demeester TR. Laparoscopic versus open repair of paraesophageal hernia: the second decade. J Am Coll Surg. 2011;212(5):813–20. https://doi.org/10.1016/j.jamcollsurg.2011.01.060.

Gastroesophageal Reflux Disease in Sleeve Gastrectomy: Pathophysiology and Available Treatments

14

Sean M. Flynn and Ryan C. Broderick

Background

Gastroesophageal reflux disease (GERD) is a common comorbidity in the obese population. Prevalence in the obese population is estimated to be around 37–72%, which greatly exceeds the 10–20% prevalence seen in normal weight individuals [1, 2]. Reflux symptoms greatly impair patients' quality of life, including disruptions of sleep and productivity, at rates comparable to backpain or headaches [3]. GERD is also linked to the development of Barrett's esophagus and esophageal adenocarcinoma [4, 5], with studies showing at least a twofold increase in the rate of esophageal adenocarcinoma in obesity-related GERD [6]. Given these impairments to quality of life and overall health, GERD has been recognized as a significant comorbidity of obesity. For every five-point increase in BMI, the DeMeester score is expected to rise by three [7]. Therefore, GERD may be preexisting or occur de novo after a bariatric operation.

GERD results from a failure of normal anti-reflux barriers, centered around the esophagus, the lower esophageal sphincter (LES), the crural portion of the hiatus, and the stomach. The pathophysiology behind obesity-related GERD appears to be the result of a multitude of anatomic and physiologic changes at the LES imposed by the central and visceral adiposity of obesity. Increasing body mass index (BMI) has been shown to correlate with increasing rates of LES hypotension and transient LES relaxation, which allows for the reflux of gastric contents into the esophagus [8]. Obesity is also associated with decreasing rates of LES length and intra-abdominal length, both of which contribute to decreased LES pressure [8]. The

S. M. Flynn
Division of Minimally Invasive Surgery, Department of Surgery, University of California San Diego, La Jolla, CA, USA

R. C. Broderick (✉)
Division of Minimally Invasive Surgery, Department of Surgery, University of California San Diego, La Jolla, CA, USA

Department of Surgery, Center for the Future of Surgery, University of California San Diego, La Jolla, CA, USA
e-mail: rbroderick@ucsd.edu

© Springer Nature Switzerland AG 2020
S. Horgan, K.-H. Fuchs (eds.), *Management of Gastroesophageal Reflux Disease*,
https://doi.org/10.1007/978-3-030-48009-7_14

increased intra-abdominal pressure seen with obesity results in an increased gastroesophageal pressure gradient, promoting gastric reflux [9, 10]. It also results in higher rates of hiatal hernias, again disrupting the normal anatomic location and function of the LES.

Gastric fundoplication has been considered the gold standard for surgical treatment of reflux disease. However, the comorbidities and increased intra-abdominal pressure associated with obesity creates unique challenges to operative options in GERD. Results of fundoplication in the obese have been demonstrated to be significantly worse than in normal weight individuals, with symptoms recurring in 31.3% of obese patients at 3 years, compared to just 4.5% with normal BMI [11]. Fundoplication failure has most commonly been attributed to hiatal hernia recurrence. Wrap failure also appears to play a significant role, with one study showing that up to 45% of obese patients who failed fundoplication had disruption of their wrap at reoperation [12].

Given the challenges with traditional anti-reflux procedures in obesity, bariatric surgery has emerged as a treatment for this population. Bariatric surgery has demonstrated proven, reliable results in achieving weight loss and resolution of a number of obesity-related comorbidities. GERD is one of those comorbidities that has been found to greatly improve postoperatively with select procedures. Currently, Roux-en-Y gastric bypass (RYGB) has shown the most promising results in postoperative GERD reduction. Studies have shown that 70% of patients have improvement or complete resolution of their reflux symptoms at one-year post procedure [13, 14]. The physiology driving the improvement in symptoms appears to be related to weight loss resulting in decreased intra-abdominal pressure, creation of a low-volume stomach remnant with low acid production capabilities, and creation of a long roux limb to prevent biliopancreatic reflux [8]. Beyond RYGB, laparoscopic sleeve gastrectomy (SG) has become the most popular primary bariatric operation, but not in the treatment of GERD. While sleeve gastrectomy has shown good results of excess weight loss, the high-pressure system of a sleeve has shown mixed results or increased rate of GERD.

The effects of SG on GERD symptoms are debated, with studies showing both improvement of GERD symptoms as well as worsening or even de novo development [15]. DuPree et al. performed a retrospective review of the Bariatric Outcomes Longitudinal Database of 4832 patients undergoing laparoscopic sleeve gastrectomy over a 3-year period. They found that the majority (84.1%) of patients with preoperative GERD symptoms had continued symptoms postoperatively. They also found that 8.6% of patients without preoperative GERD-related symptoms developed de novo reflux in the postoperative period [14]. Other studies have found the incidence of de novo GERD development in anywhere from 2.1% to 21% of patients [16, 17]. Conversely, there is also evidence to support a favorable impact of SG on GERD. Daes et al. performed a prospective evaluation of 382 patients undergoing SG and found that 94% of patients had resolution of their symptoms postoperatively [18]. Likewise, a systemic review by Chiu et al. found that seven studies showed a decrease in GERD after SG, while only four studies showed an increase [15]. Therefore, the study could not come to a definitive conclusion on the relationship between GERD and SG. Overall, evaluation of GERD after SG is also limited in part by nonstandardization of evaluation of GERD symptoms, with some studies relying only on survey reporting, while other studies performing endoscopy, esophageal pH monitoring, and/or upper gastrointestinal contrast studies.

Pathophysiology

The pathophysiologic changes resulting from SG are a complex mix of both pro- and anti-reflux factors. Postoperative improvements in GERD symptoms after SG are attributed to a number of anatomic and physiologic changes. As with RYGB, SG results in decreased BMI, which decreases intra-abdominal pressure. Through removal of the fundus and a significant portion of the stomach body, SG results in a significant decrease in the number of parietal cells and the stomach's ability to secrete acid. The post SG stomach also has a significantly reduced ability to distend, which allows for accelerated gastric emptying and overall reduction in gastric volume [19–21].

Conversely, a number of the anatomic and physiologic changes after SG are posited to perpetuate or allow for de novo development of GERD. While decreasing the fundus and compliance of the stomach decreases the stomach volume, it also results in increased intraluminal pressures. This can cause increased back pressure on the LES, as well as increased resistance to esophageal emptying; both can result in increased post prandial reflux. Performance of a SG can also result in disruption or alteration of the LES and native anti-reflux mechanisms. Disruption of the angle of His, the sling fibers, the phrenic-esophageal ligament, and the cardiac-phrenic ligament can all disrupt the natural anti-reflux barriers. A funnel shape to the final gastric sleeve may also decreased gastric emptying, increased back pressure, and ultimately reflux. Finally, intrathoracic sleeve migration can result in disruption of normal LES function. This migration may be a result of recurrent or persistent hiatal hernia, of high intragastric pressure, or of a pressure gradient between the thorax and abdomen [22].

Preoperative Evaluation

Preoperative evaluation, selection, and optimization may all help improve rates of GERD after sleeve gastrectomy, though GERD prediction can be difficult. Body mass index alone does not predict the incidence or severity of a patient's reflux symptoms [23]. However, higher preoperative BMI and higher preoperative heartburn scores can be independent factors for detecting GERD after SG [24]. A thorough history should be elicited from patients preoperatively, including review of both typical and atypical GERD symptoms.

Preoperative testing may be advisable in patients with symptoms concerning for reflux in their history. Esophageal pH testing, esophageal manometry, and upper gastrointestinal contrast series can be used to evaluate for GERD as well as esophageal dysmotility and provide insight into the severity of a patient's disease. It is the practice of the authors that all patients undergoing evaluation for bariatric surgery should have an esophagogastroduodenoscopy (EGD) and manometry, as well as patients with a reported history of GERD and on medications undergo impedance pH monitoring off PPI. Esophagogastroduodenoscopy (EGD) can be used to assess for stigmata and sequelae of GERD, including esophagitis, ulceration, and Barrett's esophagus. Findings of Barrett's esophagus or other sequelae of GERD should prompt the surgeon to reconsider proceeding with SG.

Intraoperative Considerations

A number of intraoperative techniques and considerations should be employed to help minimize GERD after SG. As mentioned previously, great care should be taken to avoid disruption of the LES and the native anti-reflux barriers, including the sling fibers, the cardiac-phrenic ligament, and the phrenic-esophageal ligament in the setting of no identified hiatal hernia. Stenosis of the sleeve results in increased intraluminal pressure and increased resistance to esophageal emptying and thus should be avoided. This includes using no smaller than a 32-Fr bougie during creation of the sleeve, as there is no improvement in weight loss with a smaller sleeve, yet there is a significantly higher rates of reflux [25]. Functional stenosis, from torsion or kinking of the sleeve, is usually a result of asymmetric resection of the anterior and posterior walls and should also be avoided. The fundus should be completely resected during the operation as a retained fundus leaves behind excess acid secreting parietal cells. It also can inhibit gastric emptying and facilitate esophageal reflux [22]. Finally, hiatal hernias result in disruption of the LES function and intrathoracic LES migration and are highly associated with GERD. Thus, hiatal hernias encountered intraoperatively should be repaired in standard fashion with full mobilization of the hiatus to achieve appropriate intra-abdominal esophagus followed by crural re-approximation.

Management of Postoperative GERD

The management of postoperative GERD should begin with dietary and lifestyle modification, similar to non-bariatric-related reflux. Patients should be advised to avoid certain dietary triggers, such as caffeine, fatty foods, spicy foods, and carbonated beverages. Tobacco and alcohol both reduce lower esophageal sphincter pressure and should be avoided. Patients with nocturnal symptoms can be advised to sleep with their head elevated, as well as to avoid eating within two to three hours of laying supine.

The staple of management of SG-related GERD symptoms begins with acid suppressive medications. While these medications will not prevent reflux, they have shown great efficacy in decreasing acid-related symptoms and complications.

Patients are typically started on daily proton pump inhibitor (PPIs) therapy, which can be increased to twice per day. While these medications are very effective, they are not without consequence and have been linked to osteoporosis and increased rates of pneumonia and other gastrointestinal infections.

Surgical options are available in patients where symptoms cannot be adequately managed with medical therapy or who are unwilling to continue lifelong medications. The gold standard for surgical correction of GERD after SG has been conversion to a RYGB. RYGB has been shown to be highly efficacious in improving and resolving GERD symptoms, with reports of greater than 80%–100% of patients having improvement in their symptoms [26, 27] and 80% of patients being able to completely stop their antacid medications after revision [26].

Alternative surgical options are also being developed if patients do not want a RYGB or if it cannot be performed. Magnetic LES augmentation (MSA) with the LINX device has shown early promise in managing severe reflux after sleeve gastrectomy [28, 29]. Endoscopic techniques have also been explored but are not yet well proven or part of standard care. The Stretta Procedure is one of the better described endoscopic options. It involves delivery of radiofrequency energy to the LES to thicken and stiffen the muscles and thus prevent reflux. It has shown promise as another minimally invasive anti-reflux procedure with good long-term results in small patient studies [30].

Conclusion

Severe GERD following sleeve gastrectomy is a well-established complication. Preoperative predictors of severe reflux should be used to have an informed discussion with patients regarding their best options for primary bariatric surgical technique. Medical therapy remains the primary therapy in worsening or de novo GERD after sleeve gastrectomy; however, surgical techniques such as conversion to RYGB or MSA are also safe and effective.

References

1. Lundell L, Ruth M, Sandberg N, Bove-Nielsen M. Does massive obesity promote abnormal gastroesophageal reflux? Dig Dis Sci. 1995;40(8):1632–5. https://doi.org/10.1007/BF02212682.
2. Anand G, Katz PO. Gastroesophageal reflux disease and obesity. Rev Gastroenterol Disord. 2008;8(4):233–9.
3. Wiklund I. Review of the quality of life and burden of illness in gastroesophageal reflux disease. Dig Dis. 2004;22(2):108–14. https://doi.org/10.1159/000080308.
4. Edelstein ZR, Farrow DC, Bronner MP, Rosen SN, Vaughan TL. Central adiposity and risk of Barrett's esophagus. Gastroenterology. 2007;133(2):403–11. https://doi.org/10.1053/j.gastro.2007.05.026.
5. Lagergren J, Bergström R, Nyrén O. Association between body mass and adenocarcinoma of the esophagus and gastric cardia. Ann Intern Med. 1999;130(11):883–90. https://doi.org/10.7326/0003-4819-130-11-199906010-00003.

6. Hampel H, Abraham NS, El-Serag HB. Meta-analysis: obesity and the risk for gastroesophageal reflux disease and its complications. Ann Intern Med. 2005;143(3):199–211. https://doi.org/10.7326/0003-4819-143-3-200508020-00006.

7. Chang P, Friedenberg F. Obesity and GERD. Gastroenterol Clin N Am. 2014;43(1):161–73. https://doi.org/10.1016/j.gtc.2013.11.009.

8. Prachand VN, Alverdy JC. Gastroesophageal reflux disease and severe obesity: fundoplication or bariatric surgery? And severe obesity: causality or. World J Gastroenterol. 2010;16(30):3757–61. https://doi.org/10.3748/wjg.v16.i30.3757.

9. De Vries DR, Van Herwaarden MA, Smout AJPM, Samsom M. Gastroesophageal pressure gradients in gastroesophageal reflux disease: relations with hiatal hernia, body mass index, and esophageal acid exposure. Am J Gastroenterol. 2008;103(6):1349–54. https://doi.org/10.1111/j.1572-0241.2008.01909.x.

10. Stenard F, Iannelli A. Laparoscopic sleeve gastrectomy and gastroesophageal reflux. World J Gastroenterol. 2015;21(36):10348–57. https://doi.org/10.3748/wjg.v21.i36.10348.

11. Perez AR, Moncure AC, Rattner DW. Obesity adversely affects the outcome of antireflux operations. Surg Endosc. 2001;15(9):986–9. https://doi.org/10.1007/s004640000392.

12. Kellogg TA, Andrade R, Maddaus M, Slusarek B, Buchwald H, Ikramuddin S. Anatomic findings and outcomes after antireflux procedures in morbidly obese patients undergoing laparoscopic conversion to Roux-en-Y gastric bypass. Surg Obes Relat Dis. 2007; https://doi.org/10.1016/j.soard.2006.08.011.

13. Hutter MM, Schirmer BD, Jones DB, et al. First report from the American College of Surgeons Bariatric Surgery Center Network. Ann Surg. 2011;254(3):410–22. https://doi.org/10.1097/sla.0b013e31822c9dac.

14. DuPree CE, Blair K, Steele SR, Martin MJ. Laparoscopic sleeve gastrectomy in patients with preexisting gastroesophageal reflux disease: a National Analysis LSG in GERD Patients LSG in GERD Patients. JAMA Surg. 2014;149(4):328–34. https://doi.org/10.1001/jamasurg.2013.4323.

15. Chiu S, Birch DW, Shi X, Sharma AM, Karmali S. Effect of sleeve gastrectomy on gastroesophageal reflux disease: a systematic review. Surg Obes Relat Dis. 2011;7(4):510–5. https://doi.org/10.1016/J.SOARD.2010.09.011.

16. Himpens J, Dapri G, Cadière GB. A prospective randomized study between laparoscopic gastric banding and laparoscopic isolated sleeve gastrectomy: results after 1 and 3 years. Obes Surg. 2006;16(11):1450–6. https://doi.org/10.1381/096089206778869933.

17. Oor JE, Roks DJ, Ünlü Ç, Hazebroek EJ. Laparoscopic sleeve gastrectomy and gastroesophageal reflux disease: a systematic review and meta-analysis. Am J Surg. 2016;211(1):250–67. https://doi.org/10.1016/J.AMJSURG.2015.05.031.

18. Daes J, Jimenez ME, Said N, Dennis R. Improvement of gastroesophageal reflux symptoms after standardized laparoscopic sleeve gastrectomy. Obes Surg. 2014;24(4):536–40. https://doi.org/10.1007/s11695-013-1117-6.

19. Sharma A, Aggarwal S, Ahuja V, Bal C. Evaluation of gastroesophageal reflux before and after sleeve gastrectomy using symptom scoring, scintigraphy, and endoscopy. Surg Obes Relat Dis. 2014;10(4):600–5. https://doi.org/10.1016/J.SOARD.2014.01.017.

20. Rebecchi F, Allaix ME, Patti MG, Schlottmann F, Morino M. Gastroesophageal reflux disease and morbid obesity: to sleeve or not to sleeve? World J Gastroenterol. 2017;23(13):2269–75. https://doi.org/10.3748/wjg.v23.i13.2269.

21. Naik RD, Choksi YA, Vaezi MF. Impact of weight loss surgery on esophageal physiology. Gastroenterol Hepatol (N Y). 2015;11(12):801–9.

22. Lee W-J. Gastro esophageal reflux disease after sleeve gastrectomy: a real issue and future perspectives OPEN ACCESS. Am J Gen GI Surg. 2018;1(1):1–7.

23. Doulami G, Triantafyllou S, Natoudi M, et al. GERD-related questionnaires and obese population: can they really reflect the severity of the disease and the impact of GERD on quality of patients' life? Obes Surg. 2015;25(10):1882–5. https://doi.org/10.1007/s11695-015-1614-x.

24. Althuwaini S, Bamehriz F, Aldohayan A, et al. Prevalence and predictors of gastroesophageal reflux disease after laparoscopic sleeve gastrectomy. Obes Surg. 2018;28(4):916–22. https://doi.org/10.1007/s11695-017-2971-4.
25. Gagner M, Hutchinson C, Rosenthal R. Fifth international consensus conference: current status of sleeve gastrectomy. Surg Obes Relat Dis. 2016;12(4):750–6. https://doi.org/10.1016/J.SOARD.2016.01.022.
26. Parmar CD, Mahawar KK, Boyle M, Schroeder N, Balupuri S, Small PK. Conversion of sleeve gastrectomy to Roux-en-Y gastric bypass is effective for gastro-Oesophageal reflux disease but not for further weight loss. Obes Surg. 2017;27(7):1651–8. https://doi.org/10.1007/s11695-017-2542-8.
27. Quezada N, Hernández J, Pérez G, Gabrielli M, Raddatz A, Crovari F. Laparoscopic sleeve gastrectomy conversion to Roux-en-Y gastric bypass: experience in 50 patients after 1 to 3 years of follow-up. Surg Obes Relat Dis. 2016;12(8):1611–5. https://doi.org/10.1016/J.SOARD.2016.05.025.
28. Broderick RC, Smith CD, Cheverie JN, et al. Magnetic sphincter augmentation: a viable rescue therapy for symptomatic reflux following bariatric surgery. Surg Endosc. 2019; https://doi.org/10.1007/s00464-019-07096-z.
29. Crawford C, Gibbens K, Lomelin D, Krause C, Simorov A, Oleynikov D. Sleeve gastrectomy and anti-reflux procedures. Surg Endosc. 2017;31(3):1012–21. https://doi.org/10.1007/s00464-016-5092-6.
30. Triadafilopoulos G. Stretta: a valuable endoscopic treatment modality for gastroesophageal reflux disease. World J Gastroenterol. 2014;20(24):7730–8. https://doi.org/10.3748/wjg.v20.i24.7730.

Magnetic Sphincter Augmentation for the Treatment of Gastroesophageal Reflux Disease

15

Ryan C. Broderick and Santiago Horgan

Introduction

The surgical treatment of gastroesophageal reflux disease can be distilled into basic components: achieving appropriate length of intra-abdominal esophagus, diaphragmatic crura re-approximation, and lower esophageal sphincter (LES) augmentation. LES augmentation traditionally has been achieved with partial or full fundoplication wraps. As an alternative to fundoplication, a magnetic lower esophageal sphincter augmentation device (LINX® Reflux Management System, Torax Medical, Ethicon US, USA) has been FDA approved for fundus-sparing treatment of GERD.

Proposed benefits of magnetic sphincter augmentation (MSA) include reduced operative time, no specialized postoperative diet, reversibility, and consistent improvement in symptom scores with less risk of dysphagia and gas bloat symptoms. These results have been shown in various cohort studies [1–4].

Indications for Surgery

The indications for surgery mirror that for traditional anti-reflux surgery, with some exclusions [5–7]. Good candidates for surgery include patients with normal esophageal motility and medically refractory reflux verified by impedance pH testing

R. C. Broderick (✉) · S. Horgan
Division of Minimally Invasive Surgery, Department of Surgery,
University of California San Diego, La Jolla, CA, USA
e-mail: rbroderick@ucsd.edu

© Springer Nature Switzerland AG 2020
S. Horgan, K.-H. Fuchs (eds.), *Management of Gastroesophageal Reflux Disease*,
https://doi.org/10.1007/978-3-030-48009-7_15

[1–4]. Hiatal hernia greater than 3 cm was not included in the FDA trial for indications in LINX placement; however, recent literature shows that the device can successfully be placed on moderate hiatal hernias, described as "expanded indications" [8–11]. One relative contraindication for use includes large paraesophageal hernias, as it is believed the fundoplication may help reduce the rate of recurrence due to bulking effect at the hiatus. Another contraindication is esophageal dysmotility, as the risk of dysphagia postoperatively is increased [7, 12, 13].

The key to this procedure is successful dissection of a plane between the posterior wall of the esophagus and the posterior vagus nerve, allowing a path for the magnetic beads to encircle the esophagus. The device is sized with the provided sizing tool in order to place the appropriate number of beads (augmentation of LES without constriction). Some, including the authors of this text, advocate for more extensive dissection of the hiatus in all patients (see Section "Minimal Dissection Versus Obligate Dissection" below).

Patient Positioning

The patient is positioned on a beanbag in supine position on the operating table. After induction of anesthesia, the patient is positioned with the arms out and legs split; each leg is secured to the table individually using circumferential padded straps. The arms are secured to each arm board, after which the beanbag is set in place while forming a saddle between the patient's legs and allowing room for strong arm retractor placement on the right side.

Surgical Technique

The operation is started by performing upper GI endoscopy to evaluate for LES location, hiatal hernia, and any unexpected esophageal or gastric lesions. Abdominal access is then obtained in the left upper quadrant, and port placement is shown in Fig. 15.1. The strong arm/Nathanson retractor is placed in the subxiphoid position for liver retraction.

Starting at the left crus, the phreno-esophageal ligament is divided and left-sided hiatal dissection performed. The pars flaccida is then divided near the right crus (above the hepatic branch of the vagus nerve) and the right hiatal dissection completed. Any hiatal hernia is reduced and the esophagus mobilized to obtain 2 cm of intra-abdominal esophagus. The crura is then closed from posterior to anterior with a zero self-retaining nonabsorbable suture (Fig. 15.2). Care is taken to allow for adequate hiatal opening for the esophagus and to not allow any "ramping" of the esophagus off of the posterior closure. The posterior vagus is then identified, and a window is created bluntly between the vagus and the posterior esophagus (Fig. 15.3a). Once the window is created, the band sizer is placed through from the left-hand port (Fig. 15.3b). After careful measuring, the appropriately sized LINX device is placed around the esophagus. The device is locked in place with the

Fig. 15.1 Port placement

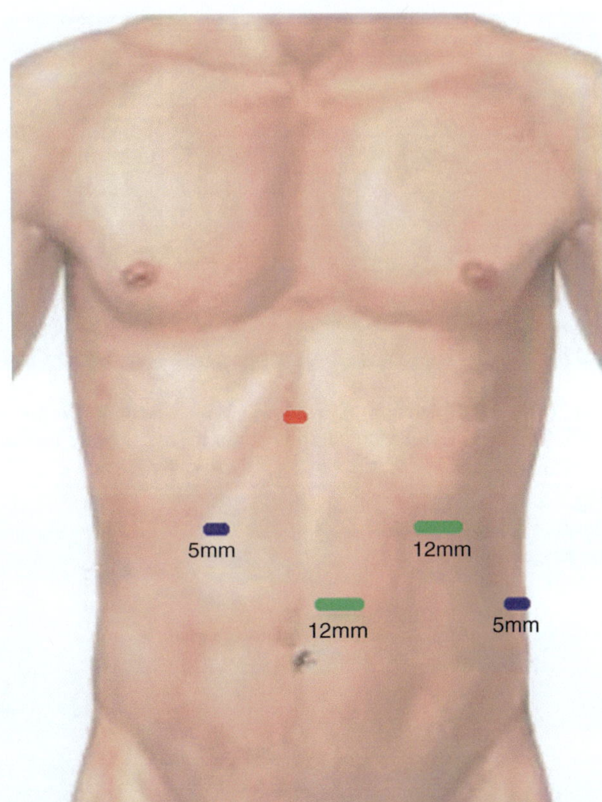

Fig. 15.2 Full hiatal dissection and cruroplasty. Adequate length of intra-abdominal esophagus

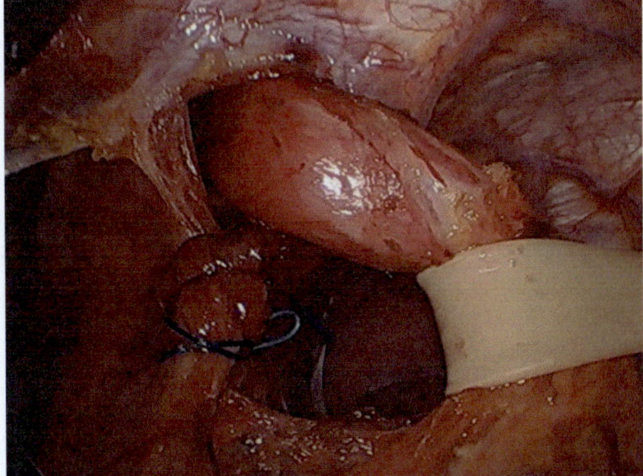

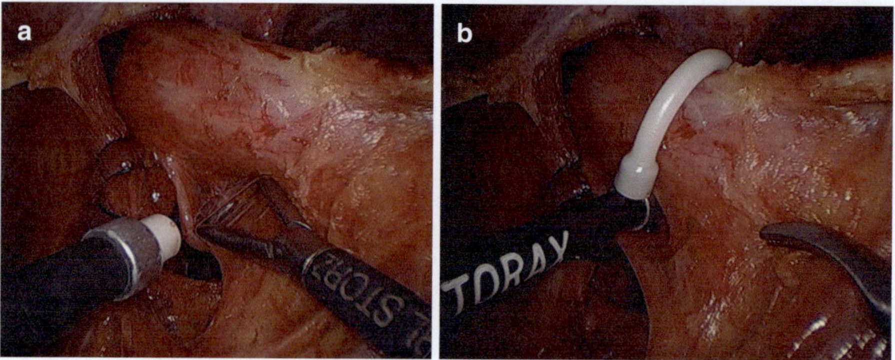

Fig. 15.3 (**a**) Dissection of window between posterior vagus nerve and the esophagus at the LES. (**b**) MSA sizer placement (number of magnetic beads indicated on device handle)

Fig. 15.4 Final LINX
position at lower
esophageal sphincter

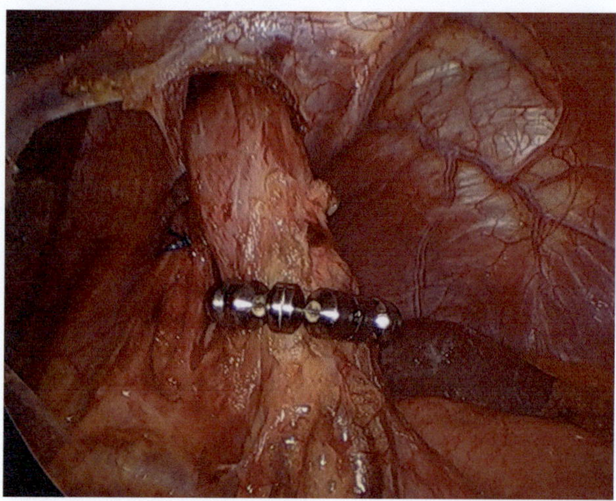

automatic locking mechanism (Fig. 15.4). The LINX is positioned below the diaphragm, on top of the hepatic branch of the vagus. Completion upper GI endoscopy is performed to verify appropriate position at the lower esophageal sphincter with good opening of the GE junction on insufflation; bead indentation can be seen on retroflexion (Fig. 15.5).

Postoperative Care

The patient is extubated in the operating room and transferred to the ward for overnight observation. A major difference in dietary management after magnetic LES augmentation is the immediate implementation of a regular diet. While liquid diet is common after fundoplication to help prevent early dysphagia and gas bloat, the

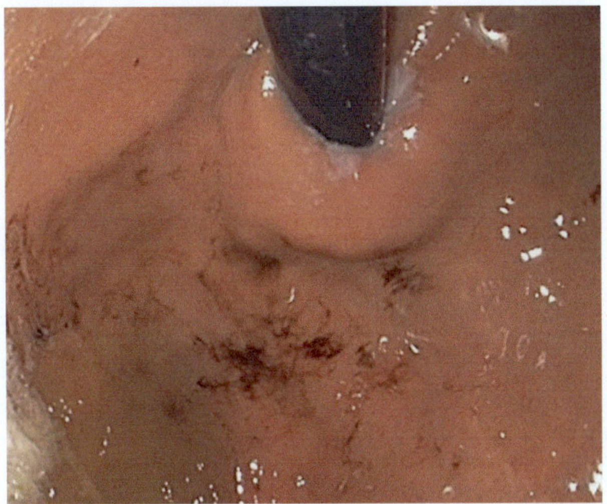

Fig. 15.5 Completion endoscopy showing augmented sphincter. GE junction traversed easily with no resistance and maintained patency

regular diet after LINX allows the patient to "exercise" the beads. It is believed that with a liquid diet after LINX, the beads do not actuate as intended and a scar capsule can form causing dysphagia; this may ultimately require endoscopic pneumatic dilation to break the scar tissue. On the other hand, regular food boluses passing through the beads allow for actuation and more normal function. Patients are discharged often on POD#1 after tolerating regular food; select patients may be amenable for discharge from the recovery unit on POD#0 (outpatient procedure).

Outcomes

Most patients undergoing MSA have favorable results with decrease in reflux symptoms and improvement of pH testing. The device decreases esophageal acid exposure, improves reflux symptoms, and allows cessation of PPI in most patients [1–4]. Studies at 3- and 5-year follow-up have shown relief of GERD symptoms, minimal long-term side effects, and ability for device removal [2–4, 7, 14, 15]. Other advantages include decreased operative time, less technical dissection (in minimal dissection cohorts), and allowing for potential reversibility or conversion to fundoplication in the future [6].

Observational cohort studies show that MSA compares well with posterior fundoplication; however, large randomized controlled trials comparing LINX with posterior fundoplication are needed to verify indications and outcomes compared to traditional anti-reflux surgery [6, 14, 16].

Expanded indications (use in large hiatal hernia, Barrett's esophagus, postbariatric surgery) are currently being studied and need to be tested long term to further compare to traditional anti-reflux surgery [6]. However, early results are positive for use in large hiatal hernia [8–11]. Additionally, positive results have been seen in small cohorts for patients receiving LINX post bariatric surgery [17].

Currently, the LINX device is not FDA approved for treatment in Barrett's esophagus, although some consider its use as an off-label indication. Further studies regarding the use of LINX in Barrett's esophagus are also needed.

Minimal Versus Obligate Hiatal Dissection

Traditional MSA placement consisted of minimal hiatal dissection with preservation of the phreno-esophageal ligament in patients without a hiatal hernia. Recent data has shown that full dissection of the hiatus with re-approximation of crura has had improved results including less recurrence of reflux and hiatal hernia, likely due to undiagnosed hiatal hernia or underlying pathology of the diaphragmatic crura in reflux disease [18].

Complications

Significant complications after MSA include dysphagia and esophageal perforation/erosion of the device. Dysphagia occurs in up to 15.5% of patients. Dilation is required in 5.6% with response to dilation around 70%, occurring usually <90 days after implantation [7, 12, 13]. Predictors of post-op dysphagia are pre-op dysphagia and esophageal dysmotility, indicating that LINX should be placed only in patients with normal esophageal motility.

Erosion overall incidence is 0.1% (29 of 9453 devices placed as of July 2017). Highest rate of erosion in undersized devices (12 beads highest rate). Erosion rates are lower than those seen in lap band placement, thought due to small size, dynamic nature of device, and no significant tissue compression [6, 19]. Devices with 12 beads have been pulled from the market. As technique and device sizes change over time, erosion rates are expected to plateau or decrease.

Removal

LINX removal, though rare, has been indicated for slippage, erosion, or conversion to another anti-reflux surgery (e.g., fundoplication). The device can be removed if necessary, and the majority of removals have been non-emergent and without long-term consequences. Device removal for any reason has been performed in 3.4% of patients (dysphagia 2.2%, GERD symptoms 0.7%, erosion 0.1%) [7]. Removal is effectively achieved in most cases with minimally invasive techniques [20].

Conclusion

Magnetic lower esophageal sphincter augmentation shows good results with respect to symptom scores and objective pH testing (reduced overall acid exposure and DeMeester scores). Magnetic LES augmentation should be another tool in the armamentarium against reflux disease for the foregut surgeon. Close follow-up with the surgeon and access to upper GI endoscopy for treating early or refractory dysphagia are necessary.

References

1. Schwameis K, Schwameis M, Zörner B, Lenglinger J, Asari R, Riegler FM, et al. Modern GERD treatment: feasibility of minimally invasive esophageal Sphincter augmentation. Anticancer Res. 2014;34:2341–8.
2. Ganz RA, Peters JH, Horgan S, Bemelman W, Dunst C, Edmundowicz SA, et al. Esophageal Sphincter device for gastroesophageal reflux disease. N Engl J Med. 2013;368:719–27.
3. Bonavina L, Demeester T, Fockens P, Dunn D, Saino G, Bona D, et al. Laparoscopic Sphincter augmentation device eliminates reflux symptoms and normalizes esophageal acid exposure. Ann Surg. 2010;252(5):857–62.
4. Ganz RA, Edmundowicz SA, Taiganides PA, Lipham JC, Smith CD, Devault KR, et al. Long-term outcomes of patients receiving a magnetic Sphincter augmentation device for gastroesophageal reflux. Clin Gastroenterol Hepatol [Internet]. 2016;14(5):671–7. Available from: https://doi.org/10.1016/j.cgh.2015.05.028.
5. Yadlapati R, Vaezi MF, Vela MF, Spechler SJ, Nicholas J, Richter J, et al. Management options for patients with GERD and persistent symptoms on proton pump inhibitors: recommendations from an expert panel. Am J Gastroenterol. 2018;113(7):980–6.
6. Asti E, Aiolfi A, Lazzari V, Sironi A, Porta ABL. Magnetic sphincter augmentation for gastroesophageal reflux disease: review of clinical studies. Updat Surg. 2018;70(3):323–60.
7. Lipham JC, Taiganides PA, Louie BE, Ganz RA, Demeester TR. Safety analysis of first 1000 patients treated with magnetic sphincter augmentation for gastroesophageal reflux disease. Dis Esophagus. 2015;28:305–11.
8. Rona KA, Tatum JM, Zehetner J, Schwameis K, Chow C, Samakar K, et al. Hiatal hernia recurrence following magnetic sphincter augmentation and posterior cruroplasty: intermediate-term outcomes. Surg Endosc [Internet]. 2018;32(7):3374–9. Available from: https://doi.org/10.1007/s00464-018-6059-6.
9. Rona KA, Reynolds J, Schwameis K, Zehetner J, Samakar K, Oh P, et al. Efficacy of magnetic sphincter augmentation in patients with large hiatal hernias. Surg Endosc. 2017;31(5):2096–102.
10. Iii FPB, Bell RCW, Freeman K, Doggett S, Heidrick R. Favorable results from a prospective evaluation of 200 patients with large hiatal hernias undergoing LINX magnetic sphincter augmentation. Surg Endosc. 2018;32(4):1762–8.
11. Kuckelman J, Philips C, Hardin MMM. Standard vs expanded indications for esophageal magnetic Sphincter augmentation for reflux disease. JAMA Surg. 2019;152(9):890–1.
12. Ayazi S, Zheng P, Zaidi AH, Chovanec K, Chowdhury N, Salvitti M, et al. Magnetic Sphincter augmentation and postoperative dysphagia: characterization, clinical risk factors, and management. J Gastrointest Surg [Internet]. 2019; Available from: https://doi.org/10.1007/s11605-019-04331-9.
13. Warren HF, Brown LM, Mihura M, Farivar AS, Aye RW, Louie BE, et al. Factors influencing the outcome of magnetic sphincter augmentation for chronic gastroesophageal reflux disease. Surg Endosc. 2018;32(1):405–12.

14. Sheu EG, Nau P, Nath B, Kuo B, Rattner DW, Nau P. A comparative trial of laparoscopic magnetic sphincter augmentation and Nissen fundoplication. Surg Endosc. 2015;29:505–9.
15. Ganz RA, Bonavina L, Saino G, Dunn DH, Fockens P, Bemelman W. The LINX reflux management system : confirmed safety and efficacy now at 4 years. Surg Endosc. 2012;26:2944–9.
16. Reynolds JL, Zehetner J, Wu P, Bildzukewicz N, Lipham JC, Shah S. Laparoscopic magnetic Sphincter augmentation vs laparoscopic Nissen fundoplication: a matched-pair analysis of 100 patients. J Am Coll Surg [Internet]. 2015;221(1):123–8. Available from: https://doi.org/10.1016/j.jamcollsurg.2015.02.025.
17. Broderick RC, Smith CD, Cheverie JN, Omelanczuk P, Lee AM, Dominguez R, et al. Magnetic sphincter augmentation: a viable rescue therapy for symptomatic reflux following bariatric surgery. Surg Endosc [Internet]. 2019; Available from: https://doi.org/10.1007/s00464-019-07096-z.
18. Tatum JM, Alicuben E, Bildzukewicz N, Samakar K, Houghton CC, Lipham JC. Minimal versus obligatory dissection of the diaphragmatic hiatus during magnetic sphincter augmentation surgery. Surg Endosc [Internet]. 2019;33(3):782–8. Available from: https://doi.org/10.1007/s00464-018-6343-5.
19. Alicuben ET, Bell RCW, Jobe BA, Iii FPB, Smith CD, Graybeal CJ, et al. Worldwide experience with erosion of the magnetic Sphincter augmentation device. J Gastrointest Surg. 2018;22:1442–7.
20. Harnsberger CR, Broderick RC, Fuchs HF, Berducci M, Beck C, Gallo A, et al. Magnetic lower esophageal sphincter augmentation device removal. Surg Endosc. 2015;29:984–6.

Endostim Implantation

16

Edy Soffer

Gastroesophageal reflux disease (GERD) is one of the most common gastrointestinal disorders. It affects up to 30% of the population in developed countries, with an increasing prevalence worldwide [1]. GERD has a major negative impact on the quality of life of affected patients [2], and its economic burden to society is substantial [3].

Non-pharmacological treatment measures involving lifestyle modifications such as raising the head of the bed and avoidance of offending foods serve primarily as an adjunct to acid suppression therapy, given their limited efficacy [4]. Pharmacotherapy for acid suppression, and proton pump inhibitors (PPI) in particular, has been the mainstay of medical therapy for GERD. This class of drugs has revolutionized the treatment of GERD, given their remarkable efficacy and overall safety. However, up to 40% of GERD patients complain of persistent symptoms while on acid suppression therapy [5, 6]. While this is a heterogeneous group, comprising patients with functional heartburn and nonacid-related etiologies, the failure to fully control symptoms is due in part to the fact that acid suppression agents only reduce the acid content of the refluxed material, but not reflux itself [6]. The importance of regurgitation as a contributing factor to partial response to PPI therapy supports this concept [7]. Incomplete control of symptoms by acid suppression therapy is one of the main reasons cited by patients who choose to undergo anti-reflux surgery [8]. Furthermore, in spite of the good safety record of PPI's [9], the ever-growing concern about adverse effects also contributes to the quest for alternative, non-pharmacological therapy for GERD. Fundoplication has been the standard anti-reflux surgery and the primary alternative to patients who are unsatisfied with pharmacological therapy because of poor symptoms control, or concerns about long-term cost and safety of PPI. Fundoplication provides an effective control of

E. Soffer (✉)
Department of Medicine, Keck School of Medicine, University of Southern California, Los Angeles, CA, USA
e-mail: Edy.Soffer@med.usc.edu

© Springer Nature Switzerland AG 2020
S. Horgan, K.-H. Fuchs (eds.), *Management of Gastroesophageal Reflux Disease*,
https://doi.org/10.1007/978-3-030-48009-7_16

GERD; however, it is associated with adverse effects, such as dysphagia, flatulence, and gas bloat, requiring a revision in a small percentage of subjects [10]. Perhaps as a result, the number of fundoplications in the United States is in decline [11]. The result is a "therapy gap" for GERD patients dissatisfied with acid suppression therapy yet reluctant to undergo surgical fundoplication because of concern of adverse effects [12]. This unmet need has been driving the search for alternative treatment modalities, surgical or endoscopic, that are effective yet less disruptive [12], the most successful of which is the magnetic sphincter augmentation devise [13]. One such alternative is application of electrical stimulation to the lower esophageal sphincter. This chapter will describe the evolution of this treatment modality, from animal studies to the human arena.

Animal Models of LES Electrical Stimulation

Studies in animal models used different techniques, pulse parameters, and protocols, but their results were comparable, showing that electrical stimulation of the LES can increase resting LES pressure. Acute experiments were performed in dogs under anesthesia, implanted surgically [14, 15] or endoscopically [16] with electrodes at the LES. These studies showed that stimulation with high-frequency pulses resulted in an increase in LES pressure. In a chronic canine model, a pair of electrodes were surgically implanted in the LES, and following recovery, animals were studied over time in an awake state. Using a variety of pulse parameters, the authors found that electrical stimulation resulted in a significant increase in resting LES pressure that was sustained beyond the termination of stimulation. Importantly, swallow-induced LES relaxation and esophageal contractile activity were not affected [15].

The results of these studies suggested that electrical stimulation of the LES and modulation of LES pressure may be used to treat patients with GERD and paved the way for subsequent application of such modality in humans.

Acute Human Studies of Electrical Stimulation of the LES

The successful results of LES electrical stimulation in animals led to two acute proof of concept studies in humans. The first study included 10 patients with symptoms of GERD and documented abnormal esophageal acid exposure, who were scheduled to undergo an elective laparoscopic cholecystectomy. At the end of the procedure, two electrodes were implanted at each side of the LES, and the lead was then exteriorized through the abdominal wall. Following recovery, patients underwent a series of intermittent stimulation for 2 days, with various pulse parameters, each lasting 30 minutes, while esophageal motor function was assessed by esophageal manometry, using a water perfused assembly. Electrical stimulation with both low- and high-frequency pulses induced a consistent and significant increase in LES pressure. As observed in the canine model, the rise in pressure was sustained beyond the end of stimulation (Fig. 16.1). There was no effect on LES relaxation in response to swallows, and none of the patients complained of dysphagia [17].

In a second study, five patients with GERD symptoms and abnormal esophageal pH were fitted with a temporary pacemaker lead, which was placed endoscopically at the level of the LES, through a 3-cm submucosal tunnel, and was exteriorized transnasally. Electrical stimulation delivered short-duration pulses of 200 microseconds, at a frequency of 20 Hz, duration of 3 msec, and current of 2–15 mA, each for 20 minutes. Comparable to the first study, stimulation resulted in consistent and significant increase in LES pressure that was sustained after the end of stimulation. Stimulation had no effect on swallow-induced LES relaxation, and none of the patients complained of dysphagia [18]. The consistent effect of LES stimulation on LES pressure, observed both in animal models and in acute human studies, prompted further assessment of this technology in GERD patients, by applying chronic stimulation using a permanently implanted system.

Chronic Human Studies

Single Center Study

The first study was an open-label trial, conducted in a single center in Santiago, Chile, and enrolled patients with symptoms of GERD and documented excessive esophageal acid exposure by intraluminal esophageal pH monitoring [19]. All patients were considering a surgical anti-reflux surgery, mostly because of

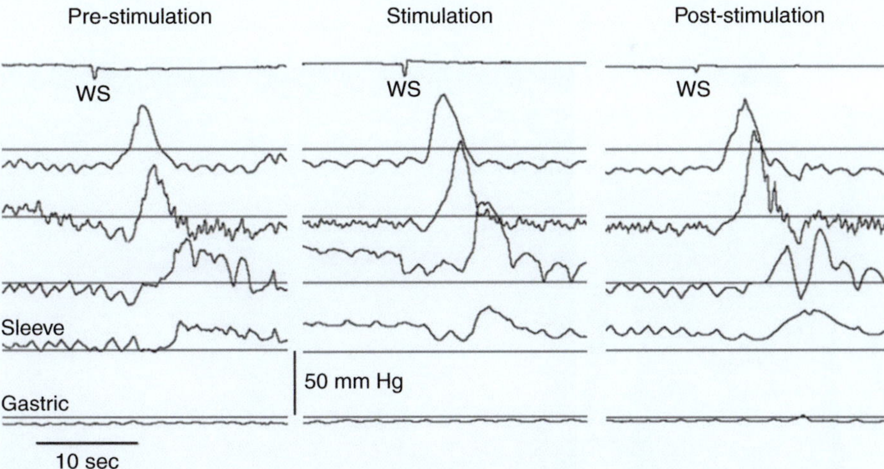

Fig. 16.1 The effect on esophageal and LES function of stimulation with pulses of 200 μsec, and 5 mA in one of the subjects. The three channels above the sleeve represent recording from the esophageal body, at 1-, 6-, and 11-cm above the sleeve. A stimulation-induced increase in resting LESP is observed at mid stimulation and after the stimulus is stopped. WS wet swallow. (Ref. [15])

incomplete response to treatment with PPI, while a few were concerned about lifelong therapy with acid suppression agents. Safety was the primary end point, determined by the incidence of device- and procedure-related adverse effects. Efficacy was evaluated by the effect of stimulation on symptoms, assessed primarily by the reduction in the GERD Health-Related Quality of Life (GERD-HRQL) composite score as well as improvement in esophageal acid exposure.

Patients were implanted with the EndoStim LES Stimulation System (Endostim BV, The Hague, the Netherlands) by conventional laparoscopy, as depicted in Fig. 16.2. In brief, 4–5 trocars are typically used, with ≥1 being a 10-mm port for introduction of the lead into the abdominal cavity; the rest were 3- or 5-mm ports. For the lead implant, the anterior right aspect of the abdominal esophagus is exposed through dissection of the paraesophageal fat and pars flaccida of the hepatogastric ligament. A rectangular longitudinal area of approximately 3 × 1 cm is needed in which the electrodes are implanted. This approach minimizes dissection of the phreno-esophageal attachment and damage to the anterior vagal nerve. The two stitch electrodes are implanted via a superficial bite into the LES muscle along the main esophageal axis with approximately 10 mm between the electrodes. Each electrode is then secured by a clip on the proximal edge of the electrode onto the nylon suture wire and also by suturing the distal anchoring "butterfly" present on the back end of the electrode. Upper gastrointestinal endoscopy is performed to verify electrode position in the LES and to confirm that no perforation of the esophageal lumen had occurred with the needle or electrode. The skin incision for the pulse generator is then performed, and a subcutaneous pocket is created by blunt dissection. After the connector is attached to the pulse generator, a functionality test is performed using the external programmer. The pulse generator is placed into its pocket, and excess lead is simultaneously pulled into the abdominal cavity and placed along the

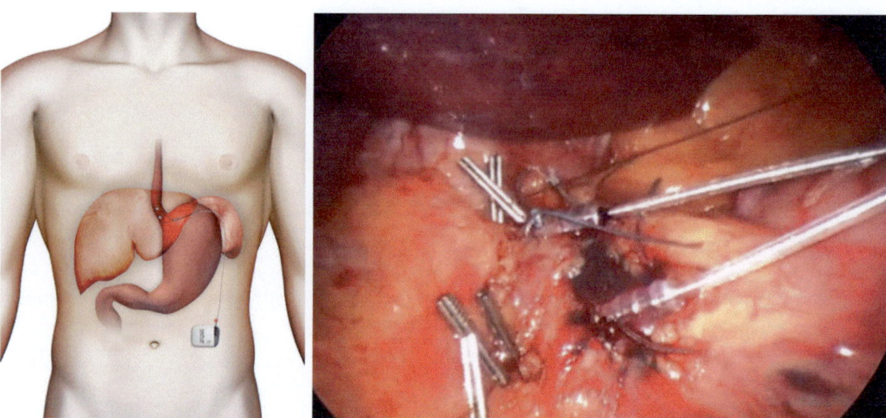

Fig. 16.2 Laparoscopic image of both electrodes in the lower esophageal sphincter. Electrode position in the lower esophageal sphincter. Bipolar stitch electrodes are placed in the abdominal esophagus 1-cm apart, away from the anterior vagus nerve. The lead is connected to the IPG that is implanted in the subcutaneous pocket in the anterior abdomen

left abdominal wall away from the midline [20]. This technique, with minor variations, was used in all chronic human studies. The LES stimulation system delivered therapy with pulse width of 215 μs and nominal amplitude of 5 mA (range 3–8 mA) at a frequency of 20 Hz. Up to twelve 30-minute sessions were delivered per day at pre-meal and pre-reflux events based on patient symptoms and baseline 24-hour pH recordings. Of the 25 implanted patients, 23 were available for evaluation at 12 months. No serious implantation or stimulation-related adverse effects or sensations were reported. Specifically, new symptoms of dysphagia were not reported. Fifteen patients reported 44 adverse effects (AEs) during the subsequent 12 months; two serious adverse effects (SAE), not related to the device or treatment; and 43 nonserious adverse effects, mostly related to postoperative symptoms. No patient reported gastrointestinal side effects or new-onset dysphagia, bloating, inability to belch, or diarrhea associated with LES stimulation. Median composite GERD-HRQL score and esophageal acid exposure were significantly improved at 12 months compared to baseline (Fig. 16.3a, b). All patients except for one were off PPI therapy. High-resolution manometry revealed no effect of LES stimulation on either esophageal body function or LES residual pressure in response to swallows, and there was no significant increase in LES resting pressure.

Fifteen patients completed their 3-year evaluation while on LES stimulation. At 3 years, the improvement in GERD-HRQL and acid exposure was still sustained with significant improvement in the scores of both metrics compared to baseline. Seventy-three percent of patients (11/15) had normalized their distal esophageal acid exposure at 3 years. All but four patients reported cessation of regular PPI use (>50% of days with PPI use). The single center studies also showed a significant reduction in the severity of regurgitation. There were no unanticipated device- or stimulation-related adverse events or untoward sensation reported during the 2–3-year follow-up. No dysphagia was reported [21].

Multicenter Study

Forty-one GERD patients with partial response to PPI were enrolled in a prospective, open-label, uncontrolled, international, multicenter study that was conducted at ten sites in eight countries. Patients were implanted with a system similar to the one used in the single center study, and stimulation was initiated with comparable pulse parameters and number of sessions [22]. Comparable to the previous study, there was a significant improvement in both GERD-HRQL and esophageal acid exposure and in daytime and nighttime episodes of regurgitation at the end of 6 months. Hiatal hernia was present in 25 of the patients, and hernia repair was left to the discretion of the surgeon in each center. Though numbers are small, esophageal acid exposure was further improved in patients who underwent a hernia repair. There were three SAEs, two of which were considered procedure or device related: one was a trocar perforation of the small bowel, which occurred during the implant procedure and was successfully laparoscopically repaired. The second SAE was an asymptomatic lead erosion, encountered at the 6-month endoscopy in a patient

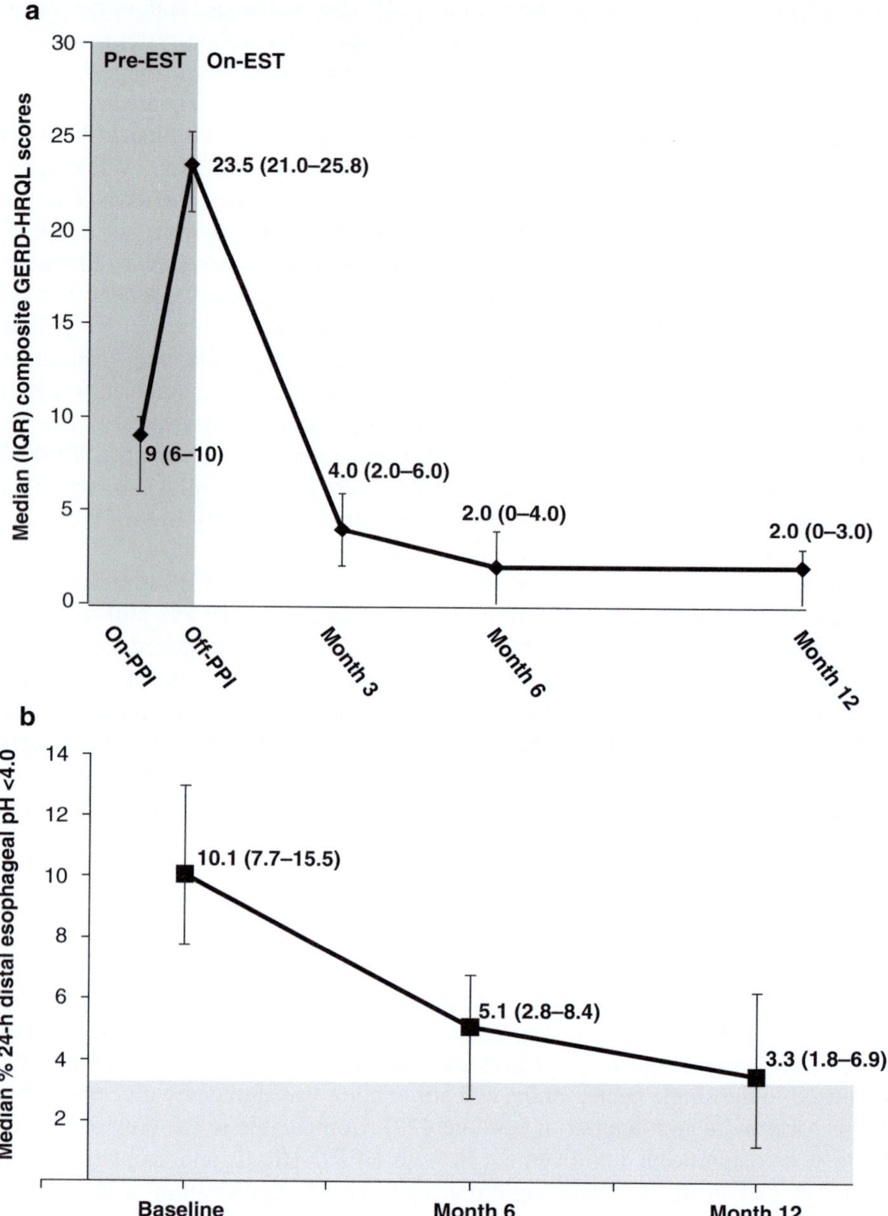

Fig. 16.3 (**a, b**) Improvement in outcomes of gastroesophageal reflux disease (GERD). (**a**) Significant improvement in median (IQR) GERD Health-Related Quality of Life (HRQL) composite score at 6 and 12 months compared with baseline scores both on and off proton pump inhibitor (PPI) therapy. (**b**) Change in median (IQR) distal esophageal pH on lower esophageal sphincter electrical stimulation therapy (LES-EST) from baseline to 3 months ($n = 23$), 6 months ($n = 23$), and 12 months ($n = 22$); $P = 0.002$ at 3 months vs. baseline and $P < 0.001$ at 6 and 12 months vs. baseline (related sample Wilcoxon Signed Rank test). The distal esophageal acid exposure had either normalized or showed >50% improvement in 77% of patients at 12 months

implanted with an investigational, modified lead that was different than the standard lead. The system was explanted, and the patient underwent a Toupet fundoplication performed during the same procedure.

Registry and Clinical Use

An ongoing, prospective international multicenter web-based registry is collecting data in patients with disruptive GERD symptoms, treated with LES electrical stimulation in clinical practice. Data are collected at baseline and at routine follow-ups for 5 years. Clinical and physiological data are collected when available. Data are available from 223 patients from 16 sites in Europe and Latin America. Paired GERD-HRQL heartburn data are presented in Table 16.1, and paired GERD-HRQL regurgitation data are presented in Table 16.2. There was a significant improvement in both metrics with electrical stimulation. Eight serious adverse events in seven patients were reported to be possibly or definitely related to the device. These included gastroparetic symptoms, lead dislodgement, palpitations, pain, and dysphagia. All events resolved; four patients had the device explanted [23].

Approximately 1400 clinical implantation has been performed worldwide thus far, most of them in Europe.

The mechanisms of action of LES-EST are not fully understood, and stimulation-induced increase in LES pressure that was observed primarily in acute and short-term studies in both animals and humans may be only one factor accounting for the beneficial effect of this intervention. In one study, electrical stimulation therapy of GERD patients reduced both the total number of postprandial transient LES relaxations (TLESRs) and the number of TLESR-associated reflux episodes in GERD patients [24]. Other potential mechanisms remain to be elucidated.

Multicenter Pivotal Study

Based on the data obtained from the open-label studies, a multicenter, randomized, double-blind, sham-controlled pivotal clinical trial was proposed and accepted by the FDA in 2016. The study enrolled patients with chronic symptoms of heartburn

Table 16.1 Paired GERD-HRQL Heartburn

	N	Pre-implant median (Q1,Q3)	Post-implant median (Q1,Q3)	Change median (Q1,Q3)	P-value
12 months	96	24 (16.50, 28.50)	6.50 (2.00, 13.00)	−14.50 (−22.50, −6.00)	<0.001
24 months	38	23.50 (17.00, 28.00)	7.00 (2.00, 12.00)	−15.50 (−21.00, −7.00)	<0.001
36 months	12	20.00 (18.50, 27.00)	3.00 (0.50, 13.50)	−16.00 (−24.00, −6.50)	0.0034

† P-values result from Wilcoxon Signed Rank Test of change from Baseline

Table 16.2 Paired GERD-HRQL Regurgitation

	N	Pre-implant median (Q1,Q3)	Post-implant median (Q1,Q3)	Change median (Q1,Q3)	*P*-value
12 months	94	18.50 (11.00, 27.00)	6.00 (1.00, 12.00)	−9.00 (−18.00, −2.00)	<0.001
24 months	37	18.00 (10.00, 24.00)	5.00 (1.00, 12.00)	−10.00 (−14.00, −4.00)	<0.001
36 months	13	17.00 (9.00, 20.00)	4.00 (0.00, 10.00)	−9.00 (−14.00, −3.00)	0.0020

† *P*-values result from Wilcoxon Signed Rank Test of change from Baseline

and/or regurgitation, documented abnormal esophageal acid exposure, and incomplete response to maximum medical therapy, assessed by a short run-in period prior to inclusion, or those intolerant to medical therapy because of adverse effects of proton pump inhibitors. All patients were implanted with the EndoStim Lower Esophageal Sphincter (LES) Stimulation System and randomized to a treatment arm (receiving electrical stimulation) or control arm (sham stimulation). All randomized subjects were to complete a 6-month double-blind phase. At the 6-month visit, control subjects are to receive electrical stimulation and complete a total of 18 months of stimulation, while treatment patients continue receiving stimulation. The primary end points were safety, assessed by the rate of occurrence of device- and/or procedure-related serious adverse events over 12 months of stimulation, and efficacy, assessed by a predetermined degree of improvement in esophageal acid exposure at the end of the 6-month randomized trial period. The trial is a Bayesian adaptive design with two-sided stopping rules (efficacy and futility) determined by an independent data monitoring committee (DMC), with interim analyses at predetermined set points. In early 2019, after 129 subjects reached the primary end point of 6 months and 160 subjects had been implanted, the DMC recommended stopping the trial for futility. The decision was based on a comparison of the primary end point between the active and control groups. The interim analysis of the 129 subjects showed that 28/62 subjects in the treatment group (45.2%) vs. 33/67 (49.3%) in the control group achieved the primary end point at 6 months ($P = 0.64$). Further analysis showed a marked difference in response based on geographic location and surgical technique between the various centers, as well as inaccuracies in the analysis process, all of which were brought to the attention of the FDA by the sponsor of the trial. As of the writing of this chapter, the FDA has indicated a willingness to consider using the existing trial data, in some form, and further discussions with the FDA are planned with a view toward possible continued recruitment of subjects in the existing trial.

Conclusion

Electrical stimulation of the LES is characterized by a number of attractive features: The surgical intervention is relatively simple, safety profile has been very satisfactory thus far, and dysphagia is essentially lacking. This latter aspect is of clinical relevance, since it suggests that patients with impaired esophageal body motor function may be particularly suitable for this therapy, as has been shown in a recent study in which patients with ineffective esophageal motility showed a significant improvement in GERD-HRQL post stimulation, without symptoms or radiological signs of dysphagia (25). The significant improvement in GERD symptoms observed in the various open-label studies, as compared to the insignificant effect observed in the pivotal trial, could be explained by a placebo effect on subjective variables. However, such effect is less likely to explain the consistent improvement in esophageal acid exposure observed in the open-label trials, as was shown in a review of several randomized control trials of procedures intended to treat GERD where placebo effect of a sham intervention on acid exposure is small or nonexistent (26). Selective enrollment criteria in all trials excluded patients with significant hiatal hernia, Barrett's metaplasia, esophageal contractile impairment, and severe erosive esophagitis. These selective criteria are comparable to ones used in initial studies of alternative interventions for GERD, endoscopic or surgical. Consequently, the applicability of electrical stimulation therapy to the wider population of GERD patients remains to be determined.

References

1. El-Serag HB, Sweet S, Winchester CC, et al. Update on the epidemiology of gastro-oesophageal reflux disease: a systematic review. Gut. 2014;63:871–80.
2. Becher A, Al-Serag H. Systematic review: the association between symptomatic response to proton pump inhibitors and health-related quality of life in patients with gastro-oesophageal reflux disease. Aliment Pharmacol Ther. 2011;34:618–27.
3. Peery AF, Crockett SD, Murphy CC, et al. Burden and cost of gastrointestinal, liver, and pancreatic diseases in the United States: update 2018. Gastroenterology. 2019;156(1):254–72.
4. Kaltenback T, Crockett S, Gerson LB. Are lifestyle measures effective in patients with gastroesophageal reflux disease? An evidence-based approach. Arch Intern Med. 2006;166:965–71.
5. El-Serag H, Becher A, Jones R. Systematic review: persistent reflux symptoms on proton pump inhibitor therapy in primary care and community studies. Aliment Pharmacol Ther. 2010;32:720–37.
6. Sifrim D, Zerbib F. Diagnosis and management of patients with reflux symptoms refractory to proton pump inhibitors. Gut. 2012;61:1340–54.
7. Kahrilas PJ, Howden CW, Hughes N. Response of regurgitation to proton pump inhibitor therapy in clinical trials of gastroesophageal reflux disease. Am J Gastroenterol. 2011;106:1419–25.
8. Fuss R, Sifrim D. Management of heartburn not responding to proton pump inhibitors. Gut. 2009;58:295–3099. Vaezi MF, Yang UX, Howden CW. Complications of proton pump inhibitor therapy. Gastroenterology. 2017;153:35–48.
9. Richter JE. Gastroesophageal reflux disease treatment: side effects and complications of fundoplication. Clin Gastro Hepatol. 2013;11:465–71.

10. Wang YR, Dempsey DT, Richter JE. Trends and perioperative outcomes of inpatient antireflux surgery in the United States. Dis Esophagus. 2011;24:215–23.
11. Ganz RA, Edmundowicz SA, Taiganides PA, et al. Long-term outcomes of patients receiving a magnetic sphincter augmentation device for gastroesophageal reflux. Clin Gastroenterol Hepatol. 2016;14(5):671–7.
12. Kahrilas PJ. Magnetic enhancement of the lower esophageal sphincter. Gastrointest Endosc. 2008;67:295–6.
13. Sanmiguel CP, Ito Y, Hagiike M, et al. Effect of electrical stimulation of the LES on LES pressure in a canine model. Am J Physiol Gastrointest Liver Physiol. 2008;295:389–94.
14. Clarke JO, et al. An endoscopically implantable device stimulates the lower esophageal sphincter on demand by remote control: a study using a canine model. Endoscopy. 2007;39:72–6.
15. Rodriguez L, Rodriguez P, Neto MG, et al. Short-term electrical stimulation of the lower esophageal sphincter increases sphincter pressure in patients with gastroesophageal reflux disease. Neurogastroenterol Motil. 2012;24:446–50.
16. Banerjee R, Pratap N, Kalpala R, et al. Effect of electrical stimulation of the lower esophageal sphincter using endoscopically implanted temporary stimulation leads in patients with reflux disease. Surg Endosc. 2014;28:1003–9.
17. Rodriguez L, Rodriguez P, Gomez B, et al. Long-term results of electrical stimulation of the lower esophageal sphincter for the treatment of gastroesophageal reflux disease. Endoscopy. 2013;45:595–604.
18. Rodriguez L, Rodriguez P, Gómez B, et al. Two-year results of intermittent electrical stimulation for the lower esophageal sphincter treatment of gastroesophageal reflux disease. Surgery. 2015;157:556–67.
19. Rodríguez L, Rodriguez P, Gómez B, et al. Electrical stimulation therapy of the lower esophageal sphincter is successful in treating GERD – long-term 3 year results. Surg Endosc. 2016;30(7):2666–72.
20. Kappelle WF, Bredenoord AJ, Conchillo JM, et al. Electrical stimulation therapy of the lower esophageal sphincter for refractory gastroesophageal reflux disease – interim results of an international multicenter trial. Aliment Pharmacol Ther. 2015;42(5):614–25.
21. Labenz J, Thattamparambil P, Gutt C, et al. Interim results of a prospective multi-center registry of lower esophageal sphincter stimulation for GERD: the Less-GERD registry. Gastroenterology. 2018;154:supplement 1 S101.
22. Rinsma NF, Kessing BF, Bouvy ND. Effect of electrical stimulation therapy of the lower esophageal sphincter on postprandial reflux mechanisms in GERD patients. Gastroenterology. 2016;150:supplement 1 S478.
23. Paireder M, Kristo I, Asari R. Electrical lower esophageal sphincter augmentation in patients with GERD and severe ineffective esophageal motility—a safety and efficacy study. Surg Endosc. 2019;33(11):3623–8.
24. Rothstein RI. Endoscopic therapy of gastroesophageal reflux disease outcomes of the randomized-controlled trials done to date. J Clin Gastroenterol. 2008;42:594–602.

Causes of Failures After Antireflux Surgery and Indication, Technique and Results of Laparoscopic Redo-Antireflux Procedures

17

Karl-Hermann Fuchs

Introduction

After the "boom" of laparoscopic antireflux surgery in the past 25 years, the necessity of revisional surgery (redo-surgery) has also increased [1–8]. It can be anticipated from large series that the average overall necessity of redo-antireflux surgery is around 5% [9]. However, this failure rate is published in literature between 5% and 60% [8–10]. One of the highest failure rates was published in a randomized trial between open antireflux surgery and proton pump inhibitors (PPI), in which this rate was determined with almost 60% [10]. Today, we know that these rates are much lower [8, 9]. In several randomized trials and meta-analyses on laparoscopic antireflux surgery, the failure rate is reported between 5% and 15% [8, 11–18]. Of course, these rates depend very much on the definition of failure [8]. In addition, the failure rates depend on several other causes, and therefore, failure rates need to be looked at in detail to be comparable. The failure after antireflux surgery can be defined as persisting, recurrent, or new onset of troublesome symptoms after the primary procedure or by results of objective testing. The most frequent symptoms are recurrent heartburn and regurgitation and persisting or new-onset dysphagia.

Overview on Causes of Failures After Primary Antireflux Surgery

Early analysis of failures has been performed by Skinner and Siewert [19, 20]. Skinner published a list of possible reasons for failures such as partial or complete loss of the antireflux barrier, a new-onset dysphagia combined with or without reflux problems due to an incorrectly placed wrap, a slipped wrap or dysphagia due to a peptic stenosis caused by reflux recurrence, or a compression of the distal

K.-H. Fuchs (✉)
University of California San Diego, Center for the Future of Surgery, La Jolla, CA, USA

© Springer Nature Switzerland AG 2020
S. Horgan, K.-H. Fuchs (eds.), *Management of Gastroesophageal Reflux Disease*,
https://doi.org/10.1007/978-3-030-48009-7_17

esophagus by para-esophageal herniation, as well as epigastric pain, cramps, and/or nausea and vomiting by gastroparesis [19]. Skinner emphasized the point that insufficient, preoperative diagnostic workup and neglecting important pathophysiologic factors that should have influenced the decision for surgery could also be a major cause of failure [19]. The latter is probably one of the most frequent mistakes in the decision process for antireflux surgery. A superficial approach necessary for diagnostic evaluations of the patient and a superficial process of therapeutic decision-making will lead to inappropriate selection of patients.

In an extensive literature review of redo-antireflux surgery, Furnee et al. analyzed causes of failures of primary antireflux surgery from 1625 publications [8]. Most frequent problems were migration of the wrap and mediastinal dislocation, a partial or complete breakdown of the wrap, a slippage of the wrap, and other anatomical changes. Several authors have analyzed their cases and determined the causes quantitatively as is demonstrated in Table 17.1 [7, 8, 21–24]. These results show that the migration of the wrap, the wrap breakdown, slippage, and para-esophageal herniation of the gastric fundus account for 70% of the causes.

The spectrum of causes demonstrates clearly that the tissue condition at the hiatus and the tendency toward migration of the stomach from its original postoperative, intra-abdominal position to the chest are the biggest problem. One could expect

Table 17.1 Causes of failures after primary antireflux surgery

	Smith 2005 [21]	Furnee 2009 [8]	Frantzides 2009 [22]	Dallemagne 2011 [7]	Awais 2011 [23]	Fuchs 2012 [24]
Study	Case control	Literature review	Case control	Case control	Case control	Case control
n	307	4509 (3175)	68	129	275	276
Gastric migration %	50.2	27.9[a] 6.1[b] 5.3[c]	33.8[a] 10.2[c]	39.0	64.0	61
Wrap breakdown	7	22.7	8.8	–	8.4	17
Slipped Nissen	11	14.1	19.7	35	–	14
Wrap in false position	10	–	23.3	–	16.4	11
Wrap too tight	–	5.3	7.3	–	9.5	10
Hiatoplasty too tight	–	–	4.4	–	–	2
Short esophagus	–	–	–	–	43.5	3
False diagnosis	–	2.0	–	3.0	–	3
Causes unclear	17	6.1	–	–	8	4

[a]Gastric migration with intact wrap
[b]Paraesophageal migration of fundus
[c]Hiatoplasty breakdown

that with the dissection of this area during the primary operation, enough adhesions would have caused a stable position of the proximal stomach within the abdomen. However, this does not happen. Clinical evidence shows that the formation of adhesions in this area can be extensive, but not firm enough to keep the stomach in the anatomical position over the years following the operation.

Furthermore, one would expect that after primary open antireflux surgery, more adhesions would be generated and therefore a better position could be achieved compared to laparoscopic approach. Based on the available analyses, this is also not the case, since breakdown of the wrap and slippage seems to occur more often after open surgery [8].

Of course, technical mistakes during the procedure can cause failures such as a wrap that is placed too tight or with an excessive length around the LES. Sometimes during a redo-procedure, one can find a wrap placed around the proximal stomach, and the esophagus has not been touched during the primary operation. These severe mistakes usually do not happen in dedicated centers of esophageal surgery with a high volume, where these technical details are performed weekly or even daily.

As mentioned above, an insufficient diagnostic workup can lead to an incorrect diagnosis and as a consequence to an incorrect indication for antireflux surgery. In the analysis, it was shown that this was the case in 2–3% [7, 8, 21–24]. Most of these patients have no GERD, but spastic esophageal motility disorders or overlapping diseases [8].

Reflecting the available literature in detail, it can be demonstrated that even prior to redo-surgery, some surgeons do not perform a necessary diagnostic workup. As a consequence, these patients may come with a second failure or third failure lacking any information about their primary functional status in 10–15% [8, 24]. Later on, the identification of the original causes of the disease and of the original functional status is impossible, and one can only speculate on the basis of current functional tests.

Special Issues Regarding Failures

The Problem of Migration

Evidence from literature and clinical evidence shows that the most frequent cause of failure is migration of the gastric fundus into the chest (Fig. 17.1) [7, 8, 21–24]. The latter will limit the functional result of the procedure and may cause new symptoms. The reasons for frequent migration upward could be an increased intra-abdominal pressure and/or an increased tension on the esophagus and stomach upward into the mediastinum. These forces can be explained by the positive pressure of the intra-abdominal environment and the negative pressure in the thoracic environment due to breathing. The level of intra-abdominal pressure is increased by breathing and physical activity due to shortening of the diaphragmatic muscle during contraction and reduction of the abdominal volume. These mechanisms lead to a continuous strain on the diaphragm and especially on the structures within the

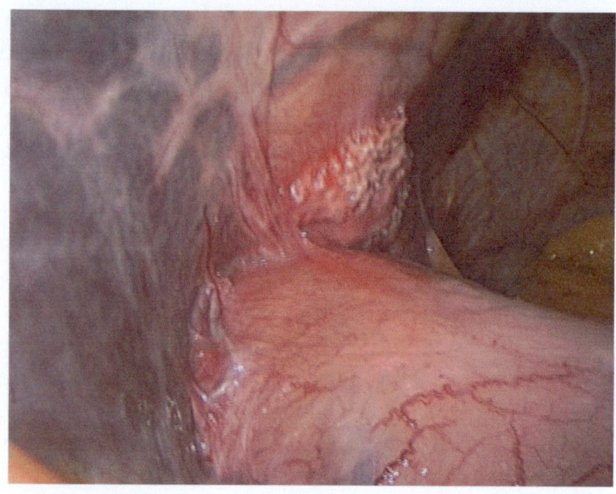

Fig. 17.1 Migration of the proximal stomach into the lower mediastinum after primary laparoscopic fundoplication and hiatal mesh enforcement

hiatal opening. As a result, it is not surprising especially in obese persons with a higher intra-abdominal pressure that migration and breakdown of the wrap can occur over time (Fig. 17.2).

This leaves the question whether migration can be prevented by any operative technical step during primary surgery. During the primary operation, it is important to mobilize the esophagus extensively to ensure a tension-free position of the LES that is approximately 2–3 cm, within the intra-abdominal pressure environment. Due to the longitudinal, esophageal muscle, there is always a tendency of the esophagus to develop a tension and shortening into the chest. This latter phenomenon has been described already by Allison in 1948 [25]. Mattioli et al. have shown the importance of a short esophagus [26–29] (see Chap. 12). Therefore, an optimal mobilization of the esophagus should be performed in all antireflux procedures [29–31].

Another technical detail is the evaluation of the presence of possible sliding areas at the hiatus, which may facilitate more easily migration and failure. Such a sliding area could be a lipoma on the anterior aspect of the aorta, which may cause an easier dislocation of the cardia in the chest. Another sliding area could be the preserved "esophageal fat pad" at the anterior aspect of the cardia. When the fat remains there and is included in the fundoplication, the interposition of fat within the fundoplication prevents a firm scaring of the anterior fundus with the cardia. The soft fat pad will enable the smooth serosa of the anterior fundus to move up and down easily and facilitate migration. As a consequence, any fat, any lipoma, or superfluous tissue such as remaining elements of the hernia sac should be removed from the cardia and esophagus in order to allow for a tight positioning of the wrap and fundus around the esophagus.

The Problem of Shaping the Wrap

Creating a fundoplication does not mean pulling some part of the fundus on the right side of the esophagus together with some part of the fundus on the left side of

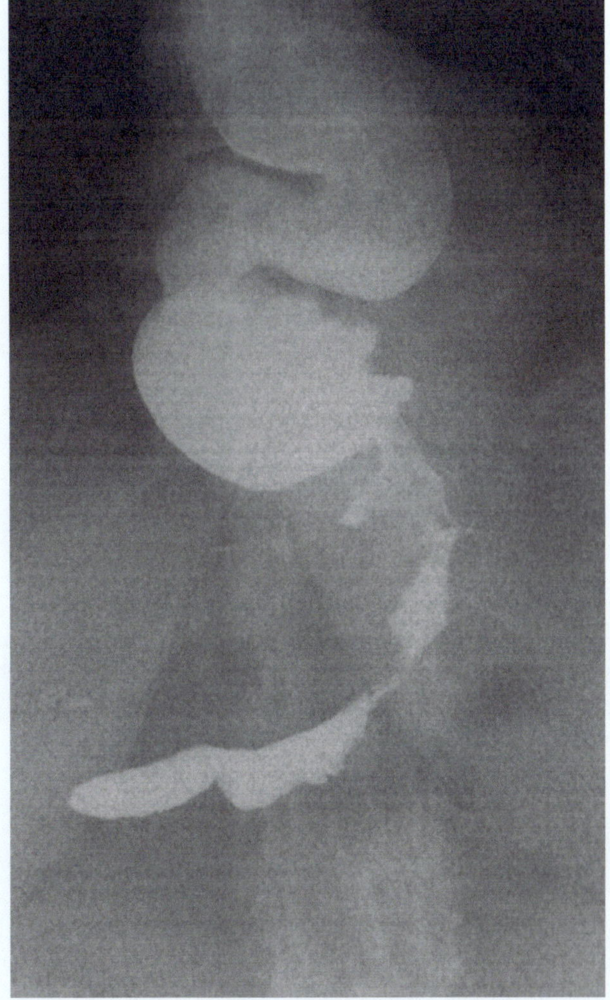

Fig. 17.2 Patient with dysphagia and thoracic pain after primary fundoplication with migration of the stomach into the lower mediastinum. Radiography with barium sandwich shows the migration and vertical compression of the esophagus due to intramediastinal tension and intra-abdominal pressure

the esophagus and then suturing it together and leaving it. Creating a fundoplication means shaping the wrap with full attention on details and best creating a symmetric wrap with similar portions of fundic flaps and placing it at the correct position at the LES. The technical details have been published several times many years ago [5, 30] (see also Chaps. 7 and 8, Standard Antireflux Surgery). This is important for redo-antireflux surgery and, of course, also best for the primary procedure.

A tight or excessive long fundoplication will cause dysphagia and even other functional problems (Fig. 17.3). An incorrectly positioned wrap will not sufficiently prevent pathologic reflux. An asymmetric wrap with a long sling formation of one of the fundic flaps will create dysphagia, maybe early satiety, unpleasant fullness, or nausea after the operation [5]. Some of these details, when not accomplished during primary surgery, will cause unspecific symptoms such as epigastric pain and

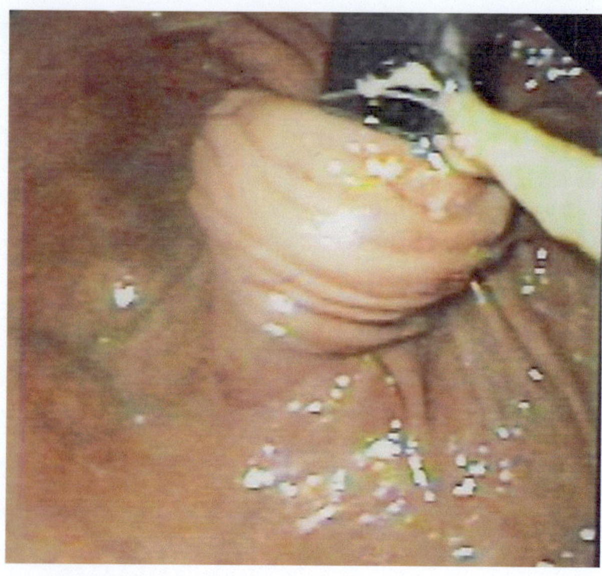

Fig. 17.3 Endoscopic view in retroflexion on tight fundoplication, causing severe and therapy refractory dysphagia

unpleasant postprandial symptoms, which are difficult to analyze and interpret. In redo-surgery, it is important to evaluate these symptoms prior to redo-surgery. During revisional procedure, the surgeon has to assess the situs for causes for these symptoms in order to correct anatomy and function.

Summary of Possible Causes of Failures

During revisional surgery, it is very important to look for these details and critically evaluate the anatomical situation. In addition, the surgeon must look for causes of the failure and also for causes of certain symptoms, which this patient was complaining about. Only this very detailed view on the operative situs will help improve the results.

A summary from the analysis of causes and their interpretation are as follows:

1. Insufficient mobilization of the esophagus in the mediastinum (facilitates migration)
2. Not realizing a short esophagus and leaving esophageal tension on the stomach toward the mediastinum (high risk for migration)
3. Insufficient mobilization of the fundus (limited mobility of the fundus postoperatively may inhibit fundic accommodation, when filling with food)
4. Excessive mobilization of the greater curvature too far down on the greater curvature (unnecessary mobility of the fundus and unnecessary redundancy of the fundic flap with risk for para-esophageal herniation)

5. Division of the complete pars flaccida at the smaller curvature allowing for an unnecessary mobility of the right side of the stomach
6. Shaping the wrap in an asymmetric fashion (no regular fundic accommodation possible with a high risk for postoperative postprandial symptoms like pain, early satiety, and dysphagia)
7. Insufficient dissection of the main anatomical landmarks leaving unnecessary tension on all these structures (risk for wrap breakdown)
8. Leaving the hernia sac and fatty tissue that will cause sliding areas with a high risk of migration and slipped fundoplication
9. Using mesh enforcement at the hiatus with no real indication (causing a risk of severe complications such as mesh penetration, rigid adhesions, secondary vagal lesions, and "frozen cardia")

Preoperative Preparations and Establishing an Indication for Redo-Antireflux Surgery

Since redo-surgery can be potentially associated with severe complications, (1) an extensive preoperative diagnostic workup should be performed; (2) a critical evaluation and interpretation of the findings should be discussed, and the indication should be established considering all these different factors; and (3) the patient should be informed also extensively about all these arguments and the potential problems and complications.

The diagnostic program should consist of an endoscopy, a dynamic radiographic investigation especially in cases of dysphagia and obstruction, an esophageal high-resolution manometry and a 24 hour impedance-pH monitoring to verify the anatomical and functional status of the patient. This program may be expanded by ultrasound investigations, computer tomography, and gastric emptying studies depending on the individual case.

There will be rarely acute situations for emergency redo-antireflux surgery; however, this situation may occur early after primary surgery in cases of early migration and incarceration of the stomach in the chest with a risk for gastric perforation. In these cases, the surgeons must be prepared to revise the situation in the abdomen and possibly expand to a transthoracic approach.

Usually, the indication for redo-surgery occurs after months or years after primary antireflux surgery, because of persisting or new-onset symptoms after a free interval. If the patient has certain "alarm symptoms" such as heavy pain, acute onset pain, bleeding, and/or increasing dysphagia with the inability to assure sufficient nutrition, immediate action is necessary with an early diagnostic workup and a quick decision for redo-surgery [32, 33].

In all other cases, there is time to schedule the necessary extensive diagnostic workup and spend time to reflect and discuss the findings. Table 17.2 demonstrates the presenting symptoms of the patients being referred for redo-antireflux surgery.

Table 17.2 Presence of major symptoms prior to indication for revisional surgery

	Furnee 2009 [7] (4584); in %	Own series (276); in %
Heartburn/regurgitation	41.7	61
Dysphagia/obstruction	16.6	23
Reflux and dysphagia	4.0	9
Gas bloat	0.7	2
Nausea/vomiting	–	7
Not determined	31	5% unclear

Technical Principles of Redo-Antireflux Surgery

The principles of antireflux redo-surgery should be based on well-established general surgical principles and in addition on the individual conditions of the patient, which are determined by the anatomical, functional, and clinical situation of these patients prior to surgery.

Choice of Surgical Team

For laparoscopic redo-antireflux surgery, it is important that there is a surgical team available with a large experience in advanced laparoscopic upper GI procedures and in addition also with any kind of possible open procedures in esophageal surgery. This may include also transthoracic esophageal surgery, because in rare cases some patients may require even esophageal or gastric resections during the process of a multiple redo-procedure [8, 34–37]. As a consequence, these procedures should be performed in centers with routine experience in upper GI and specifically esophageal and thoracic surgery. The case may start as a laparoscopic redo-procedure; however, difficulties may develop, and the procedure may emerge into a larger transabdominal and transthoracic case.

Access Technique

After the advent of minimal invasive surgery, it took many years for laparoscopic surgeons to develop sufficient experience to establish the minimal invasive approach as routine access techniques for redo-antireflux surgery [3–7]. Today, we know that the improvement of vision by magnification using modern mini-cameras during a laparoscopic procedure will enable to see details of the mediastinal structures and very adhesive areas with much greater precision than can be obtained in the mediastinum by open approach. Therefore, minimal invasive access techniques are the techniques of choice in redo-antireflux surgery [8, 33].

The necessity of a conversion must be dealt with during the procedure in a critical way. Factors, influencing a decision for conversion, should be considered well in time and should consist of the progress of the running procedure, a view on the tentative duration of the procedure, and the probability of complications. Of course, if a complication occurs, which cannot be managed by minimal invasive techniques, a conversion is required instantly. However, an experienced surgeon should do all the necessary steps to avoid such an emergency situation. He or she should sense the growing difficulties during a procedure that may lead to a complication. The experienced surgeons should, prior to these incidents of severe problems, make the decision to convert this case, if the situation can be better handled in the open technique. This is called a "calculated conversion," which should not account for a higher complication rate.

Another reason for a calculated conversion could be the necessity of increasing, time-consuming, little steps of progress in performing an adhesiolysis, which may expand the duration of the total procedure excessively. Therefore, it is always important for a surgeon to observe his own progress during such a procedure. A critical evaluation within the case may lead to a change in tactics, if the progress of laparoscopic adhesiolysis may take "forever."

Another reason for conversion may be the condition of the tissue. An example could be a tissue block after several, previous antireflux procedures with massive adhesions. If there would be a chance to dissect these structures safely with better haptic feedback from the tissue by feeling it, a conversion is justified to prevent damage during dissection. In experienced hands in esophageal centers, the conversion rate for laparoscopic redo-antireflux surgery is probably currently around 10% [8].

Laparoscopic Adhesiolysis in Redo-Cases

The initial and most important tactical step in redo-surgery is the complete dissection of the hiatal area to define the anatomy again, which may be altered substantially (Fig. 17.4) [33]. After previous laparoscopic antireflux surgery, adhesions

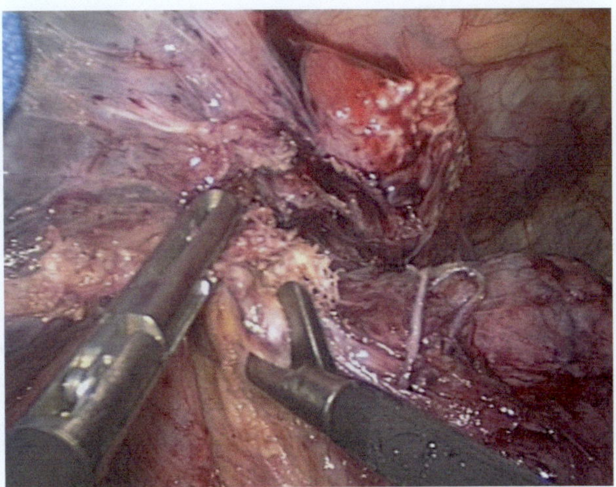

Fig. 17.4 Careful dissection and adhesiolysis of the tight tissue connections between the hiatal rim enforced by mesh and the esophagus in order to preserve the vagal trunks and the leave the esophagus intact

occur usually between the anterior gastric wall and the left liver lobe as well as within the hiatus. Therefore, it is advisable to first dissect the left liver lobe from the anterior aspect of the stomach. As clinical experience has shown, adhesions can be very different among patients. In one patient, soft adhesions may be pushed away and easily separated by scissors, while in other patients, the serosa of the liver capsule and the serosa of the stomach are grown together so tightly that no layer of separation can be identified nor dissected. In these latter cases, the surgeons have to decide whether they preserve gastric serosa or better the liver capsule. In multiple redo-surgery, it may be advisable to keep the gastric wall intact, because this wall is (due to several procedures) very fragile but is needed later for another adequate fundoplication. When separating the liver from the anterior gastric wall and dissecting in the subhepatic region, it is important to avoid any lesions to the pancreas, which may be quite adhesive to the liver.

Another problem of dissection could be the presence of a left liver artery as a branch from the left gastric artery. Such an anatomical finding may have already complicated the first procedure and may have led to bleeding and additional adhesions. It is important to stay at the liver and find as first landmark the hiatal arch and the crurae. Based on these important landmarks, dissection can be advanced into the lower mediastinum preventing lesions of the artery and the vagal nerves. An experienced surgeon will have no problems with a norm variation of the left hepatic artery, because it only needs to be pulled caudad, since the focus area of dissection is always above these structures at the right crus and the hiatal arch.

In the groove between the liver and the right crus is the vena cava, which may be covered by adhesions and may be at danger during adhesiolysis. Nevertheless, it is important to dissect the right crus completely in order to perform later a sufficient hiatoplasty.

A next challenge can be the separation of the fundic flaps of a remaining Nissen fundoplication. Sometimes the anterior and posterior fundic flap may be grown together, and it may be very difficult to separate them. Careful dissection with blunt pushing and cutting may be rewarding in separating these two structures without any perforation. Sometimes a perforation cannot be avoided. It is important that this is recognized during the procedure and oversewing is easy for an experienced surgeon. Some surgeons use a linear stapler to facilitate the separation, which may be quick but also could bear the risk for a leak, if the separation line is not met precisely.

Mobilizing the posterior fundic flap from the crurae may be very difficult, because adhesions and/or remaining sutures may fix the wrap to the crurae. The surgeon must have patience to stepwise dissect these important structures changing sites from right to left side of the stomach. Care must be taken to avoid lesions of the spleen.

Entering the mediastinum from below is usually easily done in the area of the hiatal arch, since one can find a layer between the migrated stomach and the pericardium. Of course, special attention is required for the identification of these intramediastinal structures such as the pericardium, the lung segments, and the vagal nerves. The dissection is complicated, if the previous operator has left some hernia sac in the distal mediastinum, which limits the anatomical overview in a second or third approach. Technically, the dissection of the lower mediastinum is demanding, since there is only limited space to manipulate laparoscopic instruments.

In these cases, perforations of the pleura can easily occur. This is a rather small problem, which may be not counted as a complication, since the distance between the esophagus and the pleura may be only a few millimeters. If there are adhesions between these two structures, a perforation occurs quite frequently. But it is very important to mobilize the esophagus in the lower mediastinum. Usually, no specific treatment is required, and the pleural hole can be left open. If the anesthesiologist recognizes difficulties of the respiratory function of the patient, a temporary drainage can be placed and removed at the end of the operation.

Mobilization of the Esophagus and Stomach

One of the most important technical steps in laparoscopic antireflux redo-surgery is the sufficient mobilization of the esophagus in the mediastinum to be able to place the LES tension free in the abdominal pressure environment. Nevertheless, this is the most frequent mistake, as our experience has shown in redo-procedure. Therefore, it must be emphasized to mobilize the esophagus even in the scar tissue of a previously dissected lower mediastinum with great care.

General Aspects

Furthermore, it is important to reestablish the normal anatomy of the upper quadrants as much as possible in order to create a situation similar to a preoperative situation in a primary case. Once all the landmarks and organs are freed from adhesions, the surgeons must evaluate based on the anatomical overview all possibilities to reconstruct the anatomy and the effective antireflux barrier by narrowing the hiatus and performing a new fundoplication. Once all these elements have been verified, a hiatal closure following the rules of this procedure can be performed followed by the shaping of a new fundoplication using a bougie for calibration of the cardia.

Difficult Situations

The surgeon is in a difficult situation, if the adhesions do not allow for a precise separation of the layers and a clear anatomical definition of the structures (Fig. 17.5). This may be caused by remaining hernia sac or dissection in wrong layers during the primary operation. It may consume several hours to dissect the structures and create an anatomical order, before starting the new antireflux procedure. This work is worthwhile, because without clear anatomical separations the second procedure is again doomed to fail.

After multiple previous operations with subsequent adhesions, the esophagus can shrink, and a short esophagus may develop (Fig. 17.6). The underestimated

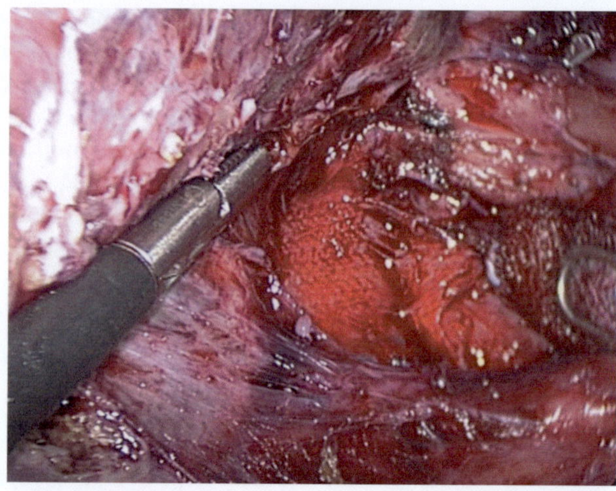

Fig. 17.5 Sometimes the esophagus and the surrounding tissue of the hiatal opening have developed into a rigid block of "wood-like" material, which can hardly be separated. We like to call this a "frozen cardia"

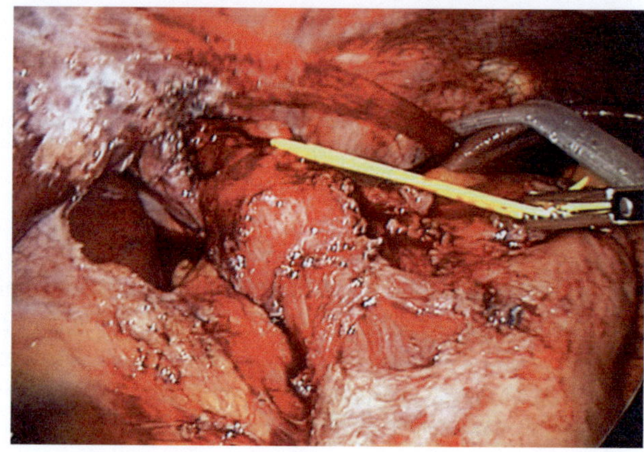

Fig. 17.6 Hiatus and the stomach after adhesiolysis of second time redo-case. The location of the previous fundoplication is visible and too low on the stomach. The anterior vagus is taped, and it shows clearly the cardia too high in the mediastinum, characterizing a short esophagus

short esophagus or a non-recognized short esophagus during the primary operation is one of the frequent reasons for failures [27–29] (see Chap. 12).

The hiatal narrowing can be a problem, if the substance of the crural muscle is reduced due to scarring and weakening or by fatty tissue. During redo-surgery, sometimes the hiatal crurae may be so weak even because of previous dissections. In these cases, a careful dissection of the remaining muscle substance is important. It may be also important to leave some scar strands on the muscle substance to use these as holding structures, when adapting and suturing the crurae. If the crurae are too weak to carry sutures, a mesh enforcement may be advisable [35, 38–41] (see Chap. 10).

Gastric motility disorders or gastroparesis may occur after damage to the vagal trunks [36, 37]. The vagal trunks around the esophagus have a constant anatomy in the lower mediastinum and therefore can be identified in primary cases of antireflux surgery very easily. Standard surgical technique is leaving the vagal trunks at the esophagus, and the fundic flaps are placed around this package. However in redo-antireflux surgery, the vagal trunks may be hidden within adhesions or gastric folds.

Any lesion of vagal trunks will cause severe gastric motility disorders and maybe even gastroparesis and diarrhea. This is a very unfavorable and troublesome situation, because the patients have seen the surgeons to improve their gastrointestinal function and now the result may be a major functional defect with severe reduction in quality of life. Therefore, during laparoscopic antireflux redo-surgery, everything possible must be done to avoid a vagal lesion [33, 36].

Only careful dissection with time-consuming steps must be performed to identify the vagal trunks and preserve them. Quite often, the vagal trunks are embodied in scar structures. Care and time must be invested to dissect these structures and preserve their function. Also care must be taken to avoid thermal lesions of the vagus, when using energy devices.

Occasionally, a patient shows after several previous procedures intraoperatively a block of adhesive tissue within the hiatus, which cannot be separated. Quite often in these cases, the previous surgery has been performed using mesh enforcement at the hiatus [35]. Of course, it is the task of the surgeon to try and dissect these structures. However, in some cases, this is not possible, and the case may end up in a major resection [35, 37]. The extent of the resection does depend on the individual case and the accompanying conditions. The decision to convert for resection may be facilitated, if these patients have some signs of delayed gastric emptying or even gastroparesis or if the esophagogastric junction is destroyed by previous operations or a long-segment Barrett's esophagus is involved. This may stimulate the decision to convert early for resection.

In cases with several previous antireflux procedures and especially in a patient with risk factors, it may be advisable to perform a partial gastrectomy with a Roux-en-Y reconstruction to reduce acid capacity and prevent biliary reflux [42].

The Results of Laparoscopic Antireflux Redo-Surgery

Table 17.3 demonstrates an overview of the results of laparoscopic antireflux redo-surgery from the past years. As these are complex procedures, there is a certain rate of mortality involved, which characterizes the difficulty of the condition and of the procedure [7, 8, 21–24]. Despite these problems and experiences, it is worthwhile to consider redo-surgery in esophageal centers, since a success rate can be achieved in 70–85% of the patients. The success rate also depends usually on the number of previous operations performed [24]. The more previous operations have been performed, the higher is the probability that a resection may be necessary. Table 17.4 demonstrates the increasing necessity of a resection in our experience, if more redo-surgery has been performed previously.

The failure rate after redo-antireflux surgery is therefore between 15% and 25% in esophageal centers [7, 8, 21–24]. In a recent study from the USA, 13,000 antireflux procedures were analyzed, and the results show that the rate of necessary redo-surgery remains between first and second procedure between 4% and 5% [9]. In

Table 17.3 Problems, complications, and results during and after antireflux redo-surgery

	Smith 2005 [21]	Wykypiel 2005 [43]	Funch-Jensen 2008 [44]	Furnee 2009 [8]	Awais 2011 [23]	Fuchs 2012 [24]	Singhal 2018 [45]
Study	Case control	Multicenter study	National registry	Review	Case control	Case control	Case control
n	307	225	113	3491	275	276	302
Intraoperative perforations %	17	6	–	13.1	–	7.0	19.9
Postoperative complication %	19.2	10.8	1.6% revisions	11.8	7.0	9.0	10
Mortality %	0.3	0.4	0.81	0.9	0	0	0.3
Good results	73–89	89.8	–	84	85	80–85%	86
Failure of redo-surgery %	10–20	–	–	15–20	11.2	16	5.3

Table 17.4 Overview of necessity of major gastric or esophageal resections during redo-surgery for GERD ($n = 151$, own experience [24])

	1. Redo	2. Redo	3. Redo	4. Redo	5. Redo
Percent of cases solved by redo-fundoplication	100	100	91	55	0
Percent of cases solved by major resection	0	0	9	45	100

case of a third necessary operation, the necessity of additional surgery rises substantially. This underlines the importance to have at least the redo-surgery done in a dedicated esophageal center.

References

1. Luostarinen ME, Isolauri JO, Koskinen MO, Laitinen JO, Matikainen MJ, Lindholm TS. Refundoplication for recurrent gastroesophageal reflux. World J Surg. 1993;17:587–93.
2. Fuchs KH, Heimbucher J, Freys SM, Thiede A. Management of gastro-esophageal reflux disease 1995. Tailored concept of anti-reflux operations. Dis Esoph. 1995;7:250–4.
3. Bonavina L, Chella B, Segalin A, Incarbone R, Peracchia A. Surgical therapy in patients with failed antireflux repairs. Hepato-Gastroenterology. 1998;45:1344–7.
4. Hunter JG, Smith CD, Branum GD, Waring JP, Trus TL, Cornwell M, Galloway K. Laparoscopic fundoplication failures: patterns of failure and response to fundoplication revision. Ann Surg. 1999;230:595–604.
5. Peters JH, DeMeester TR, Crookes P, Stefan O, de Vos Shoop M, Hagen JA, Bremner CG. The treatment of gastroesophageal reflux disease with laparoscopic Nissen fundoplication. Ann Surg. 1998;228:40–50.
6. Pointner R, Bammer T, Then P, Kamolz T. Laparoscopic refundoplications after failed antireflux surgery. Am J Surg. 1999;178(6):541–4.
7. Dallemagne B, Arenas Sanchez M, Francart D, Perretta S, Weerts J, Markiewicz S, Jehaes C. Long-term results after laparoscopic reoperation for failed antireflux procedures. Br J Surg. 2011;98:1581–7.
8. Furnée EJ, Draaisma WA, Broeders IA, Gooszen HG. Surgical reintervention after failed antireflux surgery; a systematic review of the literature. J Gastrointest Surg. 2009;13:1539–49.
9. Zhou T, Harnsberger C, Broderick R, Fuchs HF, Talamini M, Jacobsen G, Horgan S, Chang D, Sandler B. Reoperation rates after laparoscopic fundoplication. Surg Endosc. 2015;29:510–4.

10. Spechler SJ, Lee E, Ahnen D, Goyal RK, Hirano I, Williford WO. Long-term outcome of medical and surgical therapies for gastroesophageal reflux disease. JAMA. 2001;285:2331–8.
11. Dallemagne B, Weertz J, Markiewicz S, Dewandre JM, Wahlen C, Monami B, Jehaes C. Clinical results of laparoscopic fundoplication ten years after surgery. Surg Endosc. 2006;20:159–65.
12. Fein M, Bueter M, Thalheimer A, Pachmayer V, Heimbucher J, Freys SM, Fuchs KH. Ten year outcome of laparoscopic antireflux procedures. J Gastrointest Surg. 2008;12:1893–9.
13. Catarci M, Gentileschi P, Papi C, Carrara A, Marrese R, Gaspari AL, Grassi GB. Evidenced based appraisal of antireflux fundoplication. Ann Surg. 2009;239:325–37.
14. Neufeld M, Graham A. Levels of evidence available for techniques in antireflux surgery. Dis Esophagus. 2007;20:161–7.
15. Davis CS, Baldea A, Johns JR, Joehl RJ, Fisichella PM. The evolution and long-term results of laparoscopic Antireflux SUrgery fort he treatment of Gastroesophageal reflux disease. JSLS. 2010;14:332–41.
16. Fein M, Seyfried F. Is there a role for anything other than a Nissen's operation? J Gastrointest Surg. 2010;14(suppl):S 67–74.
17. Broeders JAJL, Mauritz FA, Ahmed Ali U, Draaisma WA, Ruurda JP, Gooszen HG, Smout AJPM, Broeders IAMJ, Hazebroek EJ. Systematic review and metaanalysis of laparoscopic Nissen versus Toupet fundoplication for gastro-esophageal reflux disease. Br J Surg. 2010;97:1318–30.
18. Tan G, Yang Z, Wang Z. Metaanalysis of laparoscopic total Nissen versus posterior Toupet fundoplication for GERD based on randomized clinical trials. ANZ J Surg. 2011;81:246–52.
19. Skinner DB. Surgical management after failed and reflux-operations. W J Surg. 1983;6:359–65.
20. Siewert JR, Isolauri J, Feussner H. Reoperation following failed fundoplication. W J Surg. 1989;13:791–8.
21. Smith CD, McClusky DA, Rajad MA, Lederman AB, Hunter JG. When fundoplication fails – redo? Ann Surg. 2005;241:861–71.
22. Frantzides CT, Madan AK, Carlson MA, Zeni TM, Zografakis JG, Moore RM, Meiselman M, Luu M, Ayiomamitis GD. Laparoscopic revision of failed fundoplication and hiatal hernia. J Laparoendosc Adv Surg Tech A. 2008;19:135–9.
23. Awais O, Luketich JD, Matthew J, Schuchert MJ, Morse CR, Wilson J, Gooding WE, Landreneau RJ, Pennathur A. Reoperative Antireflux Surgery for failed fundoplication: an analysis of outcomes in 275 patients. Ann Thorac Surg. 2011;92:1083–9.
24. Fuchs KH. Revisionseingriffe nach Antirefluxchirurgie. In: Fuchs KH, editor. Management der Gastroösophagealen Refluxkrankeit, vol. 183: De Gruyter Verlag Berlin; 2018. –208.
25. Allison PR. Peptic ulcer of the oesophagus. Thorax. 1948;3(1):20–42.
26. Collis JL. An operation for hiatus hernia with short esophagus. J Thorac Surg. 1957;34:768–73.
27. Gozetti G, Pilotti V, Spanaro M, Basso F, Grigioni W, Carulli N, Loria P, Felice V, Lerro F, Mattioli S. Pathophysiology and natural history of acquired short esophagus. Surgery. 1987;102:507–14.
28. Yousef YK, Shekar N, Lutfi R, Richards WO, Torquati A. Long-term evaluation of patient satisfaction and reflux symptoms after laparoscopic fundoplicatio with Collis gastroplasty. Surg Endosc. 2006;20:1702–5.
29. Mattioli S, Lugaresi ML, Costantini M, Del Genio A, Di Martino N, Fei L, Fumagalli U, Maffettone V, Monaco L, Morino M, Rebecchi F, Rosati R, Rossi M, Sant S, Trapani V, Zaninotto G. The short esophagus: intraoperative assessment of esophageal length. J Thorac Cardiovasc Surg. 2008;136:1610.
30. DeMeester TR, Bonavina L, Abertucci M. Nissen fundoplication for gastroesophageal reflux disease. Evaluation of primary repair in 100 consecutive patients. Ann Surg. 1986;204:19.
31. Fuchs KH, Breithaupt W, Fein M, Maroske J. Hammer I; laparoscopic Nissen repair: indications, techniques and long term benefits. Langenbeck's Arch Surg. 2005;390:197–202.
32. Stefanidis D, Hope WW, Kohn GP, Reardon PR, Richardson WS, Fanelli RD, SAGES Guideline committee. SAGES guidelines for surgical treatment of GERD. Surg Endosc. 2010;24(11):2647–69.

33. Fuchs KH, Babic B, Breithaupt W, Dallemagne B, Fingerhut A, Furnee E, Granderath F, Horvath OP, Kardos P, Pointner R, Savarino E, Van Herwarden-Lindeboom M, Zaninotto G. EAES recommendations for the management of Gastroesophageal reflux Disease. Surg Endosc. 2014;28:1753–73.

34. Merendino KA, Dillard DH. The concept of sphincter substitution by an interposed jejunal segment for anatomic and physiologic abnormalities at the esophagogastric junction; with special reference to reflux, esophagitis, cardiospasm and esophageal varices. Ann Surg. 1955;142:486–506.

35. Parker M, Bowers SP, Bray JM, Harris AS, Belli EV, Pfluke JM, Preissler S, Asbun HJ, Smith CD. Hiatal mesh is associated with major resection at revisional operation. Surg Endosc. 2010;24(12):3095–101.

36. Van Rijn S, Roebroek YGM, Conchillo JM, Bouvy ND, Masclee AAM. Effect of Vagus Nerve Injury on the outcome of antireflux surgery: an extensive literature review. Dig Surg. 2016;33:230–9.

37. Bhayani NH, Sharata AM, Dunst CM, Kurian AA, Reavis KM, Swanstrom LL. End of the road for dysfunctional end organ: laparoscopic gastrectomy for refractory gastroparesis. J Gastrointest Surg. 2015;19:411–7.

38. Memon MA, Memon B, Yunus RM, Khan S. Suture Cruroplasty versus prosthetic hiatal herniorraphy for large hiatal hernia: a metaanalysis and systematic review of randomized controlled trials. Ann Surg. 2016;263:258–66.

39. Koetje JH, Oor JE, Roks DJ, Van Westreenen HL, Hazebroek EJ, Nieuwenhuijs VB. Equal patient satisfaction, quality of Life and objective recurrence rate after laparoscopic hiatal hernia repair with and without mesh. Surg Endosc. 2017;31:3673–80. https://doi.org/10.1007/s00464-016-5405-9.

40. Zhang C, Liu D, Li F, Watson DI, Gao X, Koetje JH, Luo T, Yan C, Du X, Wang Z. Systematic review and metaanalysis of laparoscopic mesh versus suture repair of hiatus hernia: objective and subjective outcomes. Surg Endosc. 2017;31(12):4913–22. https://doi.org/10.1007/s00464-017-5586-x.

41. Oor JE, Roks DJ, Koetje JH, Broeders JA, van Westreenen HL, Nieuwenhuijs VB, Hazebroek EJ. Randomized clinical trial comparing laparoscopic hiatal hernia repair using sutures versus sutures reinforced with non-absorbable mesh. Surg Endosc. 2018;32(11):4579–89. https://doi.org/10.1007/s00464-018-6211-3.

42. Zehetner J, Ravari F, Ayazi S, Skibba A, Iarehzereshki A, Pelipad D, Mason RJ, Katkhouda N, Lipham JC. Minimally invasive surgical approach for the treatment of gastroparesis. Surg Endosc. 2013;27:61–6.

43. Wykypiel H, Kamolz T, Steiner P, Klingler A, Granderath FA, Pointner R, Wetscher GJ. Austrian experiences with redo antireflux surgery. Surg Endosc. 2005;19:1315–9.

44. Funch-Jensen P, Bendixen A, Iversen MG, Kehlet H. Complications and frequency of redo-antireflux surgery in Denmark: a nationwide study, 1997–2005. Surg Endosc. 2008;22:627–30.

45. Singhal S, Kirkpatrick DR, Masuda T, Gerhardt J, Mittal SK. Primary and redo antireflux surgery: outcomes and lessons learned. J Gastrointest Surg. 2018;22:177–86.

Index

© Springer Nature Switzerland AG 2020

S. Horgan, K.-H. Fuchs (eds.), *Management of Gastroesophageal Reflux Disease*,

https://doi.org/10.1007/978-3-030-48009-7